Wrong
title

Schuell's aphasia in adults

James J. Jenkins Ph.D.

*Professor of Psychology, Director of Research,
Center for Research in Human Learning,
University of Minnesota, Minneapolis, Minnesota*

Edward Jiménez-Pabón M.D., Ph.D.

*Chief of Neurology,
Veterans Administration Center,
Wood (Milwaukee), Wisconsin*

Robert E. Shaw Ph.D.

*Associate Professor of Psychology,
University of Minnesota,
Minneapolis, Minnesota*

Joyce Williams Sefer M.A.

*Clinical Speech Pathologist, Special Associate
of the Center for Research in Human Learning,
University of Minnesota, Minneapolis, Minnesota*

Schuell's
aphasia in adults

Diagnosis, Prognosis, and Treatment

Second Edition

Medical Department
Harper & Row, Publishers
Hagerstown, Maryland
New York, San Francisco, London

dedication

Hildred Schuell (1907–1970) was a remarkable woman whose life prepared her for the study of language. As a school teacher she saw the importance of communication and expression in children. As an aspiring writer and critic she devoted her early graduate training to the study of writing and to the analysis of literature. As a predoctoral student recognizing speech pathology as an area in which great needs existed, she combined her interest in language with her desire to be of service to others.

When Dr. Schuell received her doctorate from the State University of Iowa, she was asked to establish at the Minneapolis Veterans Hospital an aphasia clinic—a treatment center and a facility for basic research of the nature of the disorder. She originated a series of studies of evaluation and treatment that culminated fifteen years later in the *Minnesota Test for the Differential Diagnosis of Aphasia* and in the publication of the first edition of APHASIA IN ADULTS. At the time of her death, she was actively pursuing new lines of research with aphasics, working with Japanese colleagues to examine aphasic disorders across national, cultural, linguistic, and orthographic lines, and attempting to extend her analysis still further through studies of audiology, evoked cortical potentials, and psycholinguistics.

This record of accomplishment does not capture by any means the impact that Dr. Schuell had on those who worked with her. She was a gifted therapist with a rare ability to inspire confidence, trust, and cooperation in patients. She would win her way through the patient's initial anxiety, depression, or apathy and set him to working on his disorder instead of merely reacting to it. Her ingenuity in devising tasks and exercises to "get the language machinery going again" was unmatched and her patience and resourcefulness seemed unlimited. She was just as impressive as a researcher. She never accepted information of an "authority" without verification. She verified even her own insights, working carefully with diagnostic instruments, keeping painstaking records, following up patients, and interviewing family members in her search for firm facts about the patient and the course of the disorder. Numerous new findings about aphasia were woven together with others' knowledge in the diagnostic–prognostic–therapeutic scheme presented in this book.

As important and indispensable as were her professional skills, Dr. Schuell had still other qualities of great personal importance to those who knew her. She was a sensitive and expressive human being. She never failed to note the passings of the seasons, the joys of family and personal events, the beauty of a design, the harmony of a poem, or the meaningfulness of a person-to-person relationship. She brought out the best in all of us by responding to what was good in us and in the world we knew.

contents

preface to the second edition

Dr. Hildred Schuell was a brilliant therapist and a superb worker. She conceived this book and was responsible for the research on which it is based. The final form of the first edition came from her pen and the second would have had she lived two more years. It fell to those of us who knew her and worked with her to attempt to speak for her and set forth the fruits of her research. The deeper nature of the book—the thrust of the research, the conceptions of aphasia, and the insight into patients—truly speak for her as representations of her lasting contribution to the study of aphasia and as reflections of her varied talents.

In preparing the second edition of APHASIA IN ADULTS, we have been guided by Dr. Schuell's notes for revision, her more recent research articles, her outline of the state of the field, and her program for continuing research. Where we could, we have taken the trend of her thinking and extended it to make the view of aphasia as complete as possible. While we cannot claim that Dr. Schuell would agree *in detail* with everything we have chosen to say here, we do feel that the extension and revision is in the spirit of her thought and work. She trained all of us (with respect to aphasia), so it seems unlikely that we would agree on a position not in accord with her thinking.

The first edition was well received by professionals in the field and by students. This edition was prepared with the student as the primary focus. We have reduced technical detail where it was not central to the material. Statistics and factor analyses have been minimized. Anatomy of the nervous system appears in a technical appendix instead of a separate chapter in the text. As before, detailed data on patients also appears in an appendix. For the research worker who wants as complete data as possible, this and the first edition taken together will provide a complete description of our research on classification.

The central issue of the book is, as before, the question of how to describe the aphasic disorders. Both clinical work and research have contributed to the schema presented here. More explicitly than in the first edition we have treated with aphasia in the framework of a general theory of communication processes. The theoretical approach has been closely related to the diagnostic categories of aphasia that emerged from our 25-year research program. The diagnostic groups not only appear different but also have markedly different prognoses and require different courses of therapy. We have tried to explain the procedures for diagnosis in enough detail that students can apply them in the clinic and we have included detailed instructions concerning treatment for each classification of the disorder so that students can understand, plan and execute differential treatment programs.

We have tried to communicate our thinking about aphasia as clearly as possible to the student coming to this topic for the first time. It is our hope that these students will go on to serve both mankind and science and in their turn will advance our understanding of aphasia. Dr. Schuell demonstrated most effectively that clinical service and research work can be brought together for the benefit of both. We hope the students will continue in that tradition.

J.J.J.
E.J.-P.
R.E.S.
J.W.S.

preface to the first edition

This monograph is the outgrowth of fifteen years of systematic observation of aphasia on the Neurology Service of the Minneapolis Veterans Administration Hospital, in association with the Division of Neurology, Graduate School of Medicine, University of Minnesota. It is the result of continued efforts to increase our understanding of the nature of aphasia in order to deal more effectively with the problems it presents. We have learned about aphasia from studying some thousand aphasic patients, and much of what we have learned has been put to daily use in the clinic. Our patients have contributed willingly in the hope that their observations and their efforts might benefit other aphasic patients and other students of aphasia.

Because aphasia is a many-faceted subject we have chosen an inter-disciplinary approach for this book. One of us is a speech pathologist (H.S.), another an experimental psychologist (J.J.J.), while the third is a clinical neurologist (E.J-P.). We have studied patients together, and all of us have asked questions and made observations, which in turn have stimulated new questions and new observations, which in turn have stimulated new questions and new observations. If we have no final answers, we can at least derive comfort from Wendell Johnson's penetrating question, "What is there to scratch but the surface?"

In this book we have devoted a good deal of space to a review of the literature on aphasia, in order to show how knowledge has accumulated slowly from the time of Franz Joseph Gall to the present. At the same time, it has become evident that it is no longer tenable to think of aphasia in terms of discrete cortical lesions and isolated pure disorders. We have proposed a conceptual model for aphasia that is based on clinical and research findings and is compatible with modern neurophysiological and linguistic theory. We have described five major and two minor aphasic syndromes, with group data, prognoses for recovery from aphasia, and illustrative case material. We have presented analyses of data obtained from 157 aphasic subjects, including factor analysis and correlations with neurological findings; test-retest data for 73 subjects; and results obtained from testing 50 nonaphasic patients with a comparable age distribution. Finally, we have included a section on the management of aphasic disorders.

This is not a book for anyone who is looking for recipes or prescriptions or final truths. It is intended for all serious students of aphasia, whether their interest stems from concern with language, cerebral function, or behavior. It seems obvious that something is to be learned about all of these processes from the study of the alterations produced by cerebral injury or disease and that this kind of study is essential to both the clinician and the researcher.

H.S.

acknowledgments

We are happy to acknowledge our indebtedness to the many friends and co-workers who have helped in this work. We are especially grateful to Dr. Robert H. Brookshire, Director of the Aphasia Clinic at the Minneapolis Veterans Administration Hospital, for giving us access to the clinical records, to Mr. Bruce Schultz, E. E. G. Technician, for supplying EEG records, and to Miss Sally Hydukovich for supplying information as to final outcome and competency of many aphasic patients.

Many friends have read sections of the revision. Dr. Donald Shankweiler especially must be mentioned for his kind criticism of our theoretical efforts.

We are also happy to acknowledge the help of Mrs. Dorothy Shaw in reference work and the indispensable skills of Miss Kathleen Casey who organized our materials, old and new, and turned them into impressively clean manuscript.

It is a pleasant duty to record our debt to the Center for Research in Human Learning of the University of Minnesota where three of us have worked during the revision of this book. The Center is supported by grants from the National Institute of Child Health and Human Development (HD–01136), the National Science Foundation (GB–35703X), and the Graduate School of the University of Minnesota.

J.J.J.
E.J.-P.
R.E.S.
J.W.S.

Schuell's aphasia in adults

part one

HISTORICAL
BACKGROUND

chapter 1

"HERE SILENT SPEAK THE GREAT OF OTHER YEARS"

The ancient Egyptians reported head injuries with loss of speech between 3000 and 2500 B. C., and documented their observations in a surgical papyrus deciphered by Breasted (1930). The Egyptian surgeons believed that loss of speech resulted from "something entering from the outside," like "the breath of an outside god or death," and that the patient "was silent in sadness."

Benton and Joynt (1960) reviewed descriptions of aphasia in the literature from the time of Hippocrates to Samuel Johnson's account of his stroke in 1783. Head (1915) abstracted four cases described by Franz Joseph Gall in the early nineteenth century.

It has sometimes been forgotten that Gall was one of the leading neuroanatomists of his time. Bonin (1960) wrote that Gall "formulated the relationship between mind and body in so sharp a fashion that even a Viennese prefect of police felt the edge." Flourens (Ebstein, 1923), who opposed Gall's ideas of localization, testified that when Gall was demonstrating, it seemed to him he was looking into the brain for the first time. Bailey and Bonin (1957) pointed out that Gall's achievements were all the more remarkable in that before him the brain was generally considered a glandular organ.

It is a tragic irony that Gall's brilliant and original exploration of the brain should be forgotten while his divagations into phrenology survived and had a lasting influence upon aphasia. Gall's argument was basically that the brain imposes its configurations upon the skull. He localized language in the anterior lobes because he believed that

3

development of the orbital area produced the prominent appearance of the eyes he observed in students who excelled in oral recitation.

Marie (1906b) wrote vividly of Gall's influence upon the intellectuals of nineteenth-century Paris. He characterized Jean Baptiste Bouillaud, dean of the medical faculty of the Collège de France, as one of the most "dithyrambic" of Gall's admirers. Bouillaud did not hesitate to compare Gall to Copernicus, Gallileo, and Newton or to list him among "the great Messiahs of science."

Bouillaud was 65 years old when Broca came to Paris in 1861 to become head of the surgical service at Bicêtre. Influenced by Gall and the autopsies he himself had performed, Bouillaud localized speech in the frontal lobes anterior to the fissure of Rolando. Marie commented that this gave Bouillaud a fifty–fifty chance of being right, but fortune was against him. Bouillaud, however, was so sure of his ground that he offered a prize of 500 francs to anyone who could show him the brain of a patient with confirmed diagnosis of loss of speech without a lesion in the frontal lobes. Kussmaul (1887) said Bouillaud would never acknowledge that such a case was observed, and the prize was never awarded.

BROCA'S DISCOVERY

On March 21, 1861, Pierre Paul Broca, then 37 years old, addressed the Society of Anthropology on cerebral localization. He rejected the doctrines of phrenology but said that this did not destroy the principle of localization of function and affirmed his faith that there were in the brain "distinct regions, corresponding to the great regions of the spirit" (Marie, 1906b).

Marie later dubbed 1861 "the year of the Hegira for Aphasia." In August and November, Broca (1861a,b) published, in the *Bulletins of the Anatomical Society of Paris*, the protocols, with detailed autopsy findings, of two patients who served to establish the theory of localization of articulated speech in the third frontal convolution.

Broca labeled the observed loss of speech *aphemia*, a word he derived from the Greek deprivitive *a*, and a Greek verb meaning "to speak." He defined aphemia as loss of the faculty of articulated speech in the absence of paralysis of the tongue, impairment of comprehension, or loss of intelligence.

The first patient, Leborgne, had been an epileptic since youth. He lost his speech when he was 30 years old and had a history of progressive neurological symptoms until his death at 51. Broca argued that neither comprehension nor intelligence were impaired when Leborgne initially lost his speech but that these impairments, like the observed paralysis, had developed later.

The brain was not cut, but preserved intact in the Musée Dupuytren. Broca reported that both hemispheres were atrophied and that no part of the left was completely intact. Extensive softening involved the first, second, third, and frontal convolutions, the insula, the corpus striatum, and the first and part of the second temporal convolutions.

In accordance with the belief of his time, Broca concluded that the softening had begun in the third frontal convolution and had been propagated uniformly in all directions over a period of time. He therefore attributed aphemia, the earliest reported symptom except for seizures, to the lesion in the third frontal convolution, which he assumed to be the initial focus of softening.

The second patient, Lelong, was an 84-year-old laborer who had been confined in the infirmary at Bicêtre for eight years for senile debility. According to the history Broca obtained, Lelong lost his speech in April 1860, when he reportedly lost consciousness and fell upon a stairway. In October 1861, he fell on his left hip, bruised the neck of the femur, and was transferred to the Surgical Service, where Broca saw him.

Lelong said four words: *yes, no, always,* and *three.* He used *three* to express all numerical ideas but corrected the response by holding up the appropriate number of fingers. When asked how old he was, he held up eight fingers, then four. Except in one instance, his gestures were always correct. Broca concluded again that the patient comprehended everything that was said and that intelligence was unimpaired.

Lelong died November 8, 1861. Again, the brain was not cut. Broca judged the right hemisphere intact. The left hemisphere was atrophied, and there was an accumulation of serous fluid under the pia mater, over the left frontal lobe. Below this was a depression, about the size of a franc, in the second and third frontal convolutions. The surrounding tissue was firm, and no softening was present. Broca considered the lesion to mark the site of an old hemorrhage that had occurred when the patient lost his speech.

Marie (1906b) reexamined the brains of both patients later and reported he found no lesion in the frontal lobe of Lelong. He explained that such depressions were common in the brains of the aged and resulted from accumulations of serous fluid over atrophied convolutions, which are characteristically separated by deep gyri. He considered this a natural mistake for anyone unaccustomed to examining the brains of the aged.

Broca, however, believed his second observation confirmed the earlier one and argued earnestly that it was more correct to localize faculties by convolutions of the brain than by protuberances of the skull.

THE DOGMA OF THE THIRD FRONTAL CONVOLUTION

Forty-five years later, Marie (1906b) reviewed Broca's cases and tried to account for their impact on the period that followed. He said that Bouillaud was pleased with the demonstrations that supported his theory and "covered Broca with flowers." Bouillaud was not pleased, however, with the doctrine of the third frontal convolution.

Meanwhile, Charcot reported the autopsy of a patient seen in his clinic at Salpê-trière. Broca attended the autopsy, which showed both frontal lobes intact, with softening involving the first and second temporal convolutions and the angular gyrus.

Broca, said Marie, was shaken, since he was honest. He first questioned the diagnosis of aphemia, since he had not examined the patient himself, but went on to say that some anatomists considered all the convolutions encircling the sylvian fissure as one, and that if this view were correct, it was possible that lesions elsewhere in this area could result in loss of articulated speech. That Broca did not hold to this revision of his earlier theory Marie attributed to the authority of Bouillaud and the great popularity of the new doctrine.

In July 1863, Broca told the members of the Anatomical Society that he knew of 15 cases of aphasia with autopsy and that in all of them except the case of Charcot there was a lesion "more or less extended but always involving the left frontal convolution." Kussmaul (1887), as well as Marie, reported that in none of these cases was the damage confined to the frontal lobes.

In his lectures at the College of France in 1864, Vulpan analyzed 12 observations of aphasia gathered at Salpêtrière and reported 5 cases of lesions of the left frontal lobe with aphasia, 4 cases of lesions of the left frontal lobe without aphasia, 1 lesion of the right frontal lobe without aphasia, and 2 cases of lesions of the posterior lobes with aphasia. Marie added that almost all the brains with left frontal lobe lesions also showed lesions of Wernicke's area. He thought Broca would have taken the frequency of these temporo-parietal lesions into account had he not been so strongly influenced by Bouillaud and carried along by the strong current of localization, which was almost irresistible.

Marie (1906b) felt there were philosophical reasons for the popularity of the new doctrine, which he described as follows:

> The battle began to become heated between spiritualism on one hand, and materialism on the other, for that was the name by which they tried to brand the free-thinkers. Now, to the spiritualists, there seemed to be something that outraged the dignity of the human soul in a doctrine that tried to localize and restrict psychical functions and intellectual faculties to certain parts of the brain. . . . Political passions were aroused, also, and for a little while, among the students, faith in localization was part of the republican credo. If we have insisted a little lengthily, perhaps, on the different aspects of the question of localization, it is in order to better understand the prevailing state of mind which influenced the many and ardent partisans of Broca; how resist those who bear you in triumph!

PHYSIOLOGICAL EXPERIMENTATION IN THE LATE NINETEENTH CENTURY

THE MOTOR CORTEX

In 1870, as is well known, Fritsch and Hitzig in Berlin succeeded in mapping the motor cortex in dogs, using galvanic currents of minimal intensity. They followed the stimulation experiments with extirpation of discrete areas of the motor cortex and were able to demonstrate alterations of movements of the affected limb without loss of sensibility. Their work was considered to establish the doctrine of circumscribed cortical centers and to confirm the findings of Broca.

THE VISUAL CORTEX

Munk, of Berlin, published the results of ablation experiments with dogs and monkeys in 1881, in which he reported a visual center in the occipital lobes and described

cortical blindness resulting from bilateral extirpations of the visual cortex and homonymous hemianopsia following unilateral extirpations. Munk (1881) described the latter
as follows:

> If one extirpates the whole cortex on the one side of the occipital lobe, the monkey becomes
> hemiopic. He is blind, cortically blind for those halves of the retina which are on the side
> of the lesion. . . . As the suturing of first one eye and then the other eye shows without a
> doubt, the disturbance is the same for both eyes and this hemiopia remains for weeks and
> months. Only the monkey learns very soon to compensate his hemiopic limitation of his visual
> field by movements of head and eyes.

Munk also described loss of ability to recognize objects when vision was preserved.
Observing that his animals relearned to recognize food and other objects in the environment, he concluded that the dogs could see and form new memory images of optic
sensations. He believed these visual images were stored in an area that extended beyond
the region where ablation produced cortical blindness.

THE AUDITORY CORTEX

In 1876, Flechsig noted that the medial part of the temporal lobe received numerous
fibers from other cortical regions, and concluded it was an important association area.
In the same year Ferrier reported that laboratory animals became deaf following
bilateral temporal lobe extirpations. In 1878, Heschl traced the auditory radiations to
the superior temporal convolutions (Fulton, 1949).

In the 1881 paper on functions of the cortex, Munk reported temporal lobe ablations
in dogs previously trained to respond to spoken commands. He labeled the resulting
disturbance "psychic deafness" and reported that the dog still heard, since he pricked
up his ears at unusual sounds, but did not understand what he heard. Munk's conclusions were as follows: "Just as the place Al contains the visual images, so the place Bl
contains the acoustic images of the dog, and as the place Al is situated in the larger
visual sphere subserving visual perception, so the place Bl must be within a larger
acoustic sphere subserving acoustic perceptions. Its complete destruction must lead to
cortical deafness." He added that in the first few days after bilateral extirpations of Bl
the dog did not respond to loud sounds. When Munk extirpated the cortex of the upper
surface of both temporal lobes, he observed persisting cortical deafness, but the dogs
survived only a few days and showed such profound disturbances that he questioned
the validity of the observation.

THEODOR MEYNERT AND CEREBRAL FUNCTION

Theodor Meynert, of Vienna, was the teacher of both Wernicke and Freud. Papez
(1953) summarized Meynert's contributions to neurophysiology as follows: "Meynert's
formulation of the problem of brain structure was of historic importance. He considered the cerebral cortex as a retentive recording tissue surmounting the radial bundles,
on which the sensory and other impulses were projected by afferent paths, each
registered image being the product of a special group (pattern) of simultaneously

perceived sensations. He was the first to show that central integration was dependent on this association process."

In a paper translated by Bonin, Meynert (1881) ridiculed the theory of telegraphic transmission of cerebral impulses, which has been such a persisting fallacy in relation to aphasia that it has survived into the twentieth century. Bonin (1960) commented that Meynert sometimes seemed to be on the verge of ideas which came into general vogue only after the advent of Wiener's *Cybernetics*, although he added that in other ways Meynert was as much dated as anyone else, for nobody can go beyond his time.

THE CONTRIBUTION OF WERNICKE

Inspired by the work of Meynert, with whom he studied six months in Vienna, Carl Wernicke wrote glowingly in 1874 that everything was known that was necessary for the understanding of aphasia. His book *Der Aphasische Symptomenkomplex* (1874) was published when Wernicke was 26 years old.

Following the teaching of Meynert, Wernicke divided the cerebrum into an anterior motor and a posterior sensory region. He thought the motor cortex contained concepts of movements. Broca's aphasia was thus a loss of motor images of words. Wernicke pointed out, however, that written language was also lost and added, "I am no longer of the opinion that in pure motor aphasia the ability to understand speech always remains unimpaired."

SENSORY APHASIA

Meynert believed that the posterior cortex contained the terminal point of the auditory nerve and auditory images of words. Wernicke considered the first temporal convolution an auditory center, and was the first to describe sensory aphasia resulting from temporal lobe lesions. The symptom complex Wernicke observed consisted of loss of understanding of speech, with hearing and articulation intact, and writing severely disturbed.

CONDUCTION APHASIA

Wernicke also postulated conduction aphasia resulting from interruption of fiber tracts connecting the auditory area and the motor speech area. The chief symptom was paraphasia. His scheme also contained a concept center, which he adopted from Kussmaul. Wernicke had reservations about his model, however, for he wrote, "There are as yet few reports, and even these fail to coincide; hence it is impossible to describe a uniform clinical picture on an empirical foundation." He added, "I cannot, however, refrain from emphasizing that autopsy findings are not calculated to support the view of conduction aphasia postulated by me." He deserves to be remembered for his intellectual integrity, as well as for the classical concepts of "Wernicke's area" and "Wernicke's aphasia," which extended the observations of Broca.

IN RETROSPECT

A retrospectroscope is a scientific instrument for elimination of error. It operates on the simple principle of utilizing future information to control present events. The instrument could conceivably be adapted, by minimal readjustments, to show past events, also, in sharpened focus and reduce distortion. Regrettably, the retrospectroscope exists only as an abstract design, a distinguished medical contribution to art, but not yet an available research tool (Crosbie, 1952).

"The diagram-makers" was Head's (1926) appellation for the numerous contemporaries and successors of Broca and Wernicke who published schemata representing arrangements of centers and commissures, from which they deduced hypothetical aphasic syndromes assumed to result from hypothetical lesions at selected sites.

"Diagram-makers" has become a term of disparagement, although theoretical constructs and conceptual models remain scientifically respectable. It is true, of course, that not all the early pioneers in neurology distinguished sharply between observation and inference, and that clinical observations of aphasic patients were often extremely inadequate.

However, it is also true that we tend to remember the diagrams and not to remember the searching examinations of anatomical, pathological, physiological, and clinical materials in laboratories and clinics that preceded the diagrams. We also tend to forget the advances in methodology that occurred as a result of these studies.

The exploration of relationships between structure and function was not only a legitimate field of inquiry but also one that laid the foundation stones of neurology. The nineteenth century was a time of heuristic investigation and exciting intellectual activity. If interest in localization made one a materialist, an atheist, or a radical in Germany and France, in England Sir David Ferrier was hauled into court by the antivivisectionists (Haymaker and Baer, 1953).

It is easy to see today that cerebral processes are infinitely more dynamic and complex than the most elaborate early models of aphasia assumed. Few physiologists have ever believed completely in a motor and sensory dichotomy, which became a strangely persisting part of the dogma of aphasia.

Monokow's paper on diaschisis, which introduced the concept of remote effects of brain injury extending beyond the area of immediate damage, was not published until 1909. Bonin wrote in 1960: "But even nowadays it is not easy to be quite consistent, and to think of nervous impulses as being merely 'pips,' and not something more recondite."

Neurology has moved beyond the concept of a cortical mosaic composed of cytoarchitectural areas subserving independent processes. Psychology has progressed beyond the theory of absolute mental faculties. Language processes are known to be more complex than can be accounted for in terms of static word images or chains of associations. Experimental psychology has given us more sophisticated diagnostic tools, as well as more rigorous criteria for examination procedures. Almost all the reported findings of the early period are too incomplete to support any theory, but ingenious tests were devised by Kussmaul, Marie, Moutier, and others to explore proposed hypotheses.

Few investigators today would try to evaluate the effects of discrete lesions on performances of patients observed in extremis or in the acute period following cerebral insult. We should not attempt to correlate an obvious symptom with damage at a predicted site, ignoring less obvious symptoms and damage in areas assumed to be irrelevant. We still tend, however, to be relatively uncritical of autopsy material and not to take sufficient account of the changes that can occur in a brain between the time a reliable evaluation of performance can be obtained and the intervention of death. Surgical reports can be similarly misleading, since surgical sites frequently present few landmarks and exploration can never be complete. Surgical localizations can, of course, be dependable, but many variables need to be taken into account before this is established.

It is easy to look back and see the pitfalls into which the unwary have fallen. It is sometimes more difficult to appreciate the odds they overcame and the advances they made. It is impossible to predict what will be known in 50 years, or 10, to make present theories and methods obsolete.

With this apology for the period of schematization, we shall review the contributions of three men selected to represent characteristic elaborations and revisions of earlier formulations, and to reflect the spirit of the times.

LUDWIG LICHTHEIM

Lichtheim was professor of medicine at the University of Berne in 1884 when he published his schema for aphasia and described five cases. To Wernicke's formulation, he added a center for visual images of words and a center for movements of the hand used in writing, as postulated by Exner in 1881.

Lichtheim recognized motorial (Broca's) aphasia, sensorial (Wernicke's) aphasia, and the conduction aphasia described by Wernicke. He postulated four additional syndromes deduced from hypothetical lesions of inferred conduction tracts.

What was most remarkable about Lichtheim's paper was the unassuming honesty of his report. About Broca's aphasia, he wrote, "I have unfortunately, as was just said, not observed recently any pure cases of Broca's aphasia. . . . I always found the patients had lost the innervations of auditory representations."

About Wernicke's aphasia he simply reported, "I cannot refer to any typical instance of sensorial aphasia from my own experience."

Concerning conduction aphasia, he wrote, "Cases of this kind do not appear to be very rare, although I am not acquainted with any observation of this kind as complete as could be wished."

Of the additional derived types, he wrote, "The schema is founded upon the phenomena of the acquisition of language by imitation, as observed in the child, and upon the reflex arc which this process presupposes."

He did not consider "amnesic aphasia" a type, observing correctly that this symptom occurred in various syndromes. He maintained that difficulty recalling words was not a sign of a focal lesion, but was instead a symptom of diminished cortical activity, which seems a surprisingly modern concept.

HENRY CHARLTON BASTIAN

Bastian's (1887, 1898) schema differed in two ways from the models of Wernicke and Lichtheim.

First, Bastian rejected the idea of a concept center, proposed by Broadbent in 1872, and accepted with individual modifications by Kussmaul, Charcot, Wernicke, Lichtheim, and others. The argument concerned the relationships between thought and language. Bastian's position was that perception, conception, and revival of words were inseparable and therefore could not be relegated to different centers.

Second, Bastian held that all language centers were sensory. He considered Broca's area a glossokinesthetic center that contained kinesthetic impressions of movements executed when a word was spoken, and Exner's area a cheirokinesthetic center, registering similar impressions of movements executed by the hand when a word was written.

He postulated that language centers corresponded to kinds of verbal memory, and that each center was an area in which a particular kind of retentum was registered and stored. Primary revival of words during thought occurred subconsciously in the auditory area and was immediately followed by correlated revivals in the glossokinesthetic center.

Bastian's rationale was that revival of sensory impressions was essential for production of all voluntary movements. Although this was a relatively static concept, in that output could only be controlled by previously stored sensory impulses, it rejected a sensory and motor dichotomy and almost anticipated modern feedback theory.

Bastian distinguished between loss of memory for words, resulting from damage to the centers in which the particular retentum was stored, and loss of recall, resulting from diminished functional activity in the centers or a defect in the commissural fibers, which he regarded as associational channels. His scholarly monograph on aphasia (1898) contains more than 100 illustrative case histories culled from the literature and his own records.

Historical case material is invaluable for extending one's frame of reference in regard to aphasia. It is, however, necessary to view reported judgments with considerable skepticism. For example, the report, "He understood everything that was said," occurred again and again in the protocols. Somehow or other, this is something people always say about aphasic patients, particularly when they have no speech. It is said, again and again, about patients who cannot follow directions as simple as "Put the spoon in the cup." Perhaps the patient picked up the spoon and looked questioningly at the examiner, not knowing what to do next; perhaps he picked up the cup; perhaps he touched a pencil and a key, uncertainly.

Patients with little or no speech are usually highly motivated to communicate and to perform well. They frequently respond appropriately by making maximal use of visual cues, situational cues, and occasional words they grasp. They observe the social amenities, smile, and appear responsive when spoken to. Since they have little or no speech, they tend not to give themselves away when they misunderstand, as hard-of-hearing individuals frequently do. Sometimes when the patient makes an obvious error, the speaking person ascribes it to his own difficulty communicating with the aphasic patient. This is a very curious phenomenon.

It was Hughlings Jackson (1893) who said, "Many observers are really inferring, when they should be only looking." In reviewing historical records, it is necessary to separate inference from evidence and to determine the basis for the conclusions that were drawn.

SALOMON EBERHARD HENSCHEN

Henschen first became interested in the localization of primary sensory areas in the cortex. Working with dogs, he demonstrated that there was almost point-to-point correspondence between retinal areas and the calcarine cortex subserving vision. He contended that, in addition to the primary sensory areas, there were other sensory centers in the brain where specific sensory processes were elaborated, and that lesions had precise localizing significance.

In his monumental work, *Klinische and Anatomische Beiträge zur Pathologie des Gehirns* (1920–1922), he abstracted in detail all cases of aphasia with autopsy findings in the literature of the world and attempted to analyze them. There were more than 1500 cases, most of which he presented in the original languages. Although he found it difficult to draw conclusions because of the meagerness of description in many cases, he remained a firm believer in discrete anatomic localization of specific aspects of language.

CRITICS OF EARLY LOCALIZATION THEORY

It has been pointed out that no investigator can do more than try to understand phenomena in relation to what is known in his time. It is not surprising that as knowledge of brain structure increased, successive attempts were made to correlate anatomical knowledge with disturbances resulting from cerebral injury or disease. The remarkable thing is that so many of the distinguished pioneers in aphasia reached beyond existing knowledge in one way or another.

There were, from the beginning, some serious and original thinkers on aphasia who remained outside the main stream of localization, which Marie described so vividly. As a result, their ideas about aphasia received little contemporary recognition, and were left for the most part for future generations to discover. One of these men was Hughlings Jackson.

JOHN HUGHLINGS JACKSON

At a meeting of the Worcestershire and Herefordshire, Bath and Bristol and Gloucestershire Branches of the British Medical Association, in 1888, Hughlings Jackson said, "Empirical work must come first; it is necessary for daily practice. . . . Before we can make rational generalizations we must have made empirical observations. . . ."

Herein lay Jackson's genius. He had a fine scientific mind, but his theories grew out of searching and penetrating clinical observations, and he constantly checked one against the other. Jackson was unable to accept popular theories of localization because he observed patients continuously, and he was a sensitive and honest observer.

He repeatedly declared he was neither a localizationist nor a "universalist" (1874, 1879, 1882, 1887). He pointed out that "to locate the damage which destroys speech and to locate speech are two different things" (1874). In a letter in the *British Medical Journal* in 1864, he wrote, "M. Broca points out a particular part of the brain, where, he believes the faculty of speech resides; but I can only surmise that it is in some part of the brain supplied by the middle cerebral artery." In the same paper, he argued that to attribute errors naming objects to defects in the muscles reminded him of the excuse a gentleman once gave for bad spelling, namely, that "his pen was a bad one."

Jackson described the inability of some aphasic patients to protrude the tongue on demand, although it moved freely in eating and swallowing, and wrote, concerning this observation,

> In such cases it will certainly be better to record the fact that the patient does not put out his tongue when told than the inference it is paralyzed. I have several times seen patients put their fingers in their mouths as if to help the tongue out. Here, we shall do no harm to clinical medicine if we simply record all the facts. It is better to say that "the patient, when asked to put out his tongue, evidently knows what is wanted, as he puts his fingers in his mouth as if to help it out, and yet does not protrude it in the least," than the following: "there is total paralysis of the tongue." The first is a statement of facts and gives the reader a basis to think from; the second a theory which is, on the face of it, improbable, and if a wrong one, all the more dangerous that such a theory often passes for a fact.

Jackson continued with another caution insufficiently regarded, even today: "In a subject so wide and vague as language, it would be simple work to pile up ingenious theories, but to find a method to arrange the varying facts in many actual cases is quite a different thing" (1864).

Jackson believed that disturbances of speech should be considered within the larger framework of dissolution produced by cerebral disease. He pointed out that there was always loss of more voluntary, with preservation of more automatic, performances in disease of the hemispheres, although he was careful to add that nowhere in the nervous system were there sharp demarcations between voluntary and involuntary processes (1864).

He maintained that the aphasic patient had not lost words so much as the ability to use words to express relationships through "propositions," while more automatic uses of words were retained. He insisted that a sentence was a unit of communication consisting of words in special relationships to each other, and not a "word-heap" (1864).

Jackson argued that speechless patients did indeed use words in certain ways, and his description and analysis of utterances observed in severe aphasics is a masterpiece of clinical insight (1879).

He observed that reading and writing always suffered to some extent in aphasia, although these defects varied as much as speech defects themselves. He felt that impairment of speech, reading, and writing all reflected the same defect, in various forms, and observed that patients who could not write could usually copy correctly (1868).

Jackson believed that the processes underlying internal and external speech were the same and that the only difference between them was that in external speech the outgoing pathways were enervated, while in internal speech they were not. In his words,

"I do not mean that propositionizing occurs only when we speak to tell others what we think, but it occurs when, so to say, we are telling ourselves what to think" (1879).

He taught that the organization of the nervous system was of a hierarchical order corresponding to its evolutionary development, and that in the ascent from lower to higher levels, representation of processes increased in complexity, in specialization, and in degree of integration. The most numerous interconnections were found at the highest level, and at this level all representation was sensorimotor.

SIGMUND FREUD

In 1891, Freud wrote a brilliant critical analysis of the theory of cerebral localization in relation to aphasia, in which he acknowledged that his views were inspired by the writings of Hughlings Jackson. Freud attacked classical localization theory and the idea of speech as a cerebral reflex as follows: "We can only presume that the fibre tracts which reach the cerebral cortex after passage through other gray masses have maintained some relation to the periphery of the body, but no longer reflect a topographically exact image of it. They contain the body periphery in the same way as—to borrow an image from the subject with which we are concerned here—a poem contains the alphabet."

Freud rejected the theory of centers and conduction tracts on two grounds. First:

> What then is the physiological correlate of the simple idea emerging or re-emerging? Obviously nothing static, but something in the nature of a process. This process is not incompatible with localization. It starts at a specific point in the cortex and from there spreads over the whole cortex and along certain pathways. When this event has taken place it leaves behind a modification, with the possibility of a memory, in the part of the cortex affected. . . . Whenever the same cortical state is elicited again, the previous psychic event emerges as a memory.

He stated his second objection as follows:

> Is it (sic) possible, then, to differentiate the part of "perception" from that of "association" in the concomitant physiological process? Obviously not. "Perception" and "association" are terms by which we describe different aspects of the same process. But we know that the phenomena to which these terms refer are abstractions from a unitary and indivisible process. . . . Both arise from the same place and are nowhere static.

It is significant that Freud did not propose abandoning localization theory, any more than Broca did when he rejected phrenology. Freud formulated his revision of current doctrines as follows:

> We have rejected the assumptions that the speech apparatus consists of distinct centres separated by functionless areas, and that ideas (memories) serving speech are stored in certain parts of the cortex called centres while their association is provided exclusively by subcortical fibre tracts. It only remains for us to state the view that the speech area is a continuous cortical region within which the associations and transmissions underlying the speech functions are taking place; they are of a complexity beyond comprehension.

The theory proceeded:

> The association area of speech, into which visual, auditory, and motor (or kinesthetic) elements enter, extends for that very reason between the cortical areas of those sensory nerves and the motor regions concerned with speech. If we now imagine a movable lesion of constant size within this association area, its effect will be the greater the more it approaches one of these cortical fields, i.e., the more peripherally it is situated within the speech area. If it borders immediately on one of these cortical fields it will cut off the association area from one of its tributaries, i.e., the mechanism of speech will be deprived of the visual, or auditory, or some other element. . . . If the lesion is moved toward the interior of the association area its effect will be more indefinite.

Except that Freud was thinking in terms of cortical processes, this is a startlingly modern formulation. Freud considered the associative activity of the acoustic element to be the central part of the speech function, and pointed out that impairment of reading letters, not of reading comprehension, was characteristic of a defect of the visual element.

He defined paraphasia as "a speech disorder in which the appropriate word is replaced by a less appropriate one, which, however, still retains a certain relationship to the correct word." He pointed out that paraphasia in aphasic patients did not differ from the errors healthy persons made in conditions of fatigue, divided attention, or other kinds of disturbances. However, he asserted this did not "exclude that they may occur in most typical form as organic focal symptoms."

Finally, except for Kussmaul, Freud seems to have been the only one of the early investigators to recognize what many people still seem to overlook, despite the form of his statement: "It is hardly necessary to point out that speechlessness in the first days after the onset of an illness has no diagnostic significance. It may occur irrespective of the site of the lesion and is obviously caused by the shock to the apparatus which has previously been working with all its resources."

ADOLF KUSSMAUL

Kussmaul was interested in the origin of language, the development of language in children, in problems of philology and linguistics, and in the emotional significance of language, all of which he considered important to an understanding of aphasia. He thought the symbolic process was linked with memory, as well as with thinking.

Concerning localization, Kussmaul (1887) wrote,

> We will especially turn away with a smile from all the naive attempts to locate "a seat of speech" in this or that part of the brain. It is a priori probable that an enormous association tract in the cortex has been assigned to speech, even though the keyboard may be confined to the anterior cortical regions, through which the impulses have their outlet, since speech must be bound up with the entire tract of conscious conceptions, and this indeed stretches across the entire cortical region.

He added, "It is further very probable that the same cell can enter into very different connections. The cortex, too, is the very organ in which, after an injury to its substance, the endless interlacing of the channels contained in it guarantees to the law of substitution an intensive, though not an unlimited, application."

He cited observations to show that in aphasic patients writing was almost always more impaired than speech, and that word blindness and word deafness were usually combined with a similar loss of words in speaking and writing. In this connection he cited the case of Lordat, professor of medicine at Montpellier, who lost speech for several months after a fever. Kussmaul reported that he was at first completely unable to speak because of loss of memory for words, and commented, "In the same way the treasures of writing were closed to him as with seven seals."

Kussmaul differentiated between amnesic aphasia, characterized by loss of words, and akataphasia, characterized by disturbances of grammar and syntax. The latter he thought could not result from loss of memory, since sentences are not stored up in the memory ready for use; he pointed out that a foreign language cannot be acquired from a dictionary alone. He observed, however, that when aphasia is severe and a large number of words are forgotten, the correct construction of sentences is impossible.

PAUL PIERRE MARIE

Marie set about reopening the question of aphasia for critical examination. He reexamined the two brains Broca had deposited at the Musée Dupuytren, demonstrated that they did not constitute scientific evidence for Broca's theory (1906b), and argued controversially that the third frontal convolution played no role in aphasia (1906a).

Marie believed that there was always some impairment of comprehension in aphasia and some intellectual impairment resulting from inability to use language. His most significant contribution was his insistence that patients be examined systematically with tests of progressive difficulty, in order that mild symptoms should not be overlooked.

ARNOLD PICK

In *Die Agrammatischen Sprachstörungen* (1913), Pick reviewed the theories of his time in philology, linguistics, and psychology of speech in a scholarly and thoroughgoing manner. According to Head, Pick intended to follow this work with a second volume containing an investigation of aphasic disturbances considered in this framework. This study was never completed, although a manuscript on aphasia, by Pick and Thiele (1931), was published after Pick's death.

Pick selected disturbances of grammar and syntax to illustrate the Jacksonian principle that the word is not the unit of speech, and to demonstrate that aphasic disorders involved more than loss of images of words, although he considered a free flow of words essential for structured thought.

Pick believed it was possible to analyze processes of thought and processes of speech into orderly and successive stages. In the initial stages meaning existed for the individual but was not verbalized. Pick held that the selection of words and the final form of expression were determined by the feelings of the speaker and by those of the auditor, as well.

The temporal sequence of events consisted first of the emergence of an idea or intention, nonverbal and nonstructured. This was followed by the formulation of a proposition, in the Jacksonian sense of a relationship; this was still nonverbal. The third stage was the general grammatical arrangement of the proposition, followed by the selection of words and patterning of movements. Pick believed that in aphasia a breakdown could occur at any stage of this process. He held that language processes were on a higher level of neurological integration than sensation and recognition, and involved the entire cortex.

Not many theorists who followed Pick have agreed that thinking processes are as explicitly structured as Pick conceived them or that events in "the pathway from thought to speech" occurred as sequentially. Head, for example, contended that such stages could be separated analytically, but not temporally. The importance of Pick's contribution, however, lies in the fact that he placed aphasia in a larger context than most of his forerunners had done. In this way he extended and deepened the awareness of those who came after him.

chapter 2

THE "STEEP ASCENT FROM THE UNKNOWN TO THE KNOWN"

World War I influenced the history of aphasia almost as profoundly as the autopsies of Broca and the observations of Wernicke. Before 1917 between 90 and 96% of soldiers with penetrating head wounds died, according to statistics cited by Goldstein (1942). With advances in brain surgery and improved transportation of the wounded, percentages of survival gradually increased.

With a large population of young war-injured patients, there was a new urgency about treatment. Hospitals for the brain-injured were organized behind the lines, and distinguished neurologists and psychiatrists devoted themselves to the clinical study of aphasia, with careful exploration of symptoms and a painstaking search for effective methods of treatment. Aphasia could no longer be considered an academic problem.

Among hospitals established for treatment of brain-injured patients, Goldstein (1942) cited ones directed by Head in England, by Isserlin in Munich, Poppelreuter in Cologne, himself in Frankfurt and Hartman in Groz, Austria. Froeschels (1955) was head physician in a military hospital in Vienna with 240 beds continuously occupied by brain-injured soldiers.

In the United States, 200 head-injury cases were treated at General Hospital No. 11, Cape May, New Jersey, between October 1918 and June 1919. Residual language involvement six months or more postinjury was reported in only 16 cases (Nielsen, 1946).

SIR HENRY HEAD

Head (1926) was influenced by Hughlings Jackson, with whom he was associated as a student and a colleague. His two volumes on aphasia deserve a permanent place in the literature for the wealth of penetrating observations and insights they contain.

"Every generation," Head wrote, "has examined the manifestations afresh, armed with different general conceptions and dominated by prejudices arising from the ideas of the day. The knowledge transmitted to subsequent workers in the field has thus been a mixture of theory and fact, and it has frequently happened that the theory has survived, while the new observations have been forgotten. Many a hypothesis, based on pure conjecture, has been handed on from one authority to influence his successors, while the luminous clinical investigations of the same author have been entirely neglected or have been absorbed into the general bulk of knowledge. The world clings to theories, for they are easier to remember, can be reproduced with effect, and lead to a clarity of exposition foreign to a description of the crude experimental facts. There is in consequence a tendency to carry over the conceptions of one age on to the observations of the next. New wine is poured into old bottles with disastrous results."

Elsewhere he wrote, "The 'golden rule' upon which Dr. Jackson insisted, 'Put down what the patient *does* get at and avoid all terms such as amnesic, et cetera,' had it been habitually followed, would have saved neurologists from many years of wandering in the wilderness."

The greatness of Head's contribution lies in the fact that he carried out the injunction of Jackson, and in his own strong conviction that it was necessary to have empirical knowledge of what one wanted to localize.

HEAD'S DOCTRINES

Head felt that prevalent doctrines of aphasia still bore the imprint of the psychology of Gall, which endowed man with moral and intellectual faculties subserved by separate organs in the brain. He cited the six kinds of memories Gall postulated: the memory of things, the memory of locality, name memory, verbal memory, grammatical memory, and memory for numbers. Essentially Head was saying that, in relation to aphasia, people talked as though such faculties were separate entities and could be differentially affected by disease.

He considered the idea that there were separate centers in the brain for normal functions to be a physiological anachronism. He denied that the word was the unit of speech. He thought this fallacy was one of the most disastrous errors in classical theories of aphasia since it was responsible for the doctrine of verbal images: the auditory image of a word, the visual image of a word, and the image of the movements used in speaking and in writing a word. He denied the existence of total "pure word blindness" and "pure word deafness," isolated from other disturbances.

But Head thought there was an even greater general fallacy. "Most of the work on aphasia," he wrote, "has been vitiated by a far more subtle and deep-seated error. It was almost universally assumed that the phenomena revealed by analysis could be treated as elements which were independent and had entered into combination. Thus, speech was constructed of the direct products of articulatory, visual, and auditory activities and could be resolved into these elements by disease. All conscious processes were reduced to sensory or motor presentation and laws of association." He added that "not only is it impossible to break up a word into auditory and visual elements, but disease does not analyze a sentence into its verbal or grammatical constituents."

He pointed out that it was not enough to say that a patient could not speak, read, or write, but that it was necessary to investigate the conditions under which he could or could not perform such activities, and continued, "A disturbance of one aspect of speech is invariably associated with some other disorder in the use of language or allied functions."

Head maintained that diagnoses of isolated pure disorders resulted from false a priori assumptions combined with inadequate clinical examinations. He pointed out that patients were examined neither systematically nor comprehensively, and added that in most clinical records there was nothing to indicate that at the time of death defects were the same as those that had existed at earlier stages. This is a particularly important consideration in view of the fairly prevalent early belief that patients should be examined as soon as possible after onset of symptoms lest some of them disappear.

HEAD'S PROCEDURES

Head developed a comprehensive body of tests for aphasic behavior, which he administered systematically to 26 subjects. Because he was impressed with the variability of aphasic responses, he insisted that each item be repeated several times; because he believed that present events in the nervous system were dependent on past events, he insisted on the same order of presentation of items, in all modalities. This made the testing process a long and tedious one, as anyone who has tried to administer Head's test knows.

Head's study was based on 26 subjects, 19 of whom were World War I veterans with traumatic injuries generally resulting from gun shot or shrapnel; 4 were vascular cases; 1 a tumor case; 2 were cases of congenital aphasia observed in adulthood. Head followed some of these patients over periods of years, and reexamined them at long-term intervals. The second volume of *Aphasia, and Kindred Disorders of Speech* (1926) contains some 400 pages devoted to the clinical protocols of these 26 subjects. Besides test responses, the protocols included many searching observations reported by the patients, and by Head himself.

The account of procedures and responses constitutes a noteworthy advance in the investigation of aphasia and a valuable contribution to the literature, in spite of the understandable limitations of a pioneering study. No controls were used, and normal subjects encounter difficulties with some of Head's tests (Pearson *et al.*, 1928). Twenty-six subjects is a small number viewed in relation to the complexity of the brain and the diversity of symptoms that result from brain damage in general, and from gunshot wounds in particular.

It seems probable that if Head had been treating even 26 subjects and observing day-to-day performances he might have been less impressed with the variability of aphasic performance. It is true that there is variability of individual responses, but it is equally true that there is remarkable consistency in the kinds of errors and percentages of errors on repeated tasks. For this reason repetition and order of items are of less consequence than Head supposed. Reliability is dependent on getting an adequate sample of behavior.

Head was also impressed with the tendency of aphasic patients to confuse the names of colors even when they had no difficulty matching or sorting them, and spent an inordinate amount of time on such tests. He did not see this difficulty as related to confusions that appear between all words with strong associational linkages.

On his alphabet tests, he confined himself to investigating recognition and recall of letters in serial order. Aphasic subjects have far greater difficulty recognizing and recalling letters presented in random order, where they tend to confuse letters on the basis of contiguity, frequency, names that sound alike and, in some cases, letters with familiar visual configurations. As a result, the alphabet tests also missed the main point.

Head noted the difficulty his patients had retaining verbal sequences, and quoted various observations patients made to this effect, such as, "I like that young man; he's clever. I notice that clever people say everything in a few words, so I can understand." However, Head seemed not to appreciate the relationship between verbal retention span and the inability of patients to "grasp the full significance" of materials, in what he termed semantic aphasia.

All of this, however, is simply to say that Head's tests bear refinement in the light of present knowledge.

Head defined aphasia as impairment of "symbolic formulation and expression," substituting this term for Jackson's "propositional speech" (1926). He identified four major kinds of defects: (1) *verbal defects,* defined as defective power of forming words for both external and internal use; (2) *syntactical defects,* characterized by loss of balance and rhythm, affecting both articulation and structural forms; (3) *nominal defects,* characterized by impairment of the nominal value of words, in both comprehension and speech; (4) *semantic defects,* primarily loss of ability to appreciate or formulate the logical conclusion of a train of thought or action.

This system had the virtue of avoiding the old motor and sensory dichotomy and the concept of isolated pure disorders, which Head did not find clinically. However, there was too much overlap between categories to make them particularly meaningful, and they did not obtain general acceptance. Head's methods of localization are of historical interest only.

CONCLUSIONS

The limitations of this early empirical study do not detract from the importance of what Head was saying. He insisted on the necessity for systematic and comprehensive data. He believed that language was based on "integrated functions, standing higher in the neural hierarchy than motion or sensation." From the "facts of clinical observation," he concluded that "when a complex mode of behavior, such as the use of language, is disturbed by structural disease, the loss of function is manifested in terms of the process itself, and does not reveal the elements out of which it has been built up" (1926).

Finally, extensive observations of the behavior of aphasic subjects in a diversity of situations caused Head to believe, contrary to Marie, that general intellectual capacity was not specifically affected in aphasia, but rather "the mechanism by which certain aspects of mental activity can be brought into play" (1926). This mechanism, of course, was language.

EMIL FROESCHELS

We wish first to acknowledge the kindness of Dr. Froeschels in implementing a correspondence of many years with a resumé of his work in Vienna, where he estimated that he treated approximately 2000 brain-injured patients between 1916 and 1925. Comprehensive examinations for aphasia were administered, detailed studies were made of individual patients, and both individual and group treatment were used.

Dr. Froeschels described the scheme of examination as follows:

1. Motor speech: repetition of sounds, syllables, combined syllables, words, brief sentences, numbers; repeating syllables and words
2. Understanding: gestures and producing gestures to order; visual perception of speech movements; selecting objects and pictures to oral order; performing actions to order
3. Spontaneous speech: conversation, description, oral reports of experiences; forming sentences from given words
4. Memory: especially visual, acoustic, tactile, and taste memories
5. Generalization and specialization: What is a chicken? duck? sparrow? etc.; differentiation between hand and foot, bird and butterfly, dwarf and giant, etc.; definitions, such as, What does "blind," or "coward," mean?
6. Combinations: Sentence completion, filling in words or phrases in familiar stories; questions, such as, If a person wants to cross a river, and there is no bridge, what will he do?
7. Attention: underlining certain letters and parts of speech; correcting printed errors
8. Extensive reading and writing tests
9. Aesthetic and moral judgments

Froeschels (Froeschels et al., 1932) believes that the speech of every individual is singular and unique, and for this reason he has always been skeptical of categorizing aphasic subjects. He follows Charcot in considering mental type significant in relation to aphasia.

Charcot's idea was that some individuals tend to be strongly visual-minded, while others are auditory-minded, or motor-kinesthetic-minded, and that such predispositions play a role in initial learning of language, and consequently in symptomatology and recovery from aphasia. In 1930, Froeschels began to test school children in Vienna to determine individual mental types, his idea being that if such information were contained in school records, it would be available and useful in treating individuals who later became aphasic. This study was unavoidably interrupted in 1938. It is unfortunate that it could not have been completed, for this theory has never been tested.

Froeschels considers the speech of each individual unique, not only in production of phonemes, but also in preferences for words and grammatical forms. He has always emphasized the part played by psychological conditions in both normal and aphasic language behavior.

With Pick, Froeschels (1955) regards grammar and syntax as not "something added to the words chosen, but a matrix in which the words are embedded." He has studied verbal utterances in dreams and transition states, and reported that while neologisms were present, grammar and modulation conformed with usage in waking states. He recalls that Freud considered speech a function which helps to change unconscious into preconscious and conscious material. This was an original and penetrating study, and a significant one in that it enlarged the context of aphasic disturbances by demonstrating similar language phenomena arising in other conditions. One is reminded of observations made by Hughlings Jackson as he wandered through London hospital wards listening to the utterances of patients in delirium, in dementia, and during epileptic seizures.

Besides considering disturbances of melody and grammar in aphasia, Froeschels (1954) has noted such clinical phenomena as the sudden changes from unusual to usual modulation in pronunciation of newly learned words. He has concluded that this event is the result of the formation of an association between the newly learned pattern and the Gestalt established on original learning. He maintains that such identification may occur acoustically, when the patient's kinesthetic production is sufficiently "canalized" for him to be able to listen to himself; kinesthetically, when newly acquired kinesthetic engrams are sufficiently "canalized" for identification with old kinesthetic engrams; and when a spoken word evokes previously established engrams.

Froeschels (1954) has also described the effects of impeded feedback, and considers receptive and expressive aphasia to be theoretical constructs rarely observed in reality.

KURT GOLDSTEIN

Goldstein (1942) organized a hospital for treatment of brain-injured soldiers in Frankfurt during World War I. Facilities at Frankfurt included a hospital, a psychological laboratory, a school, a workshop, and a research institute. Goldstein estimated that he treated more than 2000 patients during this period, and had between 90 and 100 of them under continuous observation for more than 10 years. Among his important contributions to the German literature were the careful clinical studies of visual disturbances and amnesic aphasia carried on with his colleague, Gelb. In addition, Goldstein's long career in civilian neurology gave him an opportunity to study the effects of vascular, as well as traumatic, lesions.

Goldstein believed that alterations of performance with brain damage could be understood only in relation to the total organism. He elaborated this point of view in *The Organism*, published in 1939. Lashley wrote in the introduction, "Dr. Goldstein considers the problem of neural and behavioral organization from a broadly biological point of view. On such questions he is qualified to speak as one of the world's greatest authorities. His long series of studies of patients with brain injuries, less familiar than they should be to American readers, have set a new standard of careful clinical analysis combined with keen psychological insight."

In *The Organism*, Goldstein formulated many of the basic concepts which were his frame of reference for aphasia. Concerning symptomatology he wrote, ". . . If subjected to greater scrutiny than is usually the case, the classic assumption of specific separate losses of individual performances cannot be maintained. We found rather that a systematic reduction (dedifferentiation) results, a dedifferentiation which can be evaluated properly only in its relation to the whole organism. Depending on the part of the brain that is injured, this reduction affects one circumscribed performance field more than others. When the so-called peripheral areas are injured, the reduction is relatively more isolated in one motor or sensory field. When the central areas are injured, the reduction always affects all fields."

Goldstein considered the sensory and motor areas the periphery of the cortex, and the central area "those parts which are relatively independent of the projection systems and the peripheral cortex," specifically, parts of the frontal and parietal lobes and the insula.

Goldstein emphasized that the nervous system is never at rest, but instead is in a continuous state of excitation. He regarded the pattern of activity resulting from a stimulus as the foreground, or figure, and the concurrent activity in the rest of the system as the ground, in Gestalt terminology. He considered this configuration of excitation, the foreground–background relation, to be the basic form of functioning of the nervous system.

Although Goldstein regarded many of the phenomena of aphasia as disturbances of figure–ground relationships, he was critical of Gestalt theory. To him the Gestalt meant the whole organism, not phenomena in one field. A "good Gestalt" represented the organism coming to terms with the world. He considered the principle of isomorphism inadequate because it assumed a correspondence between physical Gestalt processes and mental configurations. Goldstein insisted that every past event referred to the whole, and that the whole organism supported all partitive phenomena. He considered discrepancies between Gestalt psychology and his organismic viewpoint surmountable, however, for he wrote, "In my concept of the configurational process in the organism, the figure, in the sense of the Gestalt, already represents a partitive phenomenon. If the scope of holistic events were enlarged to include the entire organism, then the Gestalt principle would become sufficiently broad to fit all the facts which may not have, as yet, been covered" (1939).

Goldstein characterized the disintegration of performance resulting from brain damage as *dedifferentiation* to emphasize the alteration from highly differentiated and articulated responses to more amorphous total behavior. He pointed out that disintegration in the central nervous system had a special structure and resulted in specific changes.

First, he cited a rise of threshold and retardation of excitation resulting in decreased receptivity and increased reaction time. Second, he listed lability of threshold, accounting for perceptual changes during stimulation, and, third, abnormal spread and duration of stimuli, which he considered the mechanism of perseveration.

Fourth, he noted that for patients deprived of functions and previous experiences, external stimuli acquired exaggerated importance. Goldstein considered this condition responsible for the distractibility reported in brain-injured patients.

Fifth, he reported a blurring of sharp boundaries between figure and ground, sometimes carried to the point of inversion so the patient said yes for no, or black for white.

Last, he held there was impairment of ability to assume abstract attitudes. The patient, bound to immediate experiences of objects and events, could only react concretely. He lacked initiative and spontaneity, and was rigid and compulsive in behavior. He was unable to assume a set voluntarily, to make a choice, to shift from one aspect of a situation to another, to keep various aspects of a situation in mind simultaneously, to grasp the essentials of a whole, to abstract common properties, to plan ahead ideationally, to assume a categorical attitude or to detach the ego from the outside world (1948).

Some of these concepts appear more valid than others. It is not necessary, for example, to infer that an opposite response represents reversal of figure and ground. Vocabulary opposites are merely associations of high strength, as are other common confusions in the language of aphasic patients, and can equally well be characterized as less differentiated responses.

Goldstein did not think there were sharp demarcations between concrete and abstract behavior, nor did he consider impairment of abstract attitude a constant finding in aphasia, as his protocols attest. Elsewhere, he reported a high incidence of frontal lobe lesions in subjects with gunshot wounds (1942). The frequency of frontal lobe damage in the population he studied may account for the emphasis he placed on concrete behavior.

We have obtained ambiguous results on the tests for abstract behavior developed by Golstein and Scheerer (1941). Tests appear to variously reflect spatial disorientation, impaired ability to comprehend or retain instructions, and inability of the patient to formulate the task to himself. Many aphasic subjects who failed the tests initially, performed them with ease a few weeks later, when they had acquired more language. Goldstein reported that patients with lesions in the left hemisphere showed more impairment of abstract attitude than patients with right-sided lesions. This would seem to give some support to the idea that ability to abstract is related to language, at least to some extent, although Goldstein does not accept this interpretation. Reservations concerning interpretation are minor, however, in comparison with the value of the observations and insights he reported.

To Goldstein, "The characteristic difference between the older and the more recent orientation in psychopathology is that the former regarded the observable symptoms simply as manifestations of changes in different functions or structures, whereas in the new approach many symptoms are seen as expressions of the change which the patient's personality as a whole undergoes as a result of disease, and also as expression of the struggle of the changed personality to cope with the defect and with the demands it can no longer meet" (1942).

"The sick man," he observed, "has a strong urge to meet all demands as well as possible; his existence is bound up with such an endeavor to a greater degree than the healthy man's (1942). He pointed out that when a patient was faced with tasks he could perform, his behavior was orderly, appropriate, and effective, and he experienced satisfaction and a sense of well-being. On the other hand, when a patient was confronted with tasks he could not perform, a "catastrophic reaction" occurred. Behavior became disordered, inconstant, inconsistent, embedded in shock, and the patient experienced intense anxiety. In Goldstein's words, he experienced "a breaking down or dissolution of the world, and a shattering of his own self" (1942).

Goldstein maintained that much of the behavior of sick people can only be understood as an unconscious defense against catastrophic situations, and that this defense results in a definite behavior pattern. Among the protective mechanisms he described are "self-exclusion" from the world, which, in extreme cases, may manifest itself in loss of consciousness. The patient tends to seek out situations which present a minimum of irritating stimuli. He avoids company. He surrounds himself with a protective fence, which he builds by constantly busying himself with something. He becomes excessively orderly: everything must be close at hand and in its place, because he can only cope with a controlled and predictable environment. In Goldstein's words, "Closer examination shows that in order to readjust itself to the world, the injured organism has withdrawn from numerous points of contact with it, and has thus attained a readjustment to a shrunken environment" (1942). Finally, the sick man is unaware of his deviations from his previous condition, the degree of such unawareness varying inversely with his ability to function with the existing deficit.

Goldstein felt that in cases where the pathology could not be removed, it was the responsibility of the physician to secure the best possible milieu for the patient. He pointed out that patients did not experience catastrophic reactions when strong transference was established with the clinician. He was not concerned about whether symptoms were organic or psychogenic, but wrote, "We must realize that the important question is whether a man is really suffering or not, really disturbed in his life and work or not. . . . Absence of organic signs does not rule out the possibility of an organic character of some of the symptoms" (1942).

Goldstein opposed quantification of test findings in aphasia. His argument was as follows: "The sequelae of a cerebral lesion rarely take the form of a complete loss of performance; more commonly the performance affected undergoes modifications. If the results are viewed, as they were formerly, as so many pluses and minuses, no real insight is gained into what the patient can still do and what he no longer can do" (1948).

This represents an extremely important kind of awareness. As Goldstein demonstrated, it is necessary to know not only the result the patient obtained, but how he obtained it. It is necessary to know not only the tasks the patient failed, but why he could not perform them. Otherwise there can be no insight into the nature of aphasic problems. It is, however, possible to construct tests so that such observations are possible, and much is to be learned from comparison of patterns of aphasic deficit that can emerge only with quantification. If Goldstein did not believe this, he would scarcely have constructed tests, or described types of aphasia as he did (Goldstein and Scheerer, 1941; Goldstein, 1948). Categories can be based only on identification of recurring patterns. However, if one compares Goldstein's searching protocols of examinations with the ambiguous and superficial reports found in much of the early literature, it is easy to understand his insistence on intensive qualitative methods.

Goldstein argued that one could not rate tests as "easy" or "hard," because tasks that were easy for normal subjects could present marked difficulties to aphasic subjects (1948). It is possible, however, to arrange given tests in order of difficulty on the basis of standardization for aphasic subjects. Difficulty is then determined by the number of aphasic subjects who pass or fail a given test. Tests that are notably easy for one segment of an aphasic population and difficult for another have a high diagnostic value. The source of difficulty is of course another problem, and usually must be explored by further tests.

Whether one agrees or disagrees with all of Goldstein's formulations is inconsequential. He was one of the great clinicians, and every student of aphasia can gain new insights through his work. In Lashley's words, "He set a new standard of careful clinical analysis."

WEISENBURG AND MCBRIDE: A CLINICAL AND PSYCHOLOGICAL STUDY

In 1935, Theodore Weisenburg, a neurologist, and Katherine McBride, a psychologist, published the results of a five-year study of aphasia supported by a grant from the Commonwealth Fund of New York. Weisenburg described the inception of the study as follows: "Six years ago while training ten graduate students in neuropsychiatry in the Graduate School of Medicine, University of Pennsylvania, two of the students, Pearson and Alpers (Pearson *et al.*, 1928) were directed to try out Head's tests for aphasia on the other students. To their amazement and mine, the results of some of the tests were similar to those obtained by Head in his aphasic patients. . . . Another series of tests was tried out with similar results. The need for adequate test methods for the study of aphasia seemed obvious, and I determined to embark on this research."

PROCEDURES

Subjects were 60 hospitalized aphasic patients (37 vascular, 15 tumor, and 8 traumatic) who were English speaking, under 60, had adequate sight and hearing and showed no signs of psychosis or advanced arteriosclerosis. A control series of 85 normal adults was obtained from surgical and orthopedic wards. In addition, 38 subjects with unilateral lesions but no aphasia were examined.

A comprehensive battery of psychological and educational achievement tests was used. Standardized tests were modified when desirable, and supplementary tests were added for further exploration. An average of 19 hours was spent examining each aphasic subject.

CLASSIFICATION OF APHASIC SUBJECTS

Weisenburg and McBride classified their aphasic subjects in four general groups:

1. *Predominantly expressive*, with the most severe disturbances in writing and speech. In some cases comprehension of both spoken and written material was seriously limited.
2. *Predominantly receptive*, characterized by a more or less serious disturbance in perception and understanding of spoken language and of printed materials. Speech was impaired and writing defective.
3. *Expressive–receptive*, with severe limitations of all language performances.
4. *Amnesic*, with the chief difficulty evoking words. There were only five subjects in this group; all of them were diagnosed as tumor cases; none of them were neurologically stable. Four continued a course of progressive deterioration; in the fifth case spontaneous recovery occurred following evacuation of an abscess.

CRITICAL COMMENTS

There are two general criticisms of the Weisenburg and McBride study. The first is the somewhat surprising fact, in view of the general sophistication of procedures, that they used subjects who were not neurologically stable, and attempted to classify them and describe the course of aphasia in various categories.

For the latter purpose they used the records of 36 subjects who received more than one examination. Nine subjects were first examined within periods of two days to a week after onset of aphasia, and eight subjects within periods of two to eight weeks. Five additional subjects were tumor cases who showed progressive deterioration, or deterioration after surgery followed by gradual improvement; one was a traumatic case who followed a similar course. Thus, 23 of the 36 subjects showed changes in performances that would be expected to reflect unpredictable physiological changes, rather than yield information about the course of aphasic syndromes. It is, of course, legitimate to study remission and progression of symptoms, but not to group subjects with acute conditions with subjects whose neurophysiological status has been unchanged over a long period of time.

The second criticism is of the classification system itself, which adds little or nothing to the value of the study. If all subjects showed both receptive and expressive impairment, these are meaningless terms in relation to aphasia. The authors reported that, "Expressive disorders free of disturbances in receptive functions were not found among the hundred-odd cases investigated in the selection of the group of aphasic patients" (1935). Similarly, descriptions of other categories showed expressive disturbances in all groups.

As a result of an admitted predilection for the "old bottles" of Broca and Wernicke,

Weisenburg and McBride discounted the evidence of their data and the excellence of their clinical observations, and settled for a classification system that can neither be regarded as informative or heuristic. The first two categories are too heterogeneous to be meaningful; the fourth has no kind of logical relation to the others. Like Head's system, the revision of Weisenburg and McBride has the virtue, however, of avoiding a motor and sensory dichotomy, and division into isolated "pure" disorders.

There is, as a matter of fact, considerable correspondence between the two classification systems, if one may assume these categories are similar:

Weisenburg and McBride	Head
Predominantly expressive	Verbal
Predominantly receptive	Syntactical
Amnesic	Nominal

The nonsimilar categories appear to represent two ends of a difficulty continuum. Head may have regarded the syndrome Weisenburg and McBride classified as expressive–receptive as a severe form of verbal aphasia. This would seem clinically and theoretically permissible, although since there is a difference in prognosis, the retention of a special category for the most severely impaired subjects is meaningful.

Weisenburg and McBride had no category corresponding to Head's semantic aphasia. It seems probable that this syndrome represents mild nominal or amnesic aphasia, and that this is really a superfluous category. Viewed in this light, the Weisenburg and McBride system represented an advance over the system of Head, which is as it should be.

WEISENBURG AND MCBRIDE'S CONTRIBUTION

The Weisenburg and McBride study is a landmark in the history of aphasia because of three important advances in methodology. It was the first study to use a normal control group, to compare performances of aphasic subjects with performances of nonaphasic subjects with cerebral lesions and to use standardized measurements.

The 22 subjects with right-hemisphere lesions and no aphasia did not equal the performance of normal subjects on any test. They performed more like normals on language tests, and less like normals on nonlanguage tests and arithmetic. The authors noted that these subjects did not perform like low normals or mild aphasics, but rather showed a characteristic pattern of deficit.

Aphasic subjects approximated normals most closely on nonlanguage tests. The performance of some aphasics was scarcely distinguishable from that of normals on these tests; others showed more deficit. In no case, however, did nonlanguage performance show the gross deterioration found in the language performances of aphasic subjects.

Some of the most valuable contributions Weisenburg and McBride made resulted from qualitative study of aphasic responses. They set out to determine not only what performances were altered but also why subjects failed specific tasks, and to examine the nature of the responses that were made and the methods by which subjects achieved results.

To Hughlings Jackson's classical description of inferior speech, Weisenburg and

McBride added a significant observation of reactive speech that was neither emotional nor automatic but was determined by external stimuli over which the patient had no control. They observed that there was no sharp line of demarcation between verbal and syntactical defects, but that, instead, one shaded off into the other. They noted reduction of auditory retention span, and that disturbances in writing tended to parallel those found in speaking. They described reversals and confusions of letters similar in form. They reported that in some cases oral spelling was less disturbed than written. They attributed this to the fact that oral spelling is a more automatic process—this seems unlikely, since the converse of this finding is often true. Nevertheless, such observations, well documented as they were, presented clinical facts of utmost importance.

After thousands of hours of observation of aphasic performance, the authors were most impressed by the regularity they found. They reported: "The widely noted irregularity in aphasic performances appears chiefly in the responses to some particular test item, naming a certain object, for instance, or reading a certain word. When the average of a number of such test items is obtained, the aphasic performance does not differ greatly from day to day or from month to month." They added that even where there was improvement or deterioration resulting from changes in pathology, "the regularity characterizing the typical aphasic disorder appears in an orderly regression or progression of symptoms. . . . There are no sudden and inexplicable spurts and no shifts from one form of the disorder to another."

They described the social adequacy of most aphasic subjects and cited the comment one aphasic patient made about another who had almost no speech, and who understood only an occasional word. "He's a sensible fellow," the first patient observed. Weisenburg and McBride added, "The typical aphasic patient is a sensible fellow, who is able to cope with the routine of everyday life insofar as it does not involve language" (1935).

CONCLUSIONS

The authors concluded, "Aphasia is first and foremost a language disorder. That is the primary conclusion which the analyses of these cases indicate." They added that aphasia is not a regression to a more primitive level of thinking, and that it represents a particular and not a general defect in intelligence.

Concerning pure forms of aphasia, the authors observed:

> The differentiation of types of aphasia according to the various forms of language—speaking, understanding, reading and writing—is, as Head pointed out, an arbitrary and unsatisfactory procedure, for actual studies do not show that one of these forms is affected to the exclusion of others, or even that the typical case manifests a predominant disturbance in one of these forms. The fact that no "pure" forms of disorder—pure motor aphasia, word-deafness, agraphia or alexia—appeared among the patients of this research is in itself a weighty argument against the existence of such forms, for the five-year survey covered a good cross section of the average run of aphasic patients. More than that, it was based on thorough examinations which would have been sufficient to reveal a pure disorder if such a phenomenon had existed. In all probability it is the thoroughness of the examination which showed each disorder in its actual complexity.

The authors did not consider it possible to localize language, or language disturbances, except in a general manner.

Good clinical observations are never dated, and in this respect theirs is a timeless study.

JOHANNES MAAGAARD NIELSEN

Nielsen was greatly influenced by the work of Henschen. In the preface of the first edition of *Agnosia, Apraxia, Aphasia: Their Value in Cerebral Localization* (Nielsen and Fitzgibbon, 1936), Nielsen wrote that "because of gross errors and unwarranted conclusions in the old teaching, the entire doctrine (of cerebral localization) has been prematurely discarded. . . . The writer is interested in the philosophy of cerebral function on the one hand and in cerebral localization in neurological diagnosis on the other. In favor of the latter he feels a diagnostic method should not be permitted to fall into discard merely because it is difficult."

This is a reasonable point of view. Uncritical rejection of a theory is as bad as uncritical acceptance, and one suspects the baby has been thrown out with the bathwater a good many times. Moreover, reexamining old theories in the light of new information is often an heuristic procedure.

Nielsen (1946) redefined engrams as "functionally educated structures over which impulses pass with much greater facility than they did the first time impulses passed over the same route." He redefined a center as "a cortical area, the functional removal of which causes a deficiency syndrome which can be recognized clinically."

In the second edition of *Agnosia, Apraxia, Aphasia: Their Value in Cerebral Localization* (1946), Nielsen distinguished 16 kinds of agnosia: 4 with highly specific localizing value and 12 localizing to some extent; 3 kinds of apraxia with highly specific localizing value, 3 with some degree, and 2 with none; and 6 kinds of aphasia all significant for localization.

In an attempt at organization, establishment of a physiological and anatomical basis of classification, and a foundation for agreement in terminology, Nielsen defined 87 specific defects, including various kinds of agraphia, alexia, acalculia, irreminiscence (impairment of recall), and aphasia, as well as agnosia, apraxia, amimia (loss of ability to mimic) and amusia (disturbance of musical sense). In most cases he stated the focus of the lesion giving rise to the defined disturbance.

In general, Nielsen accepted Dejerine's elaboration of the Freudian definition of agnosia: "Agnosia is a difficulty of recognition. Recognition is that psychological phenomenon which permits us by the use of one or another of our senses to identify an object under observation with an object previously observed and of which we have registered the memory picture in the form of a mental image." Nielsen pointed out that this loss of recognition must be confined to one sense organ, and stressed Monakow's point that only vision, hearing, and touch were involved.

Nielsen defined apraxia as "a disturbance in which a patient without dementia, incoordination, or paralysis is nevertheless, because of a motor incapacity, unable to apply his powers to a voluntary purpose" (1946). He considered Broca's aphasia a cortical motor pattern apraxia resulting from destruction of engrams for speech movements in the third frontal convolution.

Nielsen ascribed word-finding difficulties and agrammatism to lesions in Brodmann Area 37, which he considered a language formulation center. He pointed out that when Area 37 was destroyed in the dominant hemisphere only, the patient utilized the corresponding area in the nondominant hemisphere and talked volubly but incorrectly.

The theory that the nondominant hemisphere mediates retention or recovery of language in aphasia cannot be considered established. Nielsen believed that residual speech observed after hemispherectomy necessitated this conclusion. However, such cases seem only to indicate that the nondominant hemisphere may be utilized to some extent in some cases. The theory does not account for severe loss of speech, such as is sometimes produced by thrombosis of the middle cerebral artery, for example, when there is almost no residual speech or recovery of function, no indication of bilateral damage, and when angiography demonstrates an intact blood supply in the nondominant hemisphere. Neither is the theory necessary to account for recovery of functions impaired by smaller lesions, when it is at least equally probable that processes can be reintegrated in the same hemisphere.

As evidence for his theories of discrete cortical localization, Nielsen cited 94 cases from the literature, 85 of which were taken from Henschen. The latter included Broca's patient, Leborgne. In addition Nielsen described 46 cases of his own, many with autopsy findings.

The evidence is open to criticism on three major grounds:

First, too many inferences were made which were not sufficiently substantiated, as, for example, this statement from a 1937 protocol: "His general mentality was well preserved, as he helped with the housework at home" (1946). Findings reported for new patients were better documented than for the historical series, although reports were not uniform or objective enough to make comparisons between patients possible.

Second, specific defects were consistently attributed to focal lesions in patients with advanced arteriosclerosis, astrocytoma, multiple metastatic tumors, history of multiple episodes, and in patients with reported senility, dementia and mental deterioration.

Third, many patients were not neurophysiologically stable when examined. Examinations were reported that were performed during the first few days following onset of symptoms, after surgery, and preceding death. One patient incurred a cerebral infarct March first, was examined March third, and died March sixth (1946). In such cases, if it is possible to obtain reliable performances from patients, which the authors do not believe, it is certainly not possible to differentiate between disturbances resulting from a destructive lesion and disturbances resulting from temporary conditions, such as edema, unabsorbed bleeding, ischemia and diaschisis.

In other words, healing takes place in the brain after a cerebral accident. Swelling goes down, bleeding is absorbed, collateral circulation is established, and cells which were receiving insufficient nourishment may begin to function again. As a result of all these healing processes, connections may be reestablished that permit remote areas of the brain having functional relationships with areas affected to resume interrupted activity. The extent of this recovery is unpredictable. The effects of a destructive lesion cannot be assessed until such spontaneous recovery has taken place.

The importance of Nielsen's contribution lies in his insistence on considering aphasia in a neurological framework during a period when this view was relatively unpopular. While the doctrine of discrete cortical localization is no longer tenable, Nielsen was correct when he stated in 1936 that the doctrine of cerebral localization had been prematurely discarded. In the history of medicine, organic symptoms have been repeatedly referred to psychogenic sources before the neurophysiological mechanisms underlying them were completely understood. In view of the serious criticisms that must be made of his procedures and his evidence, however, his conclusions concerning types of aphasic disorders and their localization cannot be taken as established.

chapter **3**

"THE SLOW DEPOSIT OF
KNOWLEDGE"

Aphasia has always been a challenging field of inquiry. Today not only neurologists but also psychologists, speech pathologists, and linguists are concerned with its phenomena and are increasingly aware of the need for an interdisciplinary approach to the problem.

During and immediately after World War II, numerous centers for treatment of brain-injured soldiers were established. Programs of research and therapy were undertaken with new zeal and urgency, and with an unfortunate abundance of cases requiring attention and furnishing data. Most programs demonstrated that something could be done for the aphasic patient, and advances in both therapy and theory were seen. In the two decades following the war, some major investigators can be readily identified.

JOSEPH M. WEPMAN

In *Recovery from Aphasia* (1951), Wepman reported findings obtained from 68 patients treated between January 1945 and August 1946.

Wepman considers aphasia not only a language impairment, but a disturbance that affects the entire personality. He stresses the importance of psychotherapy and of treatment directed toward the individual and not the disorder. While he considers returning the individual to a useful place in society to be the goal of treatment, he also takes account of existing limitations. He writes that the aphasic adult ". . . must be looked upon as a new individual possessing the same inherited constitutional factors and the same early conditioning background, but different cortical capacity, new cortical integrative patterns, and a new concept of self. The goals of therapy must be in terms of this new individual, of his potential, of his new energy level."

In 1961 Wepman, in collaboration with Jones, published a new test called the *Language Modalities Test for Aphasia*. Language disturbances are classified as: (1) global, where little or no speech is available; (2) jargon, where speech is unintelligible; (3) pragmatic, where speech is useful, but no context can be found; (4) semantic, where the substantive language is not present; and (5) syntactic, where the syntax or grammar is not used.

In a recent article, Wepman (1972) reiterates and expands his concepts and his concern for excellent therapy. He recommends an indirect approach for some patients, a concentration on ideas in therapy rather than on just words. He maintains that it may not be a good procedure to start a patient in treatment immediately after onset, and that any therapy started soon after onset should be concerned less with specific linguistic goals than with a supportive psychological basis.

The "shutter principle" which Wepman puts forth to explain perseveration and delayed responses is defined as the time after the stimulus presentation during which the patient integrates and associates the stimulus. This is a period of involuntary inhibition when the "mind is shut off." Wepman feels this construct may be of extreme importance to the clinician who must recognize the patient's need for time to internalize and associate to the stimulus, and to formulate and practice acceptable responses.

Wepman holds that recovery from aphasia is an expanded use of previously learned behavior—the reestablishment of language usage.

JON EISENSON

Jon Eisenson is the author of a test, *Examining for Aphasia*, published in 1946, and revised in 1954. The manual presents techniques and materials found useful for examining brain-injured soldiers during the World War II, with subsequent revisions resulting from extensive clinical experience. Eisenson stresses that tests should be viewed as clinical instruments and not as rigid measuring devices. He maintains that aphasic disturbances involve symbolic disturbances, intellectual changes, and personality modifications, but that all of these are interrelated.

From the linguistic point of view, Eisenson believes that aphasic patients suffer loss of meanings more than loss of words and that nonintellectual uses of words remain relatively intact (1957). He regards intellectual and emotional changes as temporary for most aphasic patients, and as reflections of the underlying language disorder. In his view aphasia is primarily a disturbance of language rather than intelligence, and defects of attention are associated with impairment of verbalization and the resultant inability of the aphasic to "readily record and reproduce the facts and situations to which he tries to attend."

To Eisenson, difficulty in dealing with abstractions in aphasic subjects often seems to be an increased disinclination to be concerned with the abstract, together with impairment of the tools for dealing with abstractions.

Karlin *et al.* (1959) have reported reduction of specific perceptual functions in aphasia, pointing out that the practical hearing of an aphasic is usually less proficient than the results of an audiometric examination indicate.

Eisenson believes aphasia tends to modify premorbid personality instead of producing new behavior patterns. In his words, "A well-adjusted individual who becomes aphasic probably has a better chance of ultimate adjustment than a neurotic individual who becomes aphasic" (1957).

Concerning the needs of aphasic patients for psychotherapy, Eisenson (1957) makes these sensitive observations: "It is fairly obvious that any individual whose thinking and communicative ability have been disturbed and who has awareness of these disturbances must reorient and readjust himself to the modifications they impose." He goes on to observe, however, that the process of psychotherapy is precarious when the patient cannot reveal the extent to which he understands or misunderstands, and adds that "an aphasic patient is entitled to a certain number of problems because he is a human being" and when possible should be permitted to solve them himself.

Finally, Eisenson (1960) makes a distinction between early aphasic involvement and maintenance of aphasia. He considers the latter largely determined by the premorbid personality of the patient. He reports that among chronic aphasics he has found a preponderance of higher ego-orientation, better adjustment to hospital than home situations, a higher proportion of excessively withdrawn individuals, a higher proportion of so-called psychopaths or sociopaths, a higher proportion of patients who assume the privileges of the aged, a higher proportion of persons exercising the tyranny of silence, and a lower proportion of patients who have a reasonable assurance of being loved or wanted at home. Eisenson was careful to point out that there have been no studies of the premorbid personalities of patients with either transient or chronic aphasia. Even if carefully designed studies showed significant differences between these groups in the incidence of negative characteristics, further evidence would be required to establish them as causative factors. It seems possible, at least, that negative characteristics could result from conditions attendant on persisting severe aphasia, such as isolation resulting from reduced environmental stimulation or reduced capacity to receive stimulation, loss of achieved status, frustration, rejection, feelings of inadequacy, insecurity, anxiety, and ultimate hopelessness.

The latter, however, is not Eisenson's view. Among possible causes of aphasia, he lists "cerebral damage in association with a premorbid personality type for whom adjustments are difficult and whose premorbid as well as postmorbid behavioral tendencies are characterized by rigidity, ego-orientation, and concretism. Anybody can become aphasic for a while, but except for a few persons with widespread bilateral brain damage and except for those persons with progressive pathologies, some persons are more likely to maintain their aphasic involvements than others" (1960).

A. R. LURIA

Luria (1966) hypothesizes that separate regions of the cortex form complicated systems for the analysis and synthesis of visual, auditory, kinesthetic, and motor stimuli. Pavlov called these areas "cortical analyzer terminals." In the Russian literature they are commonly referred to individually as the acoustic analyzer, the visual analyzer, and the motor analyzer. Luria interprets aphasic symptoms as direct or indirect effects of impairment of one or another of these functional systems. The direct result of a focal lesion within the limits of one of these cortical areas is a disturbance of ability to differentiate incoming stimuli. However, the primary effect of such a lesion never remains an isolated one, but produces secondary effects in all functionally related systems. The pathological effect of a lesion may be selective because some language processes are more dependent than others on functions performed by specific analyzers. Consequently, the disintegration of speech varies from patient to patient, as a result of a disturbance in one analyzer system or another. This makes differential diagnosis possible.

To summarize Luria's theory of aphasia: a lesion in Wernicke's area results in impairment of phonemic discrimination, which affects articulation, vocabulary, and writing. A lesion in the parietal or parieto-occipital area results in a disturbance of simultaneous synthesis, reflected in inability to synthesize parts into wholes and difficulty in arithmetic, and in comprehending and communicating relationships expressed through the logico-grammatical forms of language. A lesion in the fronto-temporal area causes a disturbance in sequential synthesis, primarily affecting communication of events, and is characterized by impairment of syntactical usage, of internal speech, and of fluency.

Luria believes that one of the uses of language is to regulate behavior. "In Soviet psychology," he writes, "it has been established that voluntary activity does not originate from any primordial properties of an internal life, but from the relations between a child and an adult. The adult at first describes certain tasks to the child, who is later able to carry them out in response to his own verbal instructions. . . . There is no single rule in the development of a new temporary connection which does not undergo profound change as soon as the child's reactions begin to be based on information which is systematized in a verbal form. . . . This new principle involves a close association of speech and behavior and transforms man into the most advanced self-regulatory system" (1958).

Luria believes that the regulatory function of speech is disturbed in frontal lobe lesions, particularly when there is extensive or bilateral involvement. Such patients are not aphasic in any accepted sense of the term, but show lack of purposive behavior. Experimentally this disability has been shown most clearly in delayed reaction experiments. Subjects instructed to raise their hands when the examiner counted to 12, for example, could not do so, although they could identify the designated number when it occurred in sequence, and repeat test instructions afterwards. Luria argues that such a disturbance should actually be considered a form of aphasia, since it involves a disturbance of a basic language function, the use of language to regulate behavior.

Finally, Luria takes issue with Jakobson's analogy between aphasia and development of language in children. Luria writes, "It would be a mistake—though unfortunately a common one—to think that pathological states of the brain return speech to stages it has once passed through and allow one to follow out the history of its formation in reverse. Pathological changes in cerebral activity break down one or another physiological condition, indispensable for the normal existence of speech processes; therefore in fact they never reproduce any of the earlier stages of speech development."

Our view of Luria's work has been greatly enriched by his book *Higher Cortical Functions in Man* (1966) which provides the neurophysiological theory, history of research, appropriate tests, and case histories for patients with damage at various sites. His acute clinical observations and careful examination of the results of testing furnish a resource of great importance for the clinician and the researcher in aphasia. Although his neurophysiological theory does not specify mechanisms of analysis and synthesis or define these processes precisely, it does recognize the dynamic and integrative properties of perception. The theory is also compatible with modern neurophysiological theory, which holds that complex selection and integrative processes occur at all levels of the nervous system.

E. S. BEYN

Beyn (1958), of the Neurological Institute of Moscow, reported findings for 50 patients with sensory aphasia characterized by inability to differentiate speech sounds. Like Pavlov and Luria, Beyn considers the cortex of the temporal lobe an area subserving the analysis and synthesis of acoustic stimuli. She points out that to a patient with sensory aphasia different words frequently sound alike, and similar words sound different. One of her subjects observed, "If you pronounce the word 'table' three times in succession, every time I shall hear it differently." Beyn adds that this could happen to any word, whatever its grammatical category or abstraction level.

She concludes that undifferentiated perception of pronunciation results in undifferentiated perception of meaning. The word is frequently perceived in a given context only, and not in relation to other usages. This is not a tendency toward concretism since it is often the figurative or abstract meaning that is retained.

Beyn found a similar divergence of the level of generalization in word substitutions employed in naming, such as *domestic animal* for *dog; agriculture* for *tractor;* and *food* for *butter.*

Beyn observed that patients with sensory aphasia preserved an intact attitude towards the environment, and made adequate social responses. They were able to maintain intentions after interruptions. Aspiration level was not reduced in failure. Patients did not look for excuses for failures outside themselves, nor accept false evaluations of their performances. They succeeded easily in analysis and synthesis of objects presented visually, grasping and retaining principles of structure. She concludes, "The study of a number of intellectual operations in sensory aphasia confirms the opinion of some authors concerning the absence of any primary intellectual deficits in this form of aphasia." She points out that a constant "searching situation" results from the patient's basic disorder—the lability of his perception of speech—and that this determines much of the specific character of observed behavior and affect.

RUSSELL AND ESPIR

Russell and Espir (1961) reviewed the records of 1166 brain-injured patients examined at Oxford during World War II. In most cases wounds were caused by metal fragments from exploding missiles. The authors remarked that it was possible for a missile fragment to penetrate almost any area of the brain, and to cut its way through the skull or ricochet off the inner surface. In some cases showers of bone fragments were blown through the dura and into the brain.

Out of 693 patients with penetrating head wounds, 217 showed early and 135 persisting aphasic symptoms. Severe cases in which metal fragments caused damage far from the site of wounding were excluded, leaving a population of 280 aphasic subjects. Followup studies were conducted by letter, or by interview when possible.

Localization was determined by tracings from skull X-rays showing the point of entry and the position of bone fragments and foreign metal bodies. The authors assumed that remote effects of penetrating wounds were negligible and that early symptoms were the most informative. We do not agree with either premise, but patients were carefully studied, and much can be learned from the interesting observations presented.

The investigators found no evidence that left-hemisphere wounds produced aphasia oftener in right- than in left-handed subjects. Aphasia occurred in 60% of subjects with entry wounds in the left hemisphere, and in 82% of subjects with permanent weakness or sensory loss in the right extremities. Almost all cases with weakness or sensory loss in the arm showed only aphasia. There was some permanent loss of the right visual field in 31% of subjects with permanent aphasia following left-hemisphere wounds. All wounds that damaged the anterior part of the left optic radiations caused some aphasia.

The speech area defined by injuries producing aphasia included the lower half of the precentral and postcentral gyrus, the supramarginal and the angular gyrus, the inferior parietal gyrus, and a large part of the temporal lobe. The authors consider this territory "a meeting ground for cerebral mechanisms connected with the elaboration of the auditory and visual afferent systems, and with the sensorimotor organization for the muscles used for articulation and for writing." They emphasize that the physiological activity of the speech territory is dependent upon its corticothalamic connections, and that the auditory, visual, sensory, and motor components of language are so highly integrated that a wound in any part of the speech area is likely to upset all aspects of language, although small wounds might cause more disorder of one aspect than another.

Although this monograph considers aphasia in a generally modern context, the importance of discriminatory processes and feedback processes appears to be insufficiently appreciated, and some statistical treatment of the data is to be desired.

WILDER PENFIELD AND LAMAR ROBERTS*

In *Speech and Brain Mechanisms* (1959), Penfield and Roberts reported the results of a 10-year study of the neurophysiology of language. Observations were made during seizures, sodium amytal injections, electrical stimulation with mapping of the cortex in conscious and cooperating patients, and in the course of transient aphasias following circumscribed cortical excisions. The authors recognized the limitations imposed by their methodology, and scrupulously separated inference and hypothesis from conclusions supported by their data.

*This section was taken in part from a review of "Speech and Brain Mechanisms," by H. Schuell, which appeared in *Rehabilitation Literature*, 1960, and is abstracted here with the permission of the Editors.

The authors searched the records of all patients operated on for seizures from 1928 through February 6, 1951 for evidence of speech disturbance during cortical stimulation and for evidence of aphasia before and after surgery. They reviewed 663 operations in 569 patients and selected 273 operations on the dominant hemisphere and a like number on the opposite side for study. In addition, a special study was made of 72 patients tested for aphasia before and after surgery. Of the 45 patients who had surgery in the left hemisphere, 26 (58%) showed language disturbances following surgery, while 19 did not. Twenty-seven patients had surgery in the right hemisphere, and only 1 of this group had any language disturbance postsurgically.

Of the 569 patients in the original series, 47 were excluded because handedness had not been determined, and 136 because brain injury had been incurred before the age of two, making a shift of hemispheric dominance for language possible. This left a total of 386 patients without brain injury before two years of age, in whom speech arrest from electrical stimulation or postoperative aphasia was observed. Results are shown in the following table:

Occurrence of Aphasia in Right- and Left-handed Patients
After Surgery in the Left and Right Hemisphere

Surgery in the Left Hemisphere				Surgery in the Right Hemisphere				
Hand	Number of patients	Aphasic patients	Per-cent	Hand	Number of patients	Aphasic patients	Per-cent	Significant level of difference
R*	157	115	73.2	R	196	1	0.5	< .001
L*	18	13	72.2	L	15	1	6.7	< .001
TOTAL	175	128	73.1	TOTAL	211	2	0.9	< .001

*(Includes patients classified as predominantly left- or predominantly right-handed).

Thus, when patients with injury early in life were excluded, there was no difference in the incidence of aphasia after operation on the left hemisphere between the left-handed and right-handed subjects. After operation on the right hemisphere, the left-handed had aphasia 13 times as often as the right-handed, but this difference was not statistically significant, since only one left-handed and one right-handed patient were in this group. Left-handed patients had aphasia 10 times as often after operation on the left hemisphere as on the right. This difference is extremely significant and makes it necessary to revise the old theory that aphasia occurs in left-handed patients after injury to the right hemisphere.

Vocalization was obtained from stimulation of both the precentral and postcentral gyri of both hemispheres, in the same areas that yielded movements of the lips, tongue, and jaw during stimulation, and also from the supplementary motor area, including the superior and medial aspects of the precentral region in both hemispheres. Arrest of speech, if the patient was attempting to talk when the electrode was applied, as well as hesitation, repetition, distortion, and slurring, was produced by stimulation of these areas in both hemispheres.

The same negative effects, as well as inability to name with retained ability to speak, confusion of numbers while counting, perseveration, and misnaming, occurred during application of electrical current to Broca's area, the supplementary motor area, and the inferior parietalposterior temporal area in the left hemisphere. Electrical interference in a given area was effective only about 50% of the time and could not be produced in all patients, even when transient aphasia occurred postsurgically. The authors stress the fact that they observed area and not point localization, and that they were unable to differentiate the effects of the current on one language area from its effects on any other, in the left hemisphere. They conclude that these data support the previous conclusion that the left hemisphere is usually dominant for speech regardless of handedness, with the exclusion of subjects who have had cerebral injuries early in life.

Aphasia occurred immediately after surgery on the left hemisphere only 22 times in 273 operations and did not occur immediately after surgery involving the right hemisphere. The most common finding was speechlessness associated with right hemiparesis. Location of the lesion did not seem to influence the type of difficulty, except in one patient in whom temporal and frontal biopsies were done and who experienced partial auditory imperception. Absence of immediate dysarthria was observed in several cases after excision of the precentral and postcentral face area and in one instance after removal of Broca's area. The authors conclude that any limited, previously damaged area of the left hemisphere may be removed with transient, but without immediate or permanent aphasia, so long as the rest of the brain functions normally. The fact that patients with aphasia after the initial injury again had aphasia after surgery for the excision of scars is considered to indicate that the left hemisphere still functioned for speech in these cases.

The authors define the language mechanism as the three cortical areas from which they obtained cortical arrest, with their thalamic projections, and interconnections through what they term the centrencephalic system. They consider the latter the highest integrative level of cerebral function. While further studies of the centrencephalic system are needed, the hypothesis that subcortical mechanisms play an important role in language functions appears to be incontrovertible.

Some of the conclusions drawn by Roberts from his study of the aphasic subjects are as follows:

1. "Lesions in particular localities may result in specific clinical syndromes. Lesions in the region of the precentral face area and of Broca's area may cause dysphasic disorders which are predominantly expressive in type. This does not mean that a center for eupraxia, and another center for movements of the lips, etc., have been destroyed. There is no specific site where what Nielsen calls the motor engrams of speech are stored."

2. "Generally we believe that lesions near the junction of the dominant parietal and occipital lobes may produce aphasic disorders with the most pronounced difficulty in the visual sphere. But there is no localized center in the angular gyrus for the recognition of letters, numbers, or words."

3. "Terms such as those of agnosia, particularly when subdivided into visual verbal, visual literal, etc., do nothing but confuse us. There is not a single case in the literature of visual verbal agnosia without other defects, together with the ability to recognize some word at some time if the examination is detailed enough."

4. "In an individual who has learned two or more languages, if one language suffers with a cerebral lesion, all languages suffer."

5. "We believe that the most important area for speech is the posterior temporo-parietal region . . . The next important area for speech is that of Broca, including the three gyri anterior to the precentral face area. The supplementary motor area . . . is dispensable; nonetheless, lesions here can produce prolonged dysphasia, and it probably is very important if the other areas for speech are destroyed."

6. "If one of the speech areas is destroyed, then adjacent areas of cortex and the other speech areas function during speech."

7. "Persistent aphasia may occur during abnormal function or with extensive destruction of the left hemisphere. Attempts should be made to control or to excise any abnormally functioning brain to allow the patient the best chance for the recovery of language."

DIRECTIONS OF PRESENT RESEARCH

In the first edition of this book, the intent was to identify the major trends in current research. Active areas in the literature of the early 1960s were discussed, but the wisdom in selecting them for notice in a textbook can be called into question. Three of the five areas discussed seem to have "run out" in the course of the decade, and promising activity has erupted in areas unmentioned.

So many new investigators with varied approaches to aphasia have published in recent years that it is difficult to attempt a review. Given our past performance, it seems unproductive to attempt to select a new set of candidates for "major trends." In this edition we have compromised by adding a chapter that examines major ways of analzying the problems of aphasia (the next chapter) and contented ourselves here by pointing the way to the sources of current contributions.

The *Journal of Speech and Hearing Research* and the *Journal of Speech and Hearing Disorders* carry many articles each year concerning the study and observation of aphasic patients. Research that is applicable to aphasia and which supports, supplements, or refutes old ideas is being reported in such diverse areas as visual processes, auditory processes, immediate and long-term memory, and sensorimotor studies of the speech musculature. The journal *Brain* often has more technical articles concerning the neurological approach to brain damage. *Cortex* publishes many studies concerning the evaluation and treatment of aphasic patients. The *Journal of Communication Disorders*, published in Amsterdam, and the *British Journal of Disorders of Communication* often publish articles concerning brain damage and aphasia. The *Archives of Physical Medicine and Rehabilitation* also carry articles of interest to the speech pathologist working with aphasic patients.

A recent important contribution to the student of aphasia is a book edited by Martha Taylor Sarno, *Aphasia: Selected Readings* (1972). Not only does this book contain representative examples of work in aphasia, but it includes a section of recommended readings and a selected bibliography. The serious student of aphasia and related topics will find this an invaluable reference work.

part two

THEORETICAL
FRAMEWORK

chapter 4

APPROACHES TO THE STUDY OF
APHASIA

Since ancient times philosophers have tried to analyze the "essential nature" of language and its function in the communication process. Herder's essay of 1772 ushered in an age of deep concern for the anatomy of language. But at that time medical science had only the haziest notions about the anatomy of the brain and knew virtually nothing about the role of cerebral mechanisms involved in speech.

For the next century all sorts of disorders of speech and communication were often regarded as one confused and confusing disorder. What we now know as *aphasia* was lumped together with impairments of the peripheral organs involved in speech, the anomalous mutterings of the comatose patient, the impoverished speech of the demented, and the mutisms or ravings of the schizophrenic. Nor was it recognized that loss of words due to aphasia was different from general amnesia. Speechlessness was often attributed to "palsy" of the tongue. (The chief treatment for this disorder was to blister the tongue in an attempt to stimulate it to action!) Moreover, only 150 years ago was it discovered that patients whose speech failed were also unable to express themselves in writing (Critchley, 1964).

Relief from this chaotic state of affairs came almost solely from the neurologists. The pioneering work of Gall, Bouillaud, Auburtin, Broca, and Dax, in the middle to late nineteenth century, prepared the way for significant advances in aphasiology. From that time on the pace of research quickened, with the result that knowledge of malfunctions of the speech mechanism soon outstripped knowledge of the normal process.

In the last 40 years, while clinical research has continued to make great progress, the balance has been somewhat redressed by new pressures to understand the communication process itself. The emergence and explosive development of the electronic media (telegraph, telephone, radio, and television), and the employment of their "near-relatives" (radar, sonar, and the like) in sensitive detection problems, brought many new scientific disciplines to inquire into the fundamental nature of normal communication processes.

Formal theories for the communication process emerged about 35 years ago. In 1935 the British statistician Fisher proposed the first measure for the amount of information communicated by an "event." This was followed a decade later by the information theory of the physicist Gabor (1946), the engineer Shannon (1948), and finally by the computer theorist MacKay (1950).

The mathematical theory of communication has contributed greatly to rigorous attempts to describe mechanical, electrical, and electronic information processing systems. But attempts to characterize human communication processes with information theory have met with little success, even though they have been diligently pursued by some very capable investigators. The performance of a person can be described by information theory only when his inputs and outputs are extraordinarily restricted and limited to particular tasks. When one turns to normal human communication, the mathematical theory is virtually useless.

If one wants to deal with "information" as it is manipulated by a human being in some relevant, natural situation (say, involving cognition, memory, or perception), it seems to be necessary to postulate a richer theoretical base than the mathematical information theory of the 1940s and the 1950s. Efforts to characterize human information processing are now turning to theoretical notions such as *rule systems, images, schemata,* or *reverberating circuits.* Yet even with this more complex view of the processing, most researchers are attempting to investigate only simple psychological processes such as rote memory, simple concept formation, or perceptual recognition and discrimination of a limited class of stimuli.

Through hindsight, it now seems obvious to many that the earlier attempts to construe human communication processes in terms of information theories failed because they were unable to provide insights into the nature of *meaning, purpose,* and *intention.* It was no accident, of course, that scientists were unprepared to deal with these formidable terms. Most psychologists and neurologists followed in the footsteps of the logical positivists earlier in this century. In keeping with that philosophical tradition, they tried to replace all teleogical assumptions with causal ones. In an attempt to clear out misty concepts, they discarded human meanings, purposes, and intentions as well. It was, unfortunately, the proverbial case of throwing the baby out with the bath water.

Since about 1940, the computer scientists and the leaders of the "cybernetic revolution" have demonstrated that *purpose* can play a clear and important role in a hard-headed scientific field. Complex machines are more and more viewed as purposive, goal-directed, self-organizing systems, rather than as mere mechanical clockworks. Crass teleology (in which the processes of the machine are "attracted" by an external goal) is avoided in favor of a theory of machine "entelechies" or internalized goals, defined and governed by homeostatic processes. Hence, in principle at least, it seems that crass positivism can also be avoided.

Once the cybernetic approach had shown that purposive behaviors could be "left in" without losing the theoretical clarity of the mechanistic approach, psychologists and neurologists who were interested in the higher mental processes were quick to follow. They turned to the newborn field of computer science for aid in modeling behaviors and brain functions. Although scarcely a quarter of a century has passed, the wedding of the three fields has become so complete that most of us accept an hypothesis such as "the brain is a computer" as if it were a fact. Indeed, both popular books and scientific monographs have been written on just this thesis (Berkeley, 1961; Neumann, 1958; Arbib, 1964, 1972).

While some moderate progress has been made in developing theories that incorporate *purpose*, the problem of *meaning*, as a scientific concept, has been more elusive. So far no serviceable concept of meaning has been devised by philosopher, linguist, communication scientist, or psychologist. (Several notable attempts are: Katz and Fodor, 1963; Osgood, 1963; Katz and Postal, 1964; Chafe, 1970.)

Unfortunately, human *intentionality* as a scientific problem has essentially been ignored by all fields. Communication scientists do not speak to its definition, neurologists never refer to mechanisms underlying human intents, and psychologists have failed to get the notion into the laboratory where it might be systematically investigated.

The study of disordered processes of human communication cannot wait for the communication scientist (or anyone else) to present a complete scientific theory of the normal human communication process. Yet it is obvious that we are greatly in need of such a theory to organize our data and integrate our several disciplines. We must all admit that the field of aphasiology has failed to resolve its most fundamental problem; we have failed to discover a single, precise characterization of aphasia that serves the purposes of all the sciences concerned.

In this chapter we will critically review the most prominent hypotheses regarding the nature of aphasia. Although we can examine only a few "archtypical" notions, these are the ones that neurologists, linguists, psychologists, and speech pathologists have used as basic themes or metaphors. Our primary goal is to eliminate from serious contention at least two of the historically popular hypotheses regarding the nature of aphasia. We feel these approaches are factually incorrect, theoretically barren, or diagnostically misleading to the therapist.

In later chapters we will offer what we hope will be a more adequate theoretical basis on which to build a tentative science of aphasiology.

THE NEUROLOGICAL METAPHOR: LOCATIONS AND CONNECTIONS

The poet Nabokov, in his poem *Pale Fire*, provides the following poignant description of the aphasic's dilemma:

> She still could speak. She paused and groped and found
> What seemed at first a serviceable sound,
> But from adjacent cells imposters took
> The place of words she needed and her look
> Spelt imploration as she sought in vain
> To reason with the monsters in her brain.

Since the very earliest work on aphasia, neurologists have sought to find the physical location of those cerebral functions whose disturbance by disease or injury gives rise to aphasic symptoms. To quite a remarkable degree, the neurological models developed for this purpose parallel the complex mechanisms developed by the engineering and physical sciences of their time.

In Descartes' day the mechanisms believed to underlly animal behavior were patterned after the intricate mechanics of Swiss clocks. Later, after the invention of the telephone switchboard, switching mechanisms were adopted by neurologists and psychologists in order to explain the capacity of cerebral "reflexes" to become connected through maturation or learning and disconnected through injury or disease. What we now regard as "traditional" models for aphasia were based essentially on this switchboard model.

CEREBRAL REFLEX MODELS OF APHASIA

Traditional models of aphasia focus on the doctrines of Broca and Wernicke, although with some modifications and elaborations. In general, they go something like this: Streams of sensory impulses from the periphery reach "arrival platforms" or "end stations" in the cerebral cortex. These areas are usually known as the primary sensory areas. They are modality-specific; that is, each area receives impulses from one sense organ only. The primary sensory areas for vision lie along the borders of the calcarine fissure in the occipital lobes, and those for hearing lie in the region of the first transverse gyrus of Heschl on the supratemporal plane. Bilateral lesions in these areas result in cortical blindness or cortical deafness.

Adjacent to each primary sensory area, and traditionally considered to receive impulses from it through transcortical fibers, are secondary sensory areas. Visual and acoustic memory images, or engrams, are thought to be registered in the secondary sensory areas and stored for comparison with incoming patterns. This is considered the mechanism of recognition, though not of comprehension of meaning. Lesions in the secondary areas are thought to result in loss of visual or auditory recognition. This impairment was labeled imperception by Jackson, and agnosia by Freud. It was defined as inability to recognize stimuli received through a specific sensory channel. Subsequently many kinds of visual and auditory agnosias were postulated, and tactile agnosia, or astereognosis, defined as inability to recognize objects through touch, was recognized.

The secondary sensory areas are assumed to be interconnected through transcortical association fibers and conduction tracts. In some models these pathways are connected with a concept center. Operation of this association system, which includes the cortex adjacent to the secondary sensory areas, permits comprehension of "the full significance" of incoming stimuli. Lesions at various sites are considered to result in sensory aphasia, semantic alexia, and various forms of conduction aphasia.

Conduction tracts are assumed to convey impulses forward to Broca's Center in the frontal lobe, thought to contain images of movements used in speaking words, and to Exner's Writing Center, thought to contain images of movements used in writing. Impairment of Broca's area results in motor aphasia, or cortical motor pattern apraxia for speech, while impairment of Exner's area causes agraphia, or cortical motor pattern apraxia for writing.

The essentials of the traditional models are thus reception, transmission, and execution. The model is a three-system relay, which has been referred to as a reflex arc. It is often compared to a telephone relay system, with an elaborate switchboard operating between input and output mechanisms to decode, encode, and transmit messages.

INADEQUACIES OF CEREBRAL REFLEX MODELS

The cerebral reflex models appear increasingly less adequate as evidence is accumulated with respect to both the explanation of normal cerebral processes and the manner in which they can be pathologically disturbed. Not only has there been a failure to locate the neurological correlates of reflexes specific to speech, but there has been a failure to find support for the existence of cerebral reflexes associated with memory, perception, sensory, or motor activities as well.

This is *not* to argue, as Goldstein (1939) did, that the brain operates solely in terms of mass-action, for surely there is abundant evidence for the specialization of brain functions. Rather, the basic difficulty with reflex models is that no clearcut relationship has been established between psychological processes whose consequences are readily observable, and the specific underlying cerebral functions whose effective action is hidden in the integrative global activities of the brain.

Indeed, the relation between well-defined behavioral phenomena and specifiable neurological processes often seems perplexingly discrepant. We must face up to the fact that the concepts of reflexive connection or association do not have exactly the same meaning for the neurologist and psychologist. The term associative or reflexive connection as used by psychologists has no known neurological correlate. True, similar *terms* are used by neurologists such as "transcortical connections," "cortical association areas," and "commissural interconnections" between the hemispheres, but these are at best only metaphorically related to the psychological terms.

Attempts have been made to sever the relevant fiber connections following the experimental establishment of conditioned associations between stimuli of two distinct sensory modalities (e.g., Sperry, 1958). Unfortunately, severing transcortical fibers has yet to achieve the surgical extinction of conditioned associations without at the same time severely impairing general perceptual processing. Hence it is not that lesions cannot be produced which will interrupt perceptual or motor processes, but that specific types of associations cannot be selectively eliminated by surgery or other means.

Even commissurotomies, such as those performed in experiments by Sperry (1961) and his students (Myers, 1956; Downer, 1962; Trevarthen, 1962), fail to provide support for the claim that such prominent transhemispherical connections constitute the neurological correlate for the conditioned relationship between stimuli, one of which is believed to be processed in one hemisphere and one in the other. The messages transmitted across these prominent fibers seem to be concerned with "scheduling" and coordinating complex performances and have yet to be shown to collate simple stimulus information.

Lenneberg (1967) summarizes the predicament of the modern day "connectionists" who rely on current neurological research for theoretical support as follows:

> Some theorists may feel that the connectionism discussed here [in the neurological literature] is irrelevant to discussions of learning and behavior. We do not wish to argue for or against this position. But *if* behavioral 'connectionists' were to search for corroborative data produced by the new neuro-anatomical 'connectionism,' they would actually find results that are more likely to contradict their own theories of connections than to support them. (p. 210)

Since the advent of cybernetic theory and the growth of computer science, neurologists have turned to that field for theoretical inspiration. They have constructed models of the cerebral machinery which incorporate servomechanisms and multipurpose computational procedures. In doing so, however, the ideal of providing an architectonic description of the organization of cerebral functions was not relinquished. It was changed to an attempt to discover how the flexible cerebral hardware was "programmed."

The most perplexing aspect of contemporary neurological research is that the cerebral mechanisms that have been revealed empirically seem sufficiently complex and multipurpose to support almost any theory, even highly diverse ones. There are no neurological reasons to exclude, for example, switching circuits, feedback loops, or even holographic resonance fields, which have recently been postulated by Pribram (1971). In brief, what we now know about neurology is that the brain is sufficiently complicated to permit any level or kind of complexity that the researcher or theorist wishes to postulate. The brain is so resourceful and powerful that we will get little guidance in our theory-building from facts about it.

THE PSYCHOLINGUISTIC METAPHOR: REGRESSION TO SOMETHING SIMPLER

If we are unable at the present time to understand *how* language is processed by the brain, perhaps we can at least specify to some extent *what* is processed. Many theorists have turned to the fields of psychology and linguistics in an attempt to discover a functional description of the communication process. The label psycholinguistics is being used because the hypotheses reviewed are offered by psychologists who borrow significantly from linguistic theory and by linguists who borrow liberally from psychological theory.

The two hypotheses that have been most popular are both "regression" hypotheses. That is, they hold that aphasia represents a deterioration or regression from adult speech to something else. The first hypothesis holds that the regression is to an earlier developmental stage of the individual. This is referred to as *ontogenetic regression*. The second hypothesis maintains that the regression is to a logically prior, simpler stage of language processing. This is called *microgenetic regression*. The ontogenetic regression hypothesis supposes that aphasics process language (talk, comprehend, read, and write) as a child might. Sometimes the advocates of this hypothesis add that as language is recovered, the aphasic goes through all the stages of the child acquiring language for the first time. The microgenetic regression hypothesis supposes that language breaks down at the seams, so to speak, and that some components or processes function well while others are nonfunctional. (This view sometimes encourages investigators to study aphasia in order to find the basic components or fundamental processes of normal language.)

Opposed to both of these regression hypotheses is a family of hypotheses which maintain that the language deficit in aphasia is a quantitative reduction in language performance. Some of these theories hold that the reduction is restricted to special aspects of performance, while others postulate that it is a general reduction in language facility of all types. Hypotheses of these sorts may be called "language reduction" hypotheses. The hypothesis of a general reduction will be considered as a prototype.

The contrast between the quantitative hypotheses and the regression hypotheses is important not only with respect to how one describes aphasia, but also with respect to what one can learn about language from the study of aphasia. Obviously, the aphasic patient exhibits a significant reduction in his ability to perform normal language tasks. About this fact, everyone agrees. The key issue is whether the reduction of language ability should be thought of as a *qualitative* reduction of some specified sort of linguistic capacity or as a *quantitative* reduction of linguistic performance.

In order to sharpen the contrast between qualitative and quantitative hypotheses, we need to review Chomsky's distinction (1965) between linguistic *competence* and linguistic *performance*.

LINGUISTIC COMPETENCE

Linguistic competence refers to the intrinsic knowledge (but not necessarily conscious knowledge) that the normal, mature, native speaker possesses about his language. This is the knowledge which enables him to produce and comprehend linguistic utterances. All native speakers possess this intuitive functional knowledge for their native language, regardless of their intellectual endowment or educational background.

Knowledge of one's native language is assimilated from the culture in which one lives rather than learned in school or by exposure to formal methods of teaching. What can be explicitly taught is quite incidental to what the child learns implicitly through interaction with the language community from infancy through childhood. Moreover, the cognitive capacity which allows a young human to assimilate the language of his culture cannot itself be learned but is due, presumably, to the physiological structures with which his species is genetically endowed.

Linguistic competence, then, has two major distinct components: (1) a universal component (cognitive capacity) which is shared by all humans due to their physiological endowment, and (2) a more specific knowledge component acquired from the particular language culture in which one is reared. Aphasia might be either an impairment of those cognitive processes which deal with the knowledge of one's language or a severe reduction in the culturally assimilated knowledge itself. In other words, aphasia might be considered either as a failure of the cognitive processes which assemble and interpret linguistic utterances, or as a traumatic onset of ignorance about one's language. In order to clarify what might appear to be an unnecessary and wasteful distinction, let us consider Chomsky's second concept, linguistic performance.

LINGUISTIC PERFORMANCE

Chomsky (1967) distinguishes between the concepts of linguistic competence and linguistic performance in the following way:

> It is quite obvious that sentences have an intrinsic meaning determined by linguistic rule and that a person with command of a language has in some way internalized the system of rules that determine both the phonetic shape of the sentence and its intrinsic semantic content —that he has developed what we will refer to as a specific *linguistic competence*. However, it is equally clear that the actual observed use of language—actual *performance*—does not simply reflect the intrinsic sound–meaning connections established by the system of linguistic rules. Performance involves many other factors as well. We do not interpret what is said in our presence simply by the application of the *linguistic* principles that determine the phonetic and semantic properties of an utterance. Extralinguistic beliefs concerning the speaker and the situation play a fundamental role in determining how speech is produced, identified, and understood. Linguistic performance is, furthermore, governed by principles of cognitive structure—(for example, by memory restrictions) that are not, properly speaking, aspects of language. (p. 397)

In other words, linguistic competence is an idealization of *what* must be known about language structures if sentence productions and comprehension are to be perfectly realized, while linguistic performance, by contrast, refers to the psychological and physiological variables determing *how* this ideal knowledge of language is actually used. For instance, from the standpoint of the linguistic competence of the ideal native speaker there would be no practical constraints on the length or syntactic complexity of a sentence. Astronomically long sentences consisting of millions of embedded clauses would be possible, at least in principle, by a recursive application of appropriate linguistic rules. In practice, however, due to the limits on man's cognitive capacities, only utterances of a more reasonable length can be processed with any degree of reliability or communicative facility.

APHASIA: A COMPETENCE OR PERFORMANCE DEFICIT?

Now that we have made the distinction between competence and performance, we can return to the question of the value of the hypotheses introduced earlier. On the one hand we have the two regression hypotheses, both of which argue for qualitative differences in the language of aphasics, and on the other hand we have the quantitative hypotheses that argue merely for a reduction of available language. Obviously, the most important test of any hypothesis is how well it accords with and explains what we know about the phenomena in question. Let us turn to that consideration.

If the ontogenetic version of the regression hypothesis holds, the predictions are easy to make: one expects to see aphasic patients who exhibit the linguistic competence of a child at an immature stage of language development with respect to every aspect of language.

If the microgenetic version of the regression hypothesis holds, the predictions are a little less obvious. One expects to see aphasic patients with selective language errors at various levels in the hierarchical organization of linguistic structure, i.e., the levels of phonology, morphology, lesser phrase structure constituents, major phrase structure constituents, or sentence transformations. In addition, one might expect some aphasic patients to be severely limited in the types of sentences produced or understood. For instance, some patients who are regressed in their language functioning to a logically more primitive level of structure might be expected to grasp the rules for processing active sentences but not passive sentences, or questions but not imperatives, etc. Or one might expect some patients to exhibit selective dysfunctions in the appropriate use of sound patterns, various parts of speech, phrases, or clauses in sentence construction. Generally, if aphasia is a qualitative breakdown at various levels of linguistic competence, the aphasic symptoms should correspond rather exactly to defects in the patient's knowledge of linguistic rules.

(Of course, we do observe systematic structural errors in sentence formation and comprehension in both the underdeveloped language of young children and the "broken English" of nonnative speakers. This hardly proves the case, however. The question is whether or not aphasic patients show patterns of errors closely analogous to those presented by either of these two groups of deficient speakers. This question will be considered in more detail later.)

Finally, if aphasia is quantitative rather than qualitative, it implies that aphasia is a deficit in linguistic *performance*, rather than competence. One would expect this deficit to show up as an overall reduction in language facility. In this event, errors of patients should not be structurally specific but should be more or less evenly distributed over all types of sentences, parts of sentences, and sound pattern constituents. In other words, errors should reflect a general unreliability in both the production and comprehension of language. Such errors, rather than appearing to be qualitatively similar to those committed by children or nonnative speakers, should appear more like those made by the normal adult (when he is tired, hurried, or dividing his attention) but differing dramatically in their rate of occurrence.

Now that we know what we are looking for, let us turn to the evaluation of these hypotheses.

THE ONTOGENETIC REGRESSION HYPOTHESIS

The history of the ontogenetic hypothesis goes back nearly 100 years to the evolutionary philosophy of Herbert Spencer and the epoch-making introduction of evolutionary concepts into biology by Darwin. Following their lead, Hughlings Jackson (1887) proposed that ontogenetic development of individuals recapitulates the phylogenetic evolution of species in several important ways: First, he assumed that mental capacities develop concomitantly with neurological ones in accordance with the so-called Fechner–Spinoza hypothesis of psychophysical parallelism. Specifically, Jackson believed that more complex, voluntary, multipurpose mental processes developed morphologically later than simple, automatic, special-purpose ones, just as structurally more complicated, adaptively flexible species evolved later than simpler organisms capable of only a rigid repetoire of automatistic adaptive responses. Second, Jackson argued that dissolution of neurophysiological functions due to injury or disease would reverse the sequence of evolutionary development, thus resulting in a corresponding regression of mental capacities to a less mature stage of competence.

Following this line of reasoning, it is not at all surprising that Jackson and his followers would define aphasia as a regression of linguistic competence to a developmentally inferior stage as a result of neurogenic dissolution of the cerebral structures in the so-called "dominant" hemisphere.

Spreen (1968), in a review and critique of such theories, carefully traces the history of the regression hypothesis from Kussmaul (1887) through Jackson (1879), Ribot (1883) and Pitres (1895) to Freud (1891), Pick (1913), Pick and Thiele (1931), and finally Jakobson (1962). Pick (1913) first referred to the regression hypothesis as "Ribot's law" in his book on "agrammatism." In his later works, he pointed out some apparent exceptions to this "law," claiming that it applies only to chronic sequelae of the lesion rather than to the acute symptomatology exhibited by the patient.

The linguist Jakobson (1962) has presented perhaps the most extreme formulation of the hypothesis. He claims that the progressive dissolution of linguistic competence in the aphasic patient regresses him toward an early infantile stage in the disintegration of both sound patterns and syntactic structures. He proposes that reacquisition by the aphasic of sound patterns will again "mirror the child's acquisition of speech sounds."

INADEQUACIES OF THE ONTOGENETIC REGRESSION HYPOTHESIS

First, we must consider the theoretical implausibility of the ontogenetic regression hypothesis. At base, the theory supposes that all of the vast number of diverse neurological disturbances that give rise to aphasia are related to precisely the same sequence of hierarchically ordered language skills. Then it supposes that the hierarchy of skills is exactly time-dependent and that the most recently acquired skills will be the first to go. The heterogeneous defects must selectively eradicate rapidly and in precise inverse order just those neurological structures responsible for adult linguistic competence—structures which presumably took years to develop.

Although there is considerable evidence for functional separation of neurological structures, there is no conclusive evidence for the localization and separation of specific neurological structures supporting the individual rules of syntax, semantics, or phonology, much less structures that are ordered by the time that the individual rule was acquired. The coincidence of results that must be assumed to arise from cerebral injuries of diverse origins such that the ontogenetic timetable of development is reversed would rank it among nature's most miraculous mechanisms.

When we turn to the evidence in support of this remarkable hypothesis, there is little or none to be found. The major finding that could be cited in favor of the hypothesis is that significant correlations are observed between errors made by adult aphasics in the naming of common objects and the errors made by children between infancy and adolescence (Rochford and Williams, 1962, 1963). But this cannot be taken as conclusive support for the ontogenetic position, even for the restricted domain of "naming." The correlations observed may have little to do with either naming or with ontogenetic regression. For example, several investigators have shown that aphasic errors in a picture vocabulary test increase as the words decrease in frequency of occurrence in everyday language (Schuell et al., 1961; Newcomb et al., 1965). This just says that aphasics make more errors on rare words. So do children, and so do normal adults. This is scarcely evidence for regression. Furthermore, as one examines the failure to name (which used to be called "anomia"), it turns out that it is just a special case of the word frequency finding. When we try to elicit rare adjectives or rare verbs from the aphasic patient, we find that he cannot produce or comprehend them either. Thus, a more general phenomenon is at issue than a similarity to children's difficulty in naming objects. (See Sefer and Henrikson, 1966; Siegel, 1959.)

The most telling evidence for an ontogenetic theory would be examples showing that aphasic errors are of the same kind as the errors made by children. At this crucial place, the evidence seems to be against the theory. For instance, young children (three or four years old) often indicate their immature linguistic competence by committing *systematic* errors due to the *inappropriate generalization of linguistic rules.* These are obvious in the case of overextended inflectional endings, e.g., "The boy *hurted* himself," "Look at the *deers*," and "That is the *chocolatest* cake I've ever eaten."

Adult aphasics rarely show such systematic immature errors. Their errors tend to be intermittent and randomly sprinkled throughout all types of sentences—some of which are often too complex to be uttered by young children. The following errors of adult aphasics are entirely different from those of the children given above: "The banana was *breakness.*" "*Who* happened this morning?" "Tomorrow is a day that we all remember." "He stepped *on* a hole." "We cannot very spell." A collection of aphasic errors does not look like a collection of children's errors.

A close comparison of the language of aphasics and the language of children reveals merely that there is a similarity in the *quantity* of errors made on infrequent or lengthy linguistic structures. There seems to be little qualitative similarity in the pattern of errors made. Rather, the errors made by aphasics tend to reflect either a failure to apply linguistic rules reliably or, perhaps, a derangement in the system of rules which remain more or less intact in themselves.

One place in which the regression principle can be examined with considerable precision is in the area of phonetic disintegration in aphasia and its sequence in recovery. Here the developmental facts are relatively clear and the observations required are fairly straightforward and objective. Both Fry (1958) and Shankweiler and Harris (1966) failed to find evidence in favor of the ontogenetic hypothesis as stated by Jakobson.

Shankweiler and Harris studied five patients who had been selected as relatively "pure" cases of phonetic disintegration with little comprehension difficulty. The patients' task was to echo words. Pronunciation errors were tabulated. The results show that aphasics did indeed have trouble with the same sounds that Templin (1957) found to be difficult for children to articulate. However, the kinds of errors made by aphasics were different from those made by children. The children made predictable "substitution" errors; aphasics made a variety of unsystematic errors.

Shankweiler and Harris said of their aphasic patients, "Many errors can be considered neither as poor approximations to the correct phoneme nor as clearcut substitutions of related phonemes. The apparent unrelatedness of many of the substituted sounds to their targets, together with the marked lack of consistency of the substitutions, tells us much about the condition. To the extent that these features characterize a given patient's performance, the disorder must stem from disorganization of the process by which phonological units are encoded for production."

In our opinion, the ontogenetic regression hypothesis seems to have been accorded more attention than it has deserved. At present there is no reason to suppose that aphasia can be characterized in this fashion.

THE MICROGENETIC REGRESSION HYPOTHESIS

It will be recalled that the microgenetic hypothesis asserts that some sort of failure occurs in the chain of language production, either in the processes or components. Thus, it is not easy to defeat this kind of hypothesis since it has as many forms as there are theories or "sketches" of the functional organization of language processes. Spreen (1968) gives instances of some of these views, ranging from Pick's (1913) opinion that most aphasias were deficits at the final level of word finding to Werner's (1965) position which stressed the importance of prelinguistic "gestalt" formations of ideas.

The traditional psychological view, however, has stemmed from associationism. Theorists from the associationist background typically argue that aphasic errors indicate a breakdown of associative bonds between linguistic structures. The likelihood of breakdown is seen as being inversely proportional to the strength of the bond. This position then predicts that the less-frequently associated linguistic structures will be more readily lost than the more-frequently associated ones.

For instance, Howes (1964) points out that there is no true loss of vocabulary in the aphasic patient, but rather a reduction in the use of low-frequency words. Howes and Geshwind (1964) have made attempts to use such frequency measures to distinguish among various types of aphasia. Of course, all of the phenomena associated with language frequency counts and aphasic errors can be assimilated to such a theory; that is, the theory can claim success in predicting where errors will occur.

The basic shortcoming of the view lies in the theoretical inadequacy of associative mechanisms to explain language acquisition and language processing. (For an extended treatment of this assertion, see Chomsky, 1957, 1959.) For this reason, many theorists have turned to linguistic theory itself as a source of hypotheses regarding the functional organization of language processes. The general claim of this version of the microgenetic regression hypothesis is that aphasic errors are due to impairments of those processes involved in language production and comprehension at each of the various hierarchical levels of structural analysis—as those levels are designated by linguistic theory.

Although considerable empirical evidence has been amassed regarding the "psychological reality" of linguistic structures (such as phonemes, morphemes, phrase structures, and sentence transformations), no connections have been demonstrated between the nature of neurogenic disturbance and the processing of such structures. Thus, the theoretical worth of this view is still open to question. While many investigators are willing to talk about aphasia in this context, little actual research has been motivated by this point of view. (Nevertheless, as an illustration of the psycholinguistic approach to aphasia, see Schuell et al., 1969.)

In the final analysis there seems to be little to date that recommends any qualitative version of the linguistic regression hypothesis. By contrast, there seems to be ample evidence that aphasia is essentially characterized by a quantitative reduction of linguistic performance. To return to the computer analogy mentioned at the beginning of the chapter, the qualitative theories would have to argue that the program of the computer had reverted to an earlier program (ontogenetic regression) or that the program had deficient portions in it (microgenetic regression). It seems more reasonable to consider aphasics to be analogous to computers programmed to process language but whose circuits have become swamped in noise, due to faulty connections, disturbed internal signal sources, defective speech analyzers, and the general asynchronous chaos of processes whose mass action can no longer be properly coordinated. If aphasics are "fault ridden" machines whose processing components (rather than programs) are disturbed, one would expect a quantitative rather than a qualitative reduction in language processing ability.

In the next two chapters we will develop this argument and weigh the evidence in favor of the quantitative reduction hypothesis.

chapter **5**

APHASIA: AN INTERDISCIPLINARY
PROBLEM

Aphasia is a many-faceted problem which must be studied in many different scientific frameworks. The complexity of the problem accounts for the great diversity of opinion and approaches found among the investigators reviewed in the previous chapters. The realization that the problem is complex has persuaded modern investigators of the need for communication across disciplines. This theme appears repeatedly in symposia, conferences, and meetings such as: The Aphasia Research Seminar, sponsored by the Committee on Linguistics and Psychology of the Social Science Research Council (Osgood and Miron, 1963); the Symposium on Disorders of Language, sponsored by the CIBA Foundation (de Reuck and O'Connor, 1964); the Conference on Brain Mechanisms Underlying Language, sponsored by NINDB (Millikan and Darley, 1967); and the Annual Meetings of the Academy of Aphasia, begun in 1963 and continuing to the present time.

The upshot of such meetings has been a growing agreement among researchers that no one discipline can provide all the answers. Consequently, it is not surprising that many clinicians as well as researchers on aphasia have had to settle for a limited, eclectic approach to the disorder until, at some future time, the interdisciplinary approach yields sufficiently coherent information to form the groundwork for a unified theory.

Any proposed unified theory faces a series of formidable tests. It should provide a common scientific basis from which clinicians can diagnose patients with sufficient accuracy to guide them toward maximally effective treatment, neurologists can reliably infer the neurological contributions to the disorder, and researchers can design studies which truly clarify the relationship of symptoms of aphasia to impairments of normal processes. Obviously, we are a long way from such a theory. But we may still be able to make some reasonable steps toward its attainment.

Two major questions must be answered before we can entertain much hope about devising a unified theory. First, we must ask in what manner the contributions of the many disciplines involved can be made to converge on a coherent account of the disorder. Second, we must ask what specific criteria are to be satisfied by a unified theory if it is to achieve the goals we have outlined. In this chapter we will explore both of these questions, and in the next chapter we will attempt to sketch a conceptual framework in which we can work.

THE PROBLEM OF CHARACTERIZING APHASIA

In the 11 decades since 1861, the year Broca published his discoveries, no single characterization of aphasia has met with universal acceptance among clinicians, neurologists, or psychologists. In the last few chapters the most widely held views of aphasia were scrutinized critically—each failing to pass muster under one or several of the assumptions centrally important to these areas. Perhaps the most dramatic testimony against some of the views of aphasia issued from the mouths of the patients themselves, who are alone competent to give us a view from the inside. Because the evaluation of testimony from patients is more problematic than the evaluation of evidence gathered by other means—clinical tests, neurological examinations, or psychological research—we need to clarify the possible relationships among these different sources of evidence.

THE PATIENTS' INTUITIVE JUDGMENTS AS EVIDENCE

Consider, for example, the difficulty of making use of the statements of aphasic patients as evidence. The first-hand testimony of patients, although necessarily inarticulate to some degree, is too important to ignore on the grounds that it emanates from an intuitive, subjective appraisal of the disorder rather than from well-controlled objective assessment. In general, there can be no serious question about the importance of expert opinion regarding a phenomenon, regardless of its source and the difficulty of interpreting it. In the broad sense of "expertise," the patients' intuitions also provide a legitimate and important source of data for which any theory of aphasia must provide an account. Some of the aphasic patients' subjective appraisals pinpoint with eloquent accuracy the precise nature of their communication deficit (Rolnick and Hoops, 1969):

Mr. L: First, I formulate the idea in my mind, and then I try to express that idea in the language, and then I have the problem. I can get the idea real quickly . . . but to make it into language or to express it as language . . . I just couldn't do it. I just lose them. I can't express exactly the idea that I want to say. I can see them in my mind but I can't see the words.

Or

Mr. M: I know what it is . . . that's what makes me so mad . . . but I can't say it.

Or

Mr. K: I could see a lot of things but I couldn't say what it means. I knew there was something there but I couldn't say what.

One of our patients put it even more succinctly when he said, "It's as if my mind is in a locked box." What is it that the patients are trying to tell us? The search for a reasonable answer to this question is among the most exciting goals of science, for any answer one might give sheds light not only on aphasia but also on the fundamental principles governing mental processes.

The linguist Chomsky has argued that the native speaker's intuition regarding his language (e.g., his judgments regarding the acceptability of sentence constructions, their ease of comprehension, etc.) is a primary datum to be explained by linguistic theory. He regards the intuitions of the native speaker as the starting point for theory construction or as *prima facie* evidence for a theory, but of course he insists that the intuitions are not acceptable as theory themselves. If we follow this admonition, subjective reports are placed in a reasonable perspective relative to their role in scientific explanation, and we avoid the twin dangers of misusing introspective evidence as well as uncritically ignoring its worth. Indeed, psychologists as both researchers and clinicians have long realized the value of verbal reports as a legitimate thread of evidence in their attempts to weave adequate scientific theories. Similarly, physicians have always considered introspective reports of their patients about the locations and severity of discomfort as an indispensable source of diagnostic information. We argue, then, that the aphasic patient's intuitive assessment of his disorder is nothing more nor less than a native speaker's judgment concerning the nature and extent of the impairment he experiences when he attempts to communicate.

This is not to say, of course, that the reports of aphasics should be considered the only source of information useful in characterizing the disorder, or that this evidence should be accepted uncritically without independent corroboration. It serves only to remind us that the patient (like we, ourselves) often knows quite well what he can and cannot do. Moreover, it suggests that theorists and researchers, like therapists and clinicians, should try to construct theories and research projects which are sensitively directed toward use and clarification of this source of data from expert witnesses.

THE NATURE OF THE TASK

The specific question that our example raises is how this source of data is to be related to neurological, psychological, and clinical evidence in a theory of aphasia. Are we to choose one kind of evidence as basic and show that all others can be derived from it? This amounts to a reductionistic approach, reducing all the observations from each discipline to some single basic, causal level. Are there other ways in which the data are to be combined?

As we see it, the logical problems we face in trying to characterize aphasia are like those faced by a prosecuting attorney when he builds his case solely on the basis of circumstantial evidence. No single strand of evidence can be accepted as basic or conclusive or as directly implicating the culpable agent in any simple manner. Just as the testimony of the patient is biased by the very nature of his disorder, so the behavioral and physiological deficits observed by the diagnostician constitute a tangled knot of primary and secondary symptoms accompanying aphasia and its frequent complicating neurological conditions.

There is little hope that we will be rescued by neat "experiments of nature" that disclose the primary symptoms to us one by one. Isolated "pure" disorders which might reveal such primary symptoms are seldom, if ever, observed. We know of no such cases from the reports of investigators who have obtained extensive objective test results over a significantly large series of aphasic patients. Neither Head (1926) with 26 patients, Weisenburg and McBride (1935) with 60 patients, Wepman (1951) with 68 patients, nor Schuell *et al.* (1964) with 157 patients succeeded in finding a single "pure" case. Not only do complicating conditions arise from neurological involvements, but secondary symptoms also arise from social and psychological factors involved in the patients' postmorbid adjustment to his unusual state, situation, and environment.

All of the above problems pose obstacles to the serious student who hopes to find a single, simple characterization of aphasia which not only itemizes its primary symptoms but also explains them. Hence, there is need for an interdisciplinary approach which is something more than eclectic.

THE REALITY SUPPORT FOR APHASIA

The reader may object at this point that there either is or is not a disorder such as aphasia, and that we are overcomplicating an issue that will be made clear when further information is obtained. Is it not just a simple matter of gathering facts? There are two objections to this view. First, in the case of a "loose concept" such as aphasia, it is never clear at the outset what constitutes a relevant fact. Second, and perhaps less familiar to the reader, is the severe limitation on the popular notion of causal explanations.

From the standpoint of the philosophy of science, attempts to assess theories of human disorders encounter serious problems in the selection of criteria for evaluation and in proposals for causal relations. Suppose, to take an extreme example, that clinicians were successful in isolating a set of symptoms indicating a relatively unique disorder and that neurologists were to specify a nearly perfect concomitant neurological dysfunction. What could the theorist then say about the precise logical relationship between the neurogenic, psychogenic, or sociogenic factors and the clinically observed symptomatology?

We have been warned by both scientists and philosophers of science not to attribute causation to correlation. Correlated factors may not be causally related either because: (a) they are merely covariants of other unknown factors or contributing circumstances, or (b) the factors are of such a nature that they do not causally interact at all. An example of case (a) is the relation of the tuberculosis bacillus to the disease of tuberculosis. A necessary part of the symptomatology of tuberculosis is the presence of the bacillus, but many people who have the bacillus do not show the rest of the symptomatology that we identify as "having the disease." Thus, it is necessary to postulate the presence of other factors which constrain the effects of the bacillus and limit the occurrence of the disease.

Case (b) is illustrated by the early but false claim that general paresis (advanced syphilis) was due to the spine being subjected to continuous jarring or vibratory motion. This conclusion was tentatively reached by physicians who observed a high incidence of the disease among traveling salesmen, soldiers, and other men who traveled extensively by train. Obviously, the source of the correlation was more devious than suspected by the theorists. A more traditional illustration of case (b) is the perennial problem of the relation of mind to body. Philosophers have long agonized over the possibility or impossibility of a causal interaction existing between the two because of their intrinsically different natures.

Given such difficulties, we must avoid claiming any simple causal connection between the facts we may gather. We must return to the position that we stated earlier: the theorist's task is that of building a web of circumstantial evidence rather than attempting to find a strict causal explanation of the disorder we study.

Contemporary philosophers of science following Popper (1961) have rejected all logically foolproof schemes for verifying scientific theories—causal ones or otherwise. Most philosophers believe that causal explanations cannot be sufficient to account for complex biological and psychological phenomena found in nature. This does not mean that the phenomena are magical or mystical, but rather that the observed effects are the products of many constituents that are only circuitously related. Additional problems arise when the phenomena to be explained show great heterogeniety of constantly changing, loosely connected states, controlled both by earlier states, now removed in time, and current states which may be responsive to an infinitely variable set of context factors. We will call a complex system such as this a *coalition*. We believe coalitions exhibit "emergent" properties that cannot be reduced to any simple causal chain explanation.

Our situation is not unique just because we are studying aphasia. The problems we encounter here are the problems encountered in any analysis of living organisms whose nature is jointly determined by a distant evolutionary history, on the one hand, and an ever-increasing sensitivity to the biological, psychological, physical, social, and cultural context in which they function, on the other. As Simon (1969) suggests, when faced by such complexities, one who is an "in principle" reductionist might well become a pragmatic wholist. While clinicians who must treat the whole person find little difficulty with such a pragmatic view, theorists and researchers who tend to work on isolated organismic variables often fervently resist any change from an "in principle" stance for reasons of expediency.

Fortunately, we can take courage from the success of the "systems analysis" approach which has proved so useful in computer science and from the widespread recognition that such approaches are necessary in dealing with problems of complex social, political, and economic systems. The hard line of reductionist theorizing so prevalent just a few decades ago has softened appreciably in the last decade.

In addition, philosophers of science such as Kuhn (1962), Feyerabend (1970), and Lakatos (1970) have done much to clarify the history of the development of scientific explanations. They have argued convincingly that scientific progress does not pursue the pure lines described by logical principles of evaluation or discovery, but instead follows notions of conceptual economy within a framework of principles with the widest scope of application. It is fruits rather than proofs, promise rather than precision, which make one set of explanatory principles more acceptable than another. Whether scientists like it or not, they argue, this is what science has always been and will continue to be. Following their thought, we argue that the difference between researchers, theorists, and clinicians is one of degree rather than one of kind. This view of science, then, encourages closer cooperation among theorists, researchers, and clinicians since they are all engaged in what is fundamentally the same enterprise.

What we must now seek is some form of interdisciplinary approach which provides means for coordinating descriptions from several scientific domains. The recent birth of several hybrid life sciences indicates that this approach is tacitly shared by leaders in the community of such sciences. For instance, *psycholinguistics* is a comparatively new discipline that crosses the fields of psychology and linguistics. Under its stimulation a still newer discipline, *sociolinguistics*, has developed to investigate questions in linguistic enquiry which cross social and cultural lines. *Neuropsychology* has been defined as the interdisciplinary study of psychological behavior related to brain dysfunction or pathology, or more generally, the relationship of central nervous system mechanisms and behavior. *Cybernetics* has been defined as "the study of information and control in organisms and machines" (Wiener, 1961). An important focus of cybernetic science of the past two decades has been on the analogical application of mechanistic and information principles to explain the functional organization of living systems. By contrast, *bionics*, as its complementary science, attempts to apply biological principles to the design of machines.

This interdisciplinary attack has been especially vigorously applied in the fields of *computer simulation* and *artificial intelligence*. Such work is carried out by large teams of specialists from many fields according to a general systems theory approach. It is rarely, if ever, reductionistic. Although the problems are immensely difficult and success has been limited, the mere existence of such interdisciplinary teams at the Massachusetts Institute of Technology, Carnegie–Mellon University, Stanford University, and the California Institute of Technology supports the optimism many scientists feel regarding the ultimate success of such efforts.

The moral to be drawn from these contemporary trends in life sciences and communication sciences is that the precise characterization of a disorder, such as aphasia, must be given in terms of the logical, psychological, physiological, and social factors which interact to provide the reality support for that phenomenon. A *unified* theory of aphasia does not mean a *unitary* theory of aphasia. We believe that commitment to the interdisciplinary approach means that it is more accurate to speak of aphasia and other disorders as being due to a lack of adequate support of normal processing in many domains of analysis, rather than of the existence of a single cause for aphasia reduced to some single level of a particular area. This somewhat subtle distinction between *support for* versus *cause of* has great significance for how one thinks about the problems of diagnosis and treatment of any disorder.

POSITIVE AND NEGATIVE SUPPORT FOR DISORDERS

Jackson (1958) distinguishes between what he calls the positive and negative elements of a disorder with the following illustration:

> A man, from local softening of the brain, has the defect of speech which consists in uttering wrong words—he says, for one example, "chair" for "table." No one objects to the clinical statement that softening "is the cause" of the defect of speech. But strictly speaking it is simply impossible that softening of the brain can cause any wrong utterances; for softened brain is no brain; so far as function, good or bad, is concerned it is nothing at all. I submit that the wrong utterances occur during activity of parts *not* softened but healthy. Yet plainly the wrong utterances would not occur if the softening had not happened. The softening answers to the patient's negative condition, to his inability to utter the right words; the wrong utterances are owing to activity of remains of the speech nervous arrangements and hence are abnormal. Similarly, the positive elements of the several postepileptic states are not the direct results of any pathological process. But they would not have occurred had not the negative pathological condition of higher nervous arrangements been established. But it is an abuse of language to say that the negative condition is the cause of the positive phenomena, for that implies that nothing causes something. The positive manifestations are indirectly caused, or rather are "permitted." (p. 17)

Thus, the removal of adequate support for a normal process, as Jackson points out, provides means for explaining both negative and positive symptoms—those due to the removal of factors needed for the full support of normal processing, as well as those arising as an expressed function of whatever organizational structures remain in force. This means that a cerebrovascular accident, tumor, head injury, or infectious or toxic process cannot be, strictly speaking, the positive causal factor of observed symptoms; rather, such symptoms must arise from whatever residual functional integrity exists in the system.

Localization of the anatomical site of a lesion, occlusion, aneuryism, etc., is surely relevant, but it is not a sufficient explanation for why certain symptoms and not others are associated with the disorder. Such neurological "faults" are better thought of as circumstantial evidence that some of the necessary support for the process has been withdrawn at the neurological level. In this sense, the etiological contribution of a cerebral accident is negative rather than positive.

THE BRAIN AS A SELF-ORGANIZING SYSTEM

The plasticity of the brain and its tendency toward what Lashley (1951) called "equipotentiality" (the finding that diverse functions might be performed equally well at many different locales or even globally) suggests that the brain might be best considered as a "self-organizing" system. The chief property of such systems is their ability to preserve a maximum degree of organization by homeostatically adjusting to changes caused by trauma. Although the logic of the cerebral mechanism by which this can be effected is not yet understood, Ashby (1960) and others have built small-scale homeostatic devices that successfully exhibit this property. In fact, such principles have been incorporated in the design of oil refineries and are invoked in the explanation of self-supporting ecosystems and populations.

The brain is not, of course, perfectly plastic in the above sense. The high degree of specialization required for adaptation to our complex environment constitutes a major limitation on the brain's plasticity. In higher organisms the tendency toward equipotentiality decreases proportional to the maturation of the organism, especially with respect to hemispheric lateralization of functions such as speech and language. Yet the amazingly rich interconnectedness of the brain suggests that there are abundant resources by which homeostatic adjustments might be coordinated. Presumably traumatic disturbance of this complex neuronal network, say by lesions, introduces a "faulty" signal which is propagated throughout the system, altering to some degree each of the complex functional relations among all the components involved until the distorted signal is "absorbed." If, however, the functional adjustments required to absorb the fault are so great that important relations among the cerebral centers necessary for the support of normal human communication are lost, then a communication disorder arises.

Perhaps the following is what takes place during a patient's course of recovery from a cerebral accident: Immediately after the accident the patient is neurologically unstable (due to damage, swelling, edema, reduced circulation, shock, etc.). At this time he presents a bewildering array of symptoms, many of which will disappear spontaneously during the next few months. An intermediate period of adjustment follows when the patient exhibits a relatively stable core of symptoms. This is the period when, in principle, differential diagnosis becomes possible. Regular treatment of symptoms can, of course, be administered as soon as the patient is able to work at the treatment tasks, but the treatment cannot be focused nor can its results be appraised adequately until this stable period is reached. Over a period of months or even years, most patients react favorably to some degree to general stimulative therapy and experience some functional recovery from the disorder. Presumably, the effects of stimulating the functional relations among the components allows them to be reequilibrated, overcoming the faulty signal propagated, and thus restoring some of the support for the communication process.

Although this view of how communication disorders might arise is speculative and at best only descriptive, it seems to capture some of the complications involved in diagnosing and treating aphasia. In this sense the fault propagation model may prove to be of heuristic value in guiding our thinking about the etiology and development of disorders.

From this point of view we can tentatively draw the following conclusions:

1. It is not the site at which a fault originates which is the "cause" of the disorder. Rather, we say that the pattern of fault propagation (in all directions) leads to relatively global homeostatic readjustments by which both the positive and negative symptoms of a disordered process are made manifest.

2. Fault propagation may, in principle, result in either a simple or a complex symptomatology, dependent on the site of the damage, the extent of the damage, and most importantly, on the nature of the final homeostasis achieved as a consequence

of the patterns of readjustment propagated throughout the relevant portions of the system.

To elaborate the latter point we must observe that what often appears as a simple symptom, say, blindness, muteness, deafness, or paralysis, may have either a simple or complex origin, just as disorders with complex symptomatologies may also have simple or complex origins. For instance, patients suffering from disorders with complex symptomatologies, such as multiple sclerosis, may exhibit disorders of communication due to global homogeneous factors that have a simple neurological description (the breakdown in myelinization around nerve fibers). On the other hand, the schizophrenic disorder of communication might be due to global heterogeneous factors involving simultaneously the physiological, psychological, familial, and social variables believed to be important in the genesis of that disease.

FUNCTIONAL DESCRIPTION OF NORMAL PROCESSES

One of the most critical problems in understanding communication disorders arises from the difficulty of properly characterizing normal communication processes. What is the appropriate way to describe the normal so that we can precisely describe the departure from it? This is analogous to the problem of distinguishing "normally functioning" machines from those with faults in structure, components, or programs. The difficulty is that mere existence of a fault is not sufficient either to guarantee a disorder in function or to characterize one if it exists. The existence of a specific fault at the neurological level does not provide conclusive evidence for, nor a standard for measuring, the extent and nature of a resulting disorder.

As surprising as it may seem with respect to the logic of machines, there is no principled difference between a machine with faults and a so-called "normal" machine. They are both dynamic systems whose behavior is the positive expression of their respective functional organizations. They are different machines, and indeed they may be distinguishable, but not in terms of the fact that one has a fault and the other does not. They must be distinguished relative to their behaviors; that is, one produces symptoms not produced by the other. Yet behavioral differences constitute at best only circumstantial evidence that their functional organization is qualitatively different, and this only if we can specify what we mean by differences. What is different from what?

Only the criteria for "normal behavior" can tell us which behaviors of which machine constitute evidence for an existing fault. How do we select such criteria? In the case of aphasia we might argue that we can judge what normal speakers do, and we can tell when behavior departs from that norm. But we must notice that our ability to judge the normal does not in itself specify the functional principles that must govern normal processing. What we would like to be able to do is to specify the functional support that is standard for normal processing, as well as the negations of this support as departures from that standard.

This suggests that a basic understanding of a disorder of communication, such as aphasia, can only be achieved when we establish what we mean by the normal process of communication. Without a relatively explicit description of the nature of the various kinds of support required for normal communications processes, there is little hope of determining how loss of particular forms of support leads to the observed symptomatology.

What we must aim for in our attempts to construct a unified theory of aphasia is twofold: (1) a general description of the nature of the multileveled support for the normal process (the standard), and (2) a description of the functional organization of the system which when negated by fault propagation results in the observed positive and negative symptoms.

In accordance with the Jacksonian principle, we must provide a theory of aphasia which explains not only the observed disorders of communication but also the intact competencies of communication. The main problem is that of distinguishing the patterns of fault propagation which give rise to the primary symptoms of aphasia from those patterns of fault propagation which often, but not necessarily, accompany aphasia.

In the next section we attempt to provide a psychological theory of the normal communication process. Our assumption is that although the support for communication arises in many different domains, the psychological level of analysis offers the most useful language for expressing the essential functional organization. We think that the clinician, researcher, and theorist, despite their different goals, can strive for a common language here and can bring their special knowledge into fruitful interaction on this common ground.

A COGNITIVE THEORY OF COMMUNICATION

Unfortunately, there is no simple definition of the term "communication." Although we usually consider communication to be any process by which an exchange of ideas or a discourse between people takes place, it is technically quite difficult to define the principles by which linguistic, gestural, or expressive processes of communicating are distinguished from each other. Nor is it clear how these are to be distinguished from the more general perceptual processes by which information is gained through viewing objects, events, photographs, or pictures. They are all similar in that they involve understanding what is perceived. They are all different in that they involve different sources on which the perceptual information is based. Further, the differences that do exist are almost totally obscured by common statements such as the maiden's plea, "Don't just tell me you love me; show me!" or the old cliches, "Actions speak louder than words" or "A picture is worth a thousand words."

Nevertheless, for our purposes we can make a beginning by identifying that which is communicated, which we shall call a *communique*, and asking if there are some useful distinctions we can make as to the nature of its communication. (We use *communique* in a broader sense than its dictionary meaning. We want to avoid common terms like "message" and "thought" which carry too many meanings that we do not intend. The sense of *communique* will become clear in the ensuing discussion.)

COMMUNIQUES BASED ON SIGNS AND SYMBOLS

Let us consider some examples of communication in the broad sense. When a hungry child cries, he expressively communicates to his mother a need that she often understands. Even a dog can communicate the imperative, "Feed me!" by bringing his dish to his master and barking. Can we find a difference in principle between such expressive communiques and those properties of our world that signify facts about events? When we say, "Clouds are a sign of rain" or "Where there is smoke, there is fire," are we doing anything more than making explicit in linguistic form the communiques that are already implicitly understood by perceptual means?

In our attempt to understand aphasia, it is clear that we must find a principled basis for distinguishing communiques understood in the three ways discussed here:

Communiques asserted linguistically
Communiques expressed by gestures, noises, actions or, facial expressions
Implicit communiques contained in perceptual experience

We must somehow account for the fact that many aphasics who are unable to communicate adequately by linguistic means, still exhibit a nearly normal competence for doing so by gestures, acts, and facial expressions. Indeed, most patients can utter expletives such as "Damn!" or "Hell!" appropriately. Similarly, we must account for the fact that such patients show no significant deficit in perceiving nonlinguistic material. Whatever explanation we give this phenomenon must also account for the fact that deaf persons who become aphasic show comparable deterioration in using or understanding sign language, and blind persons who become aphasic show deficits in reading and writing Braille.

Philosophers of language often suggest that we distinguish between communiques expressed by *signs* and those asserted by the use of *symbols*. When we speak metaphorically of a person's face "being clouded with gloom," we are asserting a proposition of the same sort as when we say "Clouds are a sign of rain." In each case one feature of a context is taken as signifying another, less apparent one. A facial expression can be a sign of a possible emotional state just as a cloudy day can signify the possibility of rain. Thus, a sign has some "natural" relation to that which is signified. It may be a frequent concomitant of it, causally related to it, a necessary component of it, etc. For this reason it is often said that a sign is a *token* of that signified. Hence, a communique based on signs is one whose signal components are naturally related to the meaning conveyed.

A symbol, on the other hand, is a perceptual object bearing no natural relationship to that for which it stands. The relationship is specified by convention or arbitrary association. It satisfies a "naming" relation and is not in any way similar to a natural concomitant of, or causally related to, the object, event, or relationship to which it refers. In the sense we will use in this book, a *sign* is always extralinguistic while a *symbol* is by definition a unit in a linguistic or other conventional system.

It is obvious that the aphasic patient's difficulty is with symbolic communiques, not with signs. To what shall we attribute this difference? It cannot be because one is learned and the other is not. The significance of many signs must be learned just as the reference between symbols and objects must. Are more complex cognitive relationships involved in using symbols than in using signs? There does not seem to be any greater intrinsic difficulty in understanding what object is meant when its name is heard than in understanding what action is appropriate when someone crooks his finger in a "come-hither" gesture. Indeed, neither one of these seems less abstract or general than the other. Wherein lies the difference?

In order to answer these and other questions regarding the nature of the aphasic deficit, we need to examine the nature of the cognitive processes by which signal and symbolic communiques are understood and used.

KNOWLEDGE BY ACQUAINTANCE AND DESCRIPTION

Bertrand Russell (1948) argues that there are two ways by which we come to know our world and our relations to it. The most fundamental way is through our direct experience. This way includes not only what we observe and do, but also what we feel about what we observe and do. Such knowledge he calls *knowledge by acquaintance.* This knowledge has both a public and a private component. The affective component (what one feels about what he knows) is by its very nature private and can only be made public by indirect means. There is, however, a factual aspect of this form of knowledge which can be publicly indicated, e.g., "I feel sad about that." Here a private state is publicly indicated and can be either true or false, depending on whether one is telling the truth or lying. To illustrate: It is a public fact whether or not you met your friend on the street today, but a private one that you were happy or sad at doing so. If you wish to communicate the latter condition, you can do so, but only indirectly by describing the affective state experienced at the time.

This brings us to Russell's second kind of knowledge, *knowledge by description.* If you wish someone to know that you saw your friend yesterday, you may inform him through a symbolic communique, e.g., an indicative sentence stated in English. In doing so you may choose to assert the fact dispassionately or to assert it with great passion. In either case your affective state is made known to him by a signal communique. If you fear that he will take your expressive quality for something other than you intend, you may further choose to describe in detail your affection for your friend. In other words, you may, if you wish, *assert* as an additional symbolic communique what was previously only *expressed* by your signal communique.

Consequently, the distinction between what is knowable by acquaintance or by description corresponds to what we identified earlier as signal communiques and symbolic communiques (if we take "signal" in the broadest sense to include all information that is directly experienced). If aphasia is a disorder of the cognitive processes involved in understanding and using symbolic communiques, then it is obvious that we must press on to understand all that we can about the processes involved in knowledge by description.

There can be no knowledge by description except that which is based on knowledge by acquaintance. For instance, for someone to understand your symbolic report that you were happy to see your friend yesterday, he must by his own experiences be acquainted with the language you use, know what a "friend" is, what it means to "meet" somebody, what it means to recall a historical event, what it means to experience happiness, etc. We would even go so far as to say that there is no valid communication of knowledge by description without a sharing of vicarious or analogical experiences, both public and private.

For this reason, we believe that disorders of cognitive processes involved in knowing by acquaintance constitute fundamental intellectual disorders, whereas those due to impairments of the processes of knowing by description may be disorders of communication with no fundamental intellectual impairment. We must not, however, overlook the likelihood that impairment of knowledge by description may retroactively impede the more fundamental processes by which we directly experience our world. If, for instance, symbolic or verbal coding is involved in memory, then the ability to experience those aspects of the world that depend on memory will be to some degree impaired.

TWO MODES OF COGNITION*

There is a clear adaptive advantage for man to be able to distinguish between what is learned through his own direct experience and what is learned indirectly through descriptions by others. Although we rarely have any difficulty distinguishing between the two forms of knowledge on a purely phenomenological level, a precise theoretical description of how we do this is another matter. The most convincing answer to the question, and one that has been traditionally popular among philosophers, biologists, and psychologists, is that the two kinds of knowing are processes in functionally different modes.

Wigan (1847) suggested more than a century ago that, "The mind is essentially dual, like the organs by which it is exercised." Echoing this same sentiment, Jackson wrote in 1864, "If, then, it should be proved by wider evidence that the faculty of expression resides in one hemisphere, there is no absurdity in raising the question as to whether perception—its corresponding opposite—may not be seated in the other."

Bogen (1969a, b) and Bogen and Bogen (1969) recently presented an excellent compendium and critical discussion of authoritative views concerning the duality of mind and its relation to the dual structure of the brain. Bogen points out that the specialization of cerebral functions in the left and right hemispheres can be inferred from two sources: first, the effects of unilateral cerebral damage, such as found in hemiatrophies and hemispherectomies, and second, the effects of commissurotomies where there has been surgical division of the entire corpus callosum and anterior commisure (the "split-brain" operations for the purpose of preventing the spread of seizures). As a particular instance, Bogen (1969a) shows that the latter patients show an inability to write with the left hand (dysgraphia) accompanied by a disability in

*Most of the material in this section is taken from Bogen (1969a, b) and Bogen and Bogen (1969). These papers present a masterful review of the extensive literature (382 references) on the hemispheres as dual brains. We can only briefly echo salient parts of the review and analysis. Special recognition, of course, should be given to the pioneering work of Sperry and his colleagues. The interested reader should consult Gazzaniga and Sperry (1967).

copying geometric figures with the right hand (dyscopia). In split-brain patients, of course, the left hand has access only to the right hemisphere and the right hand only to the left hemisphere.

Although abundant evidence exists for attributing different functions to the two hemispheres in support of specialization, much evidence also exists for attributing equipotentiality to the whole brain. For instance, concerning the redundant functional capacities of the human brain, Glees (1961) wrote, "Even the removal of a complete hemisphere (about 400 grams of brain substance) may be said to have little effect on intellectual capacity or social behavior, producing at most a lessened capacity for adaptability and a more rapid mental exhaustion." As Bogen points out, this is not an uncommon finding.*In the 150 cases reviewed by White (1961) and the 35 cases reviewed by Basser (1962), where the number of right and left hemispherectomies is approximately equal, "there remained a 'person' no matter which hemisphere was removed." In support of this generalization in the case of split-brain patients, Sperry (1964) concludes, "Everything we have seen so far indicates that the surgery has left each of these people with two separate minds, that is, with two separate spheres of consciousness."

We should be careful, however, not to conclude from this that unilateral injuries do not express themselves in differential ways, for they obviously do. Even though the chief traits by which we identify people may remain intact when there is specific injury to only one hemisphere, major functional capabilities may be severely impaired. Alajoua-nine (1948) reports that the famous musician Ravel, who suffered an aphasic deficit at the height of his career, lost the ability to read or write musical notation although he was still able to play or sing by ear. He also reports that a prominent painter who became a severe aphasic was for the most part professionally undisturbed by the disorder. Alajouanine goes so far as to say," . . . he has even accentuated the intensity and sharpness of his artistic realization and it seems that in him the aphasic and the artist have lived together on two distinct planes."

What emerges from such evidence is a view of the brain as a redundant, flexible, multipurpose system which can reorganize itself even if greatly disturbed so as to preserve sufficient functional integrity to support persistent identity of the person. Only severe bilateral damage seems to challenge the identity of the personality.

The major functions of the brain, however, are lateralized to a great extent. These functions seem to be grouped in two major categories which we will call *symbolic* and *figural*. Teuber (1965) has characterized these major functions as being due to "differ-ent modes of organization" in the two hemispheres. Bogen (1969b) suggests that the right hemisphere recognizes stimuli (including words as labels),† apposes or collates

---

*It should be emphasized that practically all hemispherectomies are performed on patients who suffer damage to one hemisphere prenatally or quite early in life. Moreover, they are performed only when the damaged hemisphere is so dysfunctional as to impede the functioning of the good hemisphere.

†It seems reasonable to assume that the figural shape of words, as auditory and visual objects rather than just symbols, exists in both hemispheres. This assumption is necessary to explain how words as linguistic objects in the dominant hemisphere become associated with their figural reference by a process of ostensive definition. It is presumably by interhemispherical connections between the two forms of instantiation of words as figures and symbols that labeling is possible, i.e., that the evocation of words to pictures and vice versa is accomplished.

these data, and compares them with current or previous data. The right hemisphere processes much the same information as the left hemisphere, but in a different way and toward different results.

A similar view is held by other theorists. Levy-Agresti and Sperry (1968) conclude: "The data indicate that the mute, minor hemisphere is specialized for Gestalt perception, being primarily a synthesist in dealing with information input. The speaking, major hemisphere, in contrast, seems to operate in a more logical, analytic, computer-like fashion [and] the findings suggest that a possible reason for cerebral lateralization in man is basic incompatibility of language functions on the one hand and synthetic perceptual functions on the other."

Tables 5–1 and 5–2, as compiled from Bogen (1969b), summarize at a glance the consensus that has long existed among physiologists, psychologists, and philosophers regarding the characterization of the two modes of cognition. It is interesting to

TABLE 5-1. Dichotomies with Lateralization Suggested

Jackson	Expression	Perception
Jackson	Audioarticular	Retinoocular
Jackson	Propositionizing	Visual imagery
Weisenburg and McBride	Linguistic	Visual imagery
Anderson	Storage	Executive
Humphrey and Zangwill	Symbolic or propositional	Visual or imaginative
McFie and Piercy	Eduction of relations	Eduction of correlates
Milner	Verbal	Perceptual or nonverbal
Semmes, Weinstein, Ghent, Teuber	Discrete	Diffuse
Zangwill	Symbolic	Visuospatial
Hecaen, Ajuriaguerra, Angelergues	Linguistic	Preverbal
Bogen and Gazzaniga	Verbal	Visuospatial
Levy-Agresti and Sperry	Logical or analytic	Synthetic perceptual
Bogan	Propositional	Appositional

TABLE 5-2. Dichotomies without Reference to Cerebral Lateralization

C. S. Smith	Atomistic	Gross
Price	Analytic or reductionist	Synthetic or concrete
Wilder	Numerical	Geometric
Head	Symbolic or systematic	Perceptual or nonverbal
Goldstein	Abstract	Concrete
Ruesch	Digital or discursive	Analogic or eidetic
Bateson and Jackson	Digital	Analogic
J. Z. Young	Abstract	Maplike
Pribram	Digital	Analogic
W. James	Differential	Existential
Spearman	Eduction of relations	Eduction of correlates
Hobbes	Directed	Free or unordered
Freud	Secondary process	Primary process
Pavlov	Second signalling	First signalling
Sechenov (Luria)	Successive	Simultaneous
Levi-Strauss	Positive	Mythic
Bruner	Rational	Metaphoric
Akhilinanda	Buddhi	Manas
Radhakrishnan	Rational	Integral

compare the frequency with which certain polar concepts used to characterize these dichotomous modes have also been used to characterize the major functions lateralized in the two cerebral hemispheres.

There is ample evidence to attribute two distinct modes of thought to the human brain. Humphrey and Zangwill (1951) reported three patients who spontaneously reported failure to dream after their posterior brain injuries. They tentatively assert: ". . . it may be argued that just as the aphasic is unable to express his thought in propositional form, so the agnosic patient may fail to express this ideation at the lower level of fantasy and dream. While not denying that the trend and content of any given dream, or indeed of any given proposition, cannot be interpreted without reference to psychological factors, we would like at the same time to suggest that visual thinking, dreaming and imagination are liable to organic dissolution in a manner directly comparable to the dissolution of symbolic thought in aphasia."

Due to the fact that the above three patients included one left-handed patient and one with bilateral lesion, Humphrey and Zangwill were reluctant to attribute figural processes to the right hemisphere. It is widely agreed, however, that symbolic processes (with the possible exception of simple naming relations) should be attributed to the left hemisphere in most people. Patients with left hemispherectomies are unable to use words in speech or writing, although they are often able to select objects correctly with the left hand when the object is named for them.

The aphasic patient, according to Jackson (1893), has not lost words but the ability to use them in propositions. Head (1926) summarized Jackson's view as follows: "He stated that the words disturbed in consequence of unilateral lesions of the brain were those employed in the 'formation of propositions'; those which remain to the speechless patient are the same words used nonpropositionally."

It is clear that we must make a distinction between the recall of words for use as labels and the enunciation of propositions using words. If Jackson is correct, the nature of aphasia resides somewhere in this difference. We turn now to a discussion of these differences.

PSYCHOLOGICAL PROPOSITIONS

The word proposition is etymologically derived from the Latin *propositio*, which comes from *proponere*, meaning to put forth publicly. Although the notion as used in contemporary logic has taken on a highly abstract interpretation, devoid both of psychological or linguistic import, this was not always the case.

In scholastic and traditional logic, a proposition referred to a verbal statement having the meaning of an assertion. A proposition was not simply a declarative sentence in the grammatical sense, but was the sentence taken together with its meaning. There was, however, a tendency to confuse the meaning of a proposition with the particular linguistic form of the sentence enunciated. For this reason the different notion of *mental proposition* was introduced and made popular by William of Ockham. In the works of later philosophers, for instance Kant, the term "judgment" was substituted for that of proposition, and was referred to as the ideational view of propositions.

According to William of Ockham, as well as the later scholastics who followed him, the mental proposition must be formulated before its corresponding linguistic form is enunciated. Thus, the proposition was considered independent of any particular form of enunciation. Its components were considered conceptual in nature, being ideational analogues of the spoken or written forms, and sharing all aspects essential to the meaning. The mental proposition did not, according to Ockham, need to share such purely grammatical properties as particular gender, declension, or conjugation.

The more abstract usage of the term by contemporary logicians was greatly influenced by Bertrand Russell (1903). By proposition he meant only the meaning of what is linguistically formulated, rather than the psychological act (i.e., the judgment or conception) behind the formulation. Thus, Russell speaks of the possibility of propositions being unasserted. He declared that his notion of an "unasserted proposition" meant essentially the same thing as Frege's term *Gedanke*, which denotes only the sense of a declarative sentence. By this definition Russell meant to restrict the term proposition to the "indicative core of meaning" common to all possible linguistic formulations in different languages or paraphrases in a single language, as well as that which is common to all psychological modes, moods, or attitudes motivating the formulations. Thus, the concept of a proposition historically evolved from meaning particular linguistic assertions or particular judgments, to meaning only that factual import (the indicative core) capable of being true or false.

Where logic might benefit from considering propositions in such an abstract way, a psychological theory of communication must provide an account of all aspects of communiques taking place between humans.

The human communication process involves more than the mere assertion of factual communiques which make manifest the sense or indicative core of the abstract proposition intended by the speaker. Communiques once formulated can be either enunciated in the symbolic mode or enacted in the figural mode so as to assert or express respectively a variety of attitudes, in many different manners, toward the indicative core of a proposition.

Communiques can express or assert needs, intents, hopes, beliefs, doubts, commands, questions, aesthetic, affective and ethical evaluations, and fantasies. *How* a proposition is asserted is just as important as *what* is asserted. Similarly, *why* a proposition is formulated is just as important as whether it is true or not.

If we consider communiques as the manifest form of propositions, then the role that propositions play in a psychological theory of communication must be explained. The account given must be sufficiently general to include both production and comprehension of communiques, and sufficiently specific to account for the detailed symptoms of communication disorders.

In our analysis of the communication process, two major processes must be discussed —the process by which a communique is *formulated* and that by which it is *instantiated*. The first refers to the speaker's or hearer's psychological *needs, attitudes,* and *intents* surrounding the indicative core of the unasserted proposition, while the latter process refers to the *manner* and *mood* of assertion or expression which determines how the proposition is made publicly manifest as a communique. These various aspects of the psychological processes involved in the formulation and instantiation of propositions as communiques are all implicated in both production and comprehension. In this analysis we hope to find the loci of impairments which give rise to the symptoms of an aphasic deficit in the communication process.

FORMULATION

Needs.

What motivates a person to attempt to communicate? Presumably, there is a purpose behind the communication act requiring an exchange of "ideas" with other persons. The *need* to communicate and the interest to do so are quite distinct. For instance, one may feel hungry and know that he needs food, but through stubbornness or shyness refuse to make his need known to you. Here is a clear case of need or purpose without requisite *intent.*

On the other hand, a person may intend to convince you that his needs are other than what they are. The possibility of lying about his need states or goals indicates that communiques about them can be propositional in nature, since they can be either true or false. Need states may be biological or psychological; they may be inherited or acquired. Communiques asserting or expressing no need states would be devoid of purpose and thus aimless. Parrots or speech synthesizers may utter nongoal-directed communiques, or we may occasionally do so in small talk at cocktail parties. However, even in the latter cases we may consider small talk recreational or as exercise of our need for sociability. In general, we look upon a person who talks needlessly as "scatter-brained" or "addled," and those whose communiques express inappropriate need states are regarded as neurotic or, in extreme cases, even as psychotic.

Intents.

Since we often say what we do not intend, it follows that communiques about intents, like those about needs, can be propositional in nature. Intents can be considered subgoals which must be achieved if the more general goals arising from needs are to be satisfied. For instance, a youth may try out for a track team because he feels a need to be accepted by his peers. To succeed, however, he must intend to strive hard during practice; moreover, this requires that he intend to execute, with much control and vigor, the small acts involved in each exercise as he prepares for competition. Similarly, the formulation of communiques requires the integration of many intentional subgoals. To ask for food, one must intend to speak; to speak one must first think of that which needs to be said to gain food. This requires the formulation of many implicit propositions regarding the person to whom one speaks, the availability of food, etc. The factual core of propositions must be derived from the repository of cognitive structures in which knowledge gained by acquaintance or description resides.

The arrangement of intents in the service of needs, and the formulation of the individual propositions by drawing on the appropriate knowledge structures, achieves what has been called a "means–ends analysis" in the problem-solving literature. In a fundamental sense, the selection of intents and the formulation of the propositions involved in the requisite means–ends analyses require considerable intellectual competence. For this reason, we suggest that a key cognitive component in the communication process is what might be called an "executor of intents." It is here that the propositions underlying communiques are born.

Attitude, indicative core, mode.

A communique, in addition to the factual core of the proposition formulated, consists of a particular attitude which accompanies the proposition. Such attitudes are intentional qualifications placed on the assertion or expression of the indicative core of the proposition. Consider:

"There is a fire here." (assertive)
"Is there a fire here?" (interrogative)
"I want a fire here." (optative)
"There is no fire here." (negative)

The *indicative core* which expresses the sense behind each of the above statements is something like "Fire, here, now." The *attitude* toward this indicative core is assertive, interrogative, optative, or negative, as the case may be. The assertive attitude encompasses the various possible tenses (e.g., present, past, or future). The optative attitude expresses a desire rather than an intent or factual proposition. Strictly speaking it should read, "Oh, for a fire!" as a pure expression of desire rather than asserting that a particular need state exists. Since the implicit proposition entailed by the expressed optative attitude involves the assertion that a need state exists relative to object X, it differs from the other attitudes which entail assertions regarding the existence of X itself (Russell, 1948).

Formulation of a communique thus requires the marshalling of intents in the service of needs, bringing to bear one's attitudes toward the indicative core of the unasserted proposition which is selected from either the figural or symbolic *modes* of knowledge in accordance with the appropriate means–end analysis. We can schematically represent the various processes involved in the formulation of the psychological proposition behind a communique by a list of descriptors—each of which must be given some descriptive value: need, intent, attitude, mode, indicative core, etc. Neither the ordering nor the analysis of the process of formulation should be taken as more than an indication of the direction a psychological theory of propositions might take. What has been touched on here seems necessary but in no way sufficient or exhaustive as an analysis of all the alternative ingredients for psychological propositions.

INSTANTIATION

Once the propositional basis to the communique is laid, its *manner* of instantiation must be selected in order for it to be rendered publicly manifest.

Manner.

The competence to formulate a proposition is quite independent of how the communique is performed. It can be asserted as a symbolic communique or expressed figurally as a signal communique. It might even be instantiated in a mixed mode as an interlinking of both symbolic and signal communiques. We presume an ostensive definitional basis for knowledge by description, that is, we assume that the most primitive relations among symbols and objects are learned by nonverbal demonstration such as by example or pointing. This suggests that we make a clear distinction between the various manners in which signal communiques are enacted and the manners in which symbolic ones are enunciated. A verbal statement can be whispered timidly, or shouted with conviction, spoken rapidly or slowly, slurred or pronounced distinctly, directed at a particular audience, or tossed to the wind. The manner of articulation or enactment describes the performance factors involved in the public declaration of the communique.

Although manner may belie attitude, it need not. We often speak of those people whose "bark is worse than their bite," of people who appear insincere but who are honest, or vice versa. By intent to be tactful, one may ask a question rather than make an assertion, but succeed in communicating the proposition that he disagrees with your position and believes it to be in error. (For example, "Are you really going to vote for him?" may be uttered in such a sarcastic manner that the actual communique is "You are an idiot for voting for such a candidate.")

At the dinner table one may choose to enact a command to pass the salt by pointing (a signal communique) rather than asking for it (a symbolic communique). A deaf person who is finger spelling uses a different manner for enunciating symbolic communiques than does a normal speaker, while they both may use the same signal communiques (e.g., facial expressions, laughing, crying) to express their joy or sadness in response to some event.

The game of charades constitutes a lengthy chain of signal communiques when no finger spelling or other symbolic gestures are allowed. When such gestures are permitted, we have a complex mixed mode communique.

If the foregoing analysis of the communication process is correct, then Jackson's claim that "propositionizing" is carried out by the dominant hemisphere (in the symbolic mode) must be extended to cover the activities of the other hemisphere as well (the figural mode). We must admit to the possibility that "ostensive" propositionizing is as much an activity of the cerebral processes as linguistic propositionizing, since in many cases the difference between the communiques achieved is nothing more than manner of instantiation. In many cases the formulation of the enunciated proposition is little different from the proposition enacted. The main differences are those that exist between telling someone that "X is so" and showing him that it is the case.

Mood.

In order to extend the descriptor index for psychological propositionizing to include the reception of communiques as well as their production, we need to add one more term—"mood." One may participate in the communication process by assuming the "productive" or "receptive" mood, or both. A lecturer assumes the productive mood while the audience assumes the receptive mood. If the lecturer's manner of presentation is dramatic and stimulating, the audience is quite likely to choose an attentive manner in listening to his communiques. On the other hand, if the speaker is boring because his manner of delivery is repetitious and monotonic, the audience may assume a manner of listening due only to politeness. In extreme cases, members of the audience may entirely relinquish the receptive mood and daydream, chat with their neighbors, or even sleep.

We can now round out the descriptor index for psychological propositionizing to include mood:

formulation	need
	intent
	attitude
	mode
	indicative core
instantiation	manner
	mood

CRITERIA FOR COMMUNICATION

As an ideal, we will say that perfect communication has been achieved when the exact proposition intended by the producer is the proposition afforded the recipient (entailed, signified, or asserted) by the communique. This is obviously an ideal limit on normal communication since often we are mistaken in our understanding of the purpose or intent behind a communique, even though the indicative core of the proposition is well specified. At other times we clearly perceive a person's intent by the manner in which he expresses the communique, although we may, say in the heat of an argument or passionate embrace, miss much of the factual content. An example may help clarify the roles of the various components of a communique stipulated in the descriptor index.

Consider the following sentence uttered by a guilty defendant in answer to cross examination by the prosecutor:

"No, I did not murder the bookkeeper!"

The following interpretation can be given to the descriptor index for this communique: need—to preserve self; intent—to lie; attitude—negative; mode—symbolic; indicative core—"bookkeeper, murdered by me"; manner—hostile, emphatic; mood—productive. A naive matronly juror who has been taken in by the slick defendant may interpret the communique as follows (for reception we invert the order of the descriptors in the index): mood—receptive; manner—sympathetic, attentive; indicative core—"bookkeeper murdered by unknown assailant"; mode—symbolic, attitude—assertive; intent —to discover the truth; need—to see justice done.

By comparing the descriptor indices for the proposition intended by the defendant with those for the proposition afforded the naive juror, the accuracy of transmission of the communique can be evaluated. In this case, the naive juror interpreted the communique from the guilty defendant exactly as he intended; thus from his stand-point the communication was successful. However, from a more objective standpoint, since the factual content of the communique was false, communication was less than perfect. The sophisticated judge, who interprets the communique from the defendant more accurately in the context of evidence, might say to himself, "By his manner he intends to deceive us. Hence he has perjured himself." Thus the judge perfectly understood the intention of the communique.

These examples illustrate also the role that knowledge must play in the formulation or interpretation of communiques. Consequently, we might conclude that if needs are serviced by intents, then intents must be serviced by knowledge. One cannot seriously intend to do either that which he knows cannot be done or that which one does not know how to do. To intend to do something implies that one has successfully formu-lated a set of propositions which when instantiated accomplish the means–end analysis required to consummate the intent.

In the next chapter we will present a schema which uses this analysis of com-muniques as psychological propositions to account for the complex symptomatologies exhibited by communication disorders. In doing so, we hope to make a case for aphasia as an impairment of the ability to formulate propositions in the symbolic mode, rather than as a disorder of intent or impairment of the instantiation process.

SUMMARY

Aphasia is a complex problem which must be approached with the resources of many disciplines. To bring these many diverse analyses together it is necessary to find some common framework in which to represent them. This framework must be rich enough to represent the various kinds of data and specific enough to be useful to researchers, clinicians, and theorists.

The task is not one of finding a single "casual" level to which all other descriptions can be reduced. The complexity of the problem, as well as modern philosophy of science, argue against any such simple approach. The brain is viewed as a complex, self-organizing system that can adjust to a variety of changing conditions (including changes in itself) in highly interdependent ways.

A conceptual framework must indicate the kinds of *support for* communication that describe normal functioning. When communication disorders occur, we want to be able to indicate what kind of deficit of support could account for both the positive and negative symptoms observed.

In order to progress toward a framework, we have developed a cognitive theory of communication, which regards human communication as a series of *communiques* between persons. We distinguished two kinds of communiques, those involving *signs* and those involving *symbols*. We related these kinds of communiques to two modes of cognition: knowledge by *acquaintance* and knowledge by *description*. We speculated that these two kinds of cognition are fundamentally different and are (in the normal person) dominated by the separate hemispheres. *Symbolic* functions are largely in the left hemisphere and *figural* functions largely in the right hemisphere.

Finally, we developed a view of the propositionalizing functions underlying communication. Psychological propositions can be divided into the stages of *formulation* and *instantiation*. Formulation involves *needs, intents, attitudes,* and *modes of knowledge*. The *indicative core* is, roughly, what the communique is about. Instantiation deals with the performance of the communique and has to do with the *manner* in which the communique is asserted or expressed. *Mood* has to do with the productive or receptive role taken by the participant. Specifying these variables (descriptors) provides a functional description of the communique.

chapter **6**

A FUNCTIONAL SCHEMA FOR
APHASIC SYMPTOMATOLOGY

In our attempts to work toward a unified theory of aphasia, we found that our thinking was greatly facilitated by the use of an heuristic scheme that we call a *functional schema for the communication process*. This schema is diagrammed in Figure 6–1.

Using this schema, we have attempted to provide systematic characterizations of a wide range of symptoms associated with communication disorders. We can ask what variation in the functional integrity of the schema could produce the symptoms we see in aphasia, in the complicating conditions that accompany aphasia, and in the nonaphasic disorders. Conversely, we can arbitrarily assume faults in the components of the schema and ask if we know of clinical patterns of symptoms that reflect such presumed impairment.

Our mode of operation has been essentially (though not viciously) circular. We began with the psychological analysis presented in Chapter 5 and with our knowledge of the general nature of the clinical evidence concerning major patterns of aphasia. We generated the schema as a visual reminder of the functional processes involved. Then we turned to the information on communication disorders and revised (and simplified) the schema. Functions that we had postulated but which seemed to have no reasonable projection onto the communication disorders were eliminated, and our notions about the nature of some of the functional unities were altered as we came to understand better the inferred unities of the disorders we encountered. The schema presented here is still in the process of revision, and of course we expect future changes. We offer it as a preliminary guide in the hope that it will be of assistance to clinicians, researchers, and theorists.

We cannot stress too strongly, however, that this schema should *not* be considered a model depicting the number or arrangement of physiological structures involved in communication, nor is it meant to represent the temporal organization of the psychological processes involved in communication. Rather, it is an heuristic scheme that we can use in discussing the logically interdependent, functional components supporting the communication process and in trying to organize the related but distinct symptomatologies of various communication disorders.

In denying that the schema is a model, we do not mean to claim that it has no explanatory value. To the extent that it proves useful in characterizing aphasia, it moves us closer to an adequate model of the functional systems supporting human communication. The reader should recall that we do not mean to characterize the site from which the faulty signals originated, nor do we mean to give a diagrammatic tracing of the paths followed by divergent signals. Rather, we wish to characterize the support for normal communication and the new state of functional organization of the system after trauma. We wish to be able to say how a disordered communication differs from a normal one, rather than how it got that way.

In a sense our task is analogous to attempts to characterize a city before and after a major breakdown of electrical facilities. A description of the burned-out coil in the solenoid controlling the master relay (the "causal site") provides no characterization of the trouble experienced by the population due to the failure of radios, televisions, elevators, subways, ovens, refrigerators, and other electrical devices throughout the city. On the other hand, giving a real process model entails describing the entire distribution network and all its intermediate transitory states in addition to the before-and-after picture of the disordered system—an incredible wealth of detail.

Our schema, then, represents an intermediate level of analysis. It is neither a causal model nor a process model; in fact, it is not a model in the usual scientific sense at all. It is a scheme for talking about communication disorders while we try to assemble relevant data from all the disciplines involved on our way to building a true model.

THE USE OF MODELS IN SCIENCE

A *model* is a system used to represent another system because it is either conceptually simpler to study than the original system, due to its abstract nature, or practically more convenient to explore, due to its smaller scale. For example, the study of model airplanes in a wind tunnel is convenient for both of these reasons. It is a small-scale simulation of real flight conditions as well as being sufficiently simple to allow for the test and application of the principles of aerodynamics.

While convenience is a sufficient justification for the use of models, explicitness is a necessary requirement for their effective use. One of the most important uses of models is as a testing ground for the adequacy of the principles they embody. These principles are borrowed by analogy from familiar, well-understood phenomena and applied to a less well-understood one. In order to evaluate the explanatory adequacy of the borrowed principles, the new phenomenon under study must be sufficiently characterized so that the points of the analogy can be explicitly stated. Since an analogic model, like any other analogy, is valid in some ways but not in others, saying exactly in what respects the model matches the phenomenon to be modeled is an absolute necessity.

Given that our current knowledge of aphasia does not provide a precise characterization of the disorder, there is little chance that an explanatory model can be developed at this time. We believe that the schema presented here moves us a little closer to such a characterization of aphasia and should help provide the prerequisites for a model.

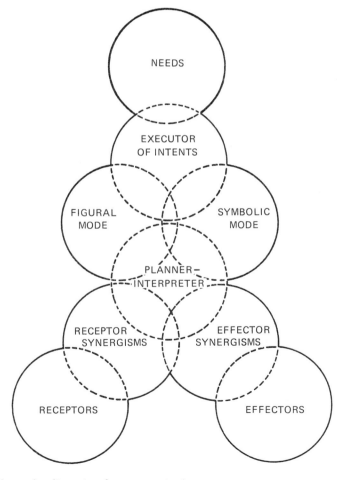

Fig. 6–1. Schema for discussing the communication process.

THE SCHEMA

The functional schema for human communication provides the framework for our discussion of communication disorders in general, and aphasia in particular. Brief descriptions of the components of the schema follow.

PROPOSITION FORMULATION

Needs.

This component represents the source of purposes or goals that a person must continually satisfy if well-being is to be maintained. Some of the need states are biological in origin (e.g., food, oxygen, sleep, activity, optimal stimulation, etc.); other need states are probably acquired (e.g., love, communication, social dominance, etc.).

Executor of intents.

This component executes all decisions required for formulating "means–ends" propositions directed toward the satisfaction of needs. Attitudes toward the indicative core of propositions are selected, as well as the cognitive mode in which the proposition is to be formulated.

Figural mode of knowledge.

We regard this as the most primitive (basic) mode of cognition. Signal communiques are formulated in this mode. It is also the repository of information gained from signal communiques and from direct experience of objects and events. Definitions of symbols through pointing, acting out, demonstrating, etc. (ostensive definitions), must also be processed and stored in this mode.

Propositions formulated in this mode may be expressed by gesture, facial expressions, or actions. Such propositions are true or false by virtue of whether or not what they express is also a component of what they signify. For instance, a smile is a true expression of a happy mood, if it originates from such a mood, rather than being shammed. The expressed proposition is part of the meaning of what it signifies.

Symbolic mode of knowledge.

This is the mode in which knowledge by description is processed and stored. Symbolic communiques are formulated in this mode. It is the primary repository of knowledge derived from languages of all types, including mathematical, musical, and chemical notations and artificial codes of any kind.

Propositions formulated in this mode are asserted via symbolic representations. These propositions have derivative meaning only. They are true or false by virtue of whether what they assert satisfies either conventional relations (e.g., "A circle is round.") or ostensive relations (e.g., "That is a dog.").

PROPOSITION INSTANTIATION

Let us now consider the lower portion of our schema, which refers to the functions of those components that make the implicit proposition evident to others. This deals with the appropriate patterns of activation of the effector systems of the body by which the proposition is enacted as either a signal or symbolic communique. The arguments for the specific subdivisions we have chosen will follow later. Brief descriptions of the functions carried out by the subsystems involved in the enunciation or enactment of communiques may be sketched first.

Planner–Interpreter.

The planner is the first stage in a three-stage command system by which the effector organs are activated appropriately for the proposition formulated. Although we do not understand how, the implicitly formulated proposition provides a "model" or higher-order pattern by which complex sets of motor activities can be integrated into speech or other molar action sequences. The planner component, following directives originating from the means–end analysis performed by the executor of intents, has as its primary function the synthesis of a program by which the effector action is controlled.

The interpreter functions similarly on the side of reception. Note that we assume here that higher-order plans for the analysis of incoming signals are necessary for comprehension of either symbolic or signal communiques.

Effector synergisms.

A synergism is a preprogrammed sequence of coordinated activities which, once initiated, runs off automatically to completion. Effector synergisms were once thought to be simple chains of reflexes, but since the manner in which they are executed can be varied by higher control processes (here, the planner), the reflexive definition is no longer appropriate.

The evidence for the existence of synergisms is abundant. The chief theoretical argument for assuming their existence arises from attempts to explain highly integrated, complicated motor activities, such as those involved in speech, playing musical instruments, dancing, and sports. The rapidity with which such activities must occur defies explanation in terms of voluntary response patterns or response sequences controlled by sensory or neural feedback. Preprogramming or "prepackaging" seems absolutely necessary.

Receptor synergisms.

Although the evidence for receptor synergisms is more indirect than for effector synergisms, we believe that analogous arguments can be made for their existence. For the present we will simply assume the existence of preprogrammed subroutines for the analysis of incoming communiques to account for the efficiency with which rapidly occurring and incompletely specified signals are processed.

It is tempting to suggest that the receptor synergisms are closely related to the effector synergisms, although this cannot be demonstrated at the present time in any strong manner. We believe, as a first guess, that the output of the receptor synergisms is at least "written in the same code" as the input to the effector synergisms. In the case of speech at least, there is a good deal of evidence in support of this hypothesis, as we shall see later.

Effector organs.

These are the systems of body action at the end of the production process. Their activation provides the instantiation of communiques as an explicit enactment of publicly observable behaviors.

Receptor organs.

These are the sensory systems involved in the pickup of the physical energy patterns supporting the manifest form of the communique.

Overall organization.

The functional components listed above are not presumed to be related in a simple hierarchical form. Neither are they a disconnected set of independent parts. Taken together they form a *coalition* in which to varying degrees each functional component influences, and is influenced by, the others. This is a difficult notion to convey and is best understood in the context of examples of their interaction. Such examples follow later in the chapter. For the present, it is enough to point out that the components are not only productively and receptively interrelated but also interconnected by a variety of forms of feedback and "feedforward" controls.

It is important to note that the figure representing the schema is simplified in several important ways. The most important simplification to note now is that the components in the lower half of the figure are represented by single structures on the diagram. Of course, the reader is expected to elaborate this flat scheme into parallel layers of components. For example, when we are considering a speech act, the effectors involved are those of the speech musculature; when we consider an act of writing, the effectors are the arm, hand, and fingers. The effector synergisms are correspondingly different in the two cases. On the receptive side the same kinds of parallel structures exist. For reading, the visual receptors and visual analyzing systems are implicated; for listening, the auditory receptors and the auditory analysis systems are involved. One can imagine many special systems pressed into service of communication functions—gesturing in sign language, reading words by touching raised letters or Braille, writing with a pencil held in one's teeth or lashed to one's foot, etc. We do not suppose that the specific aspect of these diverse systems are represented in the same functional component: thus, the schema must not be so interpreted. Obviously, at some point the various systems converge on language and the analysis is in common. However, at the periphery in both production and perception the systems may be very different, alike only in performing the same kind of function for the overall communication system.

In the next section we will discuss some of the arguments that led us to postulate the components in the lower half of the chart having to do with the instantiation of propositions.

PROBLEMS IN ENACTING COMMUNIQUES

In 1951 Lashley posed the problem of serial order in behavior as a challenge to both psychological and physiological theorists. In this provocative paper he argued that the organization of complex motor events (speaking, typewriting, playing the piano) could not be explained by reflexes or associative chains of responses. The speed, the diversity, and the integrated assembly of the component responses simply prohibited the traditional interpretations. Since that time many other theorists have joined Lashley in urging the notion of some kind of higher-order planning component as a necessary part of any explanatory scheme (e.g., Miller *et al.*, 1960; Lenneberg, 1967; Pribram, 1971). Such a component must be capable of organizing individual effector synergisms into diverse programs for the control of complex motor activities.

Although most psychological theories have not yet progressed to the point of incorporating such planning components in a meaningful way, there appears to be little objection to the arguments for such a component. In the case of speech sound production, however, Wickelgren (1969) has argued that a proliferation of particular responses (up to the level of 1,000,000 or so) might save an associative production model. In reply, Halwes and Jenkins (1971) have argued that such a model is unsuitable and loses more in explanatory power than it gains in simplicity of production. Aside from this one instance, theorists in most fields seem to agree that such a productive component is required.

In regard to interpreter programs, the agreement is not so great because the phenomena are even less well understood. Yet it seems to us that one must argue for such a component. For example, research on speech perception over the last 20 years has destroyed any hope of finding simple one-to-one correspondence between the acoustic signal and the linguistic elements that are crucial in the interpretation of that signal. In different contexts a specific acoustic pattern may be heard as different phonemes. And in some contexts different acoustic patterns are heard as the same phoneme. In general, however, the interaction of the stimulus pattern and the context are predictable from higher-order rules using linguistic and articulatory constructs. This latter finding seems to argue for an interpreter component that is closely tied to the planner component, if not identical to it.

Such primary arguments aside, the justification of the planner–interpreter component can also rest on the evidence that can be adduced in favor of the existence of synergisms. If synergisms can be clearly demonstrated, then it is obvious that they must be programmed or interpreted by another functional component.

EVIDENCE FOR THE EXISTENCE OF SYNERGISMS

The evidence for synergisms is derived from the study of too many diverse biological phenomena to be reviewed here. (For an excellent discussion of the various synergisms involved in speech, see Lenneberg, 1967, from whom much of our discussion is derived.) Rather than attempt a survey, we will illustrate the characteristic nature of synergisms involved in communication by selecting a few exemplary cases.

Respiratory synergisms.

Draper, *et al.* (1957, 1959, 1960) have shown that the mean subglottal pressure may remain fairly constant during steady-state phonations (e.g., in uttering a prolonged "a-a-a-a-a-ah"). An analysis of this phonation process indicates that a very complicated coordination must be maintained among abdominal muscles and those used in inspiration and expiration. Lenneberg (1967) provides the following description of this process:

> At the beginning of phonation (that is, while air is already escaping), the tonus of the inspiratory muscles continues, from which it must be inferred that these muscles at first prevent the thorax from slumping back too fast and thus seem to be counteracting the elastic contractile forces. At a certain point, the inspiratory muscles suddenly relax, and some expiratory muscles come into action at once; gradually other expiratory muscles become active until the speaker has to catch his breath. Now the expiratory muscles become electrically silent and inspiratory muscles take over again. (p. 82)

If simple steady-state phonation requires such complicated coordinations of different muscle groups, imagine the degree of complication of those coordinated muscular movements involved in the complex phonation patterns required for articulated speech.

Penfield and Roberts (1959) offered corroborating evidence in support of the independent existence of synergisms involved in speech. They showed that direct stimulation of the cortex near the Rolandic fissure would occasionally elicit fractions of the motor speech act. Vowel sounds were typically emitted such that if the patient ran out of breath he would quickly inhale and continue phonation. They reported that the patient was usually aware that he was phonating but was unable to bring this activity under voluntary control. In addition to voicing, pursing of the lips and movements of the tongue and jaw were observed. These movements were not mere random contractions of muscles but appeared as well-integrated synergistic acts that might be involved in speaking, chewing, or swallowing.

Articulatory synergisms.

Adult speakers of English are quite capable of producing about 500 syllables per minute, while a more normal rate which includes hesitation pauses is more like 210 to 220 syllables per minute (Goldman-Eisler, 1954). Although the precise number of muscles required for speech is not known, a reasonable estimate can be made. If we assume that the muscles that are ordinarily involved in speech are those of the thoracic and abdominal walls, the neck and face, the larynx, pharynx, and the oral cavity, then it is obvious that over 100 muscles must somehow be controlled by some higher-order command structure.

In changing from one speech sound to another, complex muscular adjustments must be made about 14 times per second. These readjustments cannot occur simultaneously for all muscles involved since the various muscle groups have different characteristic roles to play in articulation; some must be activated before phonation, others during, and still others shortly after. Similarly, some muscles are activated for very short durations while others must hold their tonus for a relatively long period. A rough calculation suggests that something of the magnitude of several hundred effector events must take place every second to achieve ordinary speech (Lenneberg, 1967).

Given the complex reorganization of synergisms involved each time a novel sentence is uttered, there can be little credence given to explanations in terms of the learning of simple chains of reflexes or associated responses. Nor is it likely, given the rate at which these complex patterns of motor events must be accomplished, that the system issuing commands can be under the control of voluntary decision processes. The automatic nature of such motor processes can be satisfied only by assuming the existence of effector synergisms, while the variety and flexibility of their reorganization in uttering new sentences requires a higher-order control component to achieve the reprogramming. Hence the evidence for the existence of synergisms implies a planner component by which the synergisms may be reorganized. (For more on this viewpoint, see Bernstein, 1967.)

Receptive Synergisms.

It is difficult to collect direct evidence on receptive synergisms, but four lines of evidence lead us to believe that such synergisms must be postulated for speech perception.

First, it is abundantly clear that natural speech signals are "privileged" signals. Arbitrary codes (e.g., Morse code) and substitutions of noises for natural speech sounds cannot be processed by listeners at rates that are at all comparable to the rates at which they can process speech. Even after years of practice in listening to such codes, the rate of transmission of communiques remains at a low level, about 30 words per minute. In contrast, natural speech and carefully contrived synthetic speech can be heard at rates more than 10 times that of the arbitrary codes (Liberman *et al.*, 1967).

Further, it appears that even natural speech segments cannot be assembled or compiled into new sequences without great losses in effective communication. If we collect speech sounds, syllables, or even words, and then call them out in new orders and try to butt them together, they have low intelligibility and little communicative power (Harris, 1953).

Thus, it is clear that there is something special about the processing of speech signals themselves. This observation suggests that speech perception relies on special machinery or special processing routines in the nervous system.

The second line of evidence stems from the unusual nature of findings from studies of the perception of highly encoded speech sounds, such as stop consonants. Such studies have convincingly demonstrated the phenomenon of "categorical perception" (Liberman *et al.*, 1967). Briefly, this means that as one changes some of the acoustic parameters of a speech sound, the perception does not change until a critical region is reached. Then, at this critical point, a further small change produces a different speech percept. For example, in English, as the experimenter manipulates the cue for voicing (voice-onset time), the subject reports hearing /ba/ for values over a 100-millisecond range, but a further change of 5 to 10 milliseconds results in the subject hearing /pa/. Further, the subject is very poor in discriminating between /ba/ sounds that differ in voice-onset time but excellent at hearing the tiny differences that produce the difference between /ba/ and /pa/. The evidence has led Stevens (1971) to conclude, ". . . the auditory mechanism must be endowed with 'property detectors,' each of which responds to an acoustic attribute corresponding to a feature of language." Furthermore, these detectors are not likely to respond to simple acoustic changes but rather, ". . . will generally correspond to a more complex pattern of events in time and frequency. . . ."

The third line of evidence comes from the recent studies of speech perception in infants. In such studies experimenters habituate the infant to a repeated speech sound and then play a different speech sound. The experimenter observes some index of habituation, like heart rate or sucking rate, and looks for evidence of a sharp change of rate to indicate that the infant has "noticed" the change in the signal. Moffitt (1968) demonstrated that four-month-old infants detected the difference between the speech sounds /ba/ and /ga/. Eimas and his colleagues (1971) showed that four-week-old infants detected the difference between /ba/ and /pa/ but did not detect the same difference in voice-onset time when it was within the range that adults hear as /ba/ or within the range that adults hear as /pa/. Such dramatic studies not only suggest the presence of receptor synergisms but also imply that some speech property detectors may be part of the innate equipment of the human being.

The fourth line of evidence, the studies of dichotic listening, is more direct but adds weight to the argument (Shankweiler, 1971). These studies show that the analysis of highly encoded speech sounds seems to be most effectively performed in the left hemisphere. The evidence extends over a range from distinctive feature analysis (subphonemic level) to the processing of strings of words. This implies (although only weakly) that specialized processing mechanisms for several levels of speech analysis are available in that hemisphere.

As in the case of effector synergisms, the postulation of receptor synergisms argues for an interpreter component. If batteries of receptor synergisms are firing, they must somehow be "composed" at some level for further processing. If one considers that not all information gets properly encoded in the acoustic stream, and that not all that is encoded gets reliably extracted, there is need for a component that can operate on this input. Returning to Stevens (1971) again, "The listener most certainly will be required to resort to higher-level information such as constraints imposed by the phonological rules of language, the lexicon, and syntax and semantic rules, in order to decode the signal."

Finally, we must mention that the "motor theories" of speech perception such as advanced by Liberman et al. (1967) make the additional supposition that there is some kind of equivalence between the planner and response synergisms, on the one hand, and the interpreter and receptor synergisms, on the other. While most motor theories are vague, and no one at present has any idea how to spell out a motor theory in detail, we feel the suggestion of a correspondence is very important. Stevens (1971) tries to be as specific as possible. After reviewing the evidence, he comments, "The evidence would suggest that such property detectors are matched to the property-generating capabilities of the articulatory mechanism, and that the common acoustic properties correspond to features of language."

Comment.

The lines of argument are sketched above to justify our inclusion of the planner–interpreter and effector and receptor synergisms in our schema for communication. The arguments do not, of course, explain how these components might work; they simply lead us to postulate such components. But this is all that our schema is meant to be at this time—namely, a description of *what* is done, not a model indicating *how* it is done.

USING THE SCHEMA TO DISCUSS DISORDERS

In this section we attempt to illustrate our earlier claim that the primary symptoms for a wide range of communication disorders can be explained as the failure of specific functional components to provide necessary support for the normal communication process. In the following analyses we assume that the disorders discussed are relatively free of any complicating conditions. The symptoms that interest us most are those that arise from dysfunctions of language-relevant components alone.

DISORDERS OF FORMULATION

Disorders of need states.

Dysfunctions of this component are among the most debilitating of all communication disorders. A person whose need priorities are so radically deranged that he cannot communicate with others is usually diagnosed as psychotic or severely retarded. His language is typically classified as bizarre, incoherent, or even babbling, and fails to exhibit the goal direction that typifies normal discourse. Since intents are recruited by need-specific goals, and the modes of cognition draw their guidance from intents, disorders of need states permeate all the components, shattering the functional integrity of the cognitive systems needed for communication.

Disorders of intent.

Impairments of this component interfere either with the basic ability to formulate propositions appropriate to the satisfaction of needs or with the urge to do so. The most severe forms of disturbance to the executor of intents impede the formulation of the means–end analyses necessary to normal problem-solving activities. A person so afflicted may exhibit perceptual disorientation, disorganized thought processes, general amnesia, an inability to sustain attention, or be subject to "flights of ideas." These symptoms often arise from a wide range of disorders such as psychotic reactions, especially hebephrenia and Korsakoff's syndrome, and generalized brain damage as caused by trauma, toxic agents, or arteriosclerosis. In catatonia and depressive reaction there seems to be a total failure of urge to communicate (psychotic mutism).

Exclusive of the above, there are two disorders, not involving psychoses or generalized brain damage, which exhibit as primary symptoms the inability to execute appropriate intents necessary to achieve communication—what has been called "superfluency" or logorrhea and psychological mutism.

Superfluency.

This is a volitional disorder involving an inability to control the direction or rate of flow of speech. The patient continues to speak once he begins in spite of an awareness that his discourse violates the rules of syntax or is inappropriate to the social context. His speech is rambling, interminably long, improperly begun, filled with cliches and repetitive phrases, and often so loosely connected in theme that it is quite incomprehensible to others. When asked the simplest question, the patient may begin answering but switches rapidly to numerous irrelevant topics.

The superfluent patient differs from the simple aphasic in that he does not appear to have word-finding difficulties. He differs also from the "tachyphemic" patient as found in some neurological diseases such as Parkinson's disease, who appears to have a disordered speech "pace-maker." (Lenneberg, 1967) (In this latter patient, what appears to be an increase in the rate of speech is due to the interpolation of irrelevant, nonspeech sounds. In fact, the articulators are moving at normal rate so that the semantic density of discourse is normal.) The superfluent patient also differs from the aphasic and tachyphemic patients in his inability to achieve the goals of social communication. This suggests that an underlying thought disorder may be present.

Psychological mutism.

If superfluency is due to a pathology of the intent to speak, then mutism can be defined as its complementary volitional disorder, namely, a pathological lack of the intent to speak. Although mutism is often a symptom of psychotic disorders, it need not be merely psychogenic in origin. It may be traceable to a neurogenic interference with what Lenneberg has called "the activating system" for language. Van Buren (1963), for example, has reported an apparent arrest of the impulse to speak when the head of the caudate nucleus is electrically stimulated.

Patients afflicted with this disorder can be distinguished from the aphasic by the fact that most aphasic patients exhibit a highly motivated desire to speak even though they do not. These patients may surprise themselves and hospital personnel by a temporary ability to speak normally when placed under severe emotional stress.

Disorders of the figural mode.

The term agnosia was introduced by Freud to mean "disturbances in the recognition of objects" in spite of apparently intact sensory processes. In other words, agnosia was meant to refer to a deficit in noticing or interpreting what is seen, not in seeing itself. Bay (1953, 1962) has disputed this claim, and argues that some sensory impairment can always be found associated with visual agnosia if rigorous tests are made. Brain (1961), however, points out that Ettlinger (1956) and others, using tests similar to those suggested by Bay, found that some patients exhibit symptoms of visual agnosia without any symptoms of sensory impairment being present.

Agnosia has also been used to refer to the failure to perceive spatial relations. Indeed, this kind of agnosia seems to be much more common than "object agnosia." Other descriptions of agnosia have included inability to identify objects tactually or to interpret tonal stimuli in the auditory realm.

Because our experience with such patients is very limited and because the word "agnosia" has taken on so many meanings, we are reluctant to use it, even descriptively. In the absence of tests for aphasia, the loss of ability to name or describe objects may be misinterpreted. Inferring the nature of such a disorder requires the gathering of data that permit the separation of sensory from perceptual deficits, and both of these from memory deficits and from the variety of response deficits that may be present. In aphasic patients we have frequently seen the impairment of visuospatial processes and have often found such problems associated with bilateral or diffuse brain damage. In extreme cases of disturbance of spatial relations a patient exhibits a general disorientation to his surroundings, being unable in some cases even to find his way around his home or neighborhood in which he has lived for years. With thorough testing, such problems can readily be separated from aphasia itself.

We think it is reasonable to suppose that there are disorders of figural information, regardless of modality of input or output. It has been reported (Bogen, 1969b) that some left hemiplegic patients fail to recognize their disorder and exhibit "a delusion of body scheme," in the face of evidence from *several* sensory domains. We further suppose that some kinds of information may be restricted by this very nature to specialized systems (e.g., pitch perception). For example, Nielsen and Sult (1939), Brain (1941) and Spreen *et al.* (1965) have documented cases of "auditory agnosia" existing without aphasia in patients with unilateral right-hemisphere injury.

Reviewing the evidence, Critchley (1953) suggests, "Such a combination of defects in gnosis argues strongly in favor of some general defect rather than a circumscribed 'pure' disability." It seems reasonable to us to consider seriously the possibility that what has been called "agnosia" is a functionally complementary disorder to aphasia—being a disorder of the figural mode of knowledge while aphasia is a disorder of the symbolic mode. Thus, if aphasia is an impairment of the ability to handle symbolic communiques, then agnosia is an impairment of the ability to handle signal communiques.

Although we have used the terms "figural" and "symbolic" to refer to functional rather than structural concepts, we must note, as in the previous chapter, that there is considerable evidence that these functions are for the most part lateralized in the right and left hemisphere, respectively.

In any event, the existence of the varieties of disorders that are grouped under the rubric of agnosia gives strong reason for the postulation of deficits of the figural mode, and must sensitize us to the careful exploration of those disorders as impairments of that mode. The kind of research to which aphasia has been subjected must be applied to the figural deficits.

Disorders of the symbolic mode.

We view aphasia as synonymous with dysfunctions of processing in the symbolic cognitive mode. It is in the symbolic mode that the knowledge that a person has gained through description rather than by direct experience must be formulated. It should be especially noted that we expect that the ability to process symbolic communiques will be impaired with respect to both receptive and productive aspects of communication. The defect is in symbolic processing itself, and such processing is basic to symbolic communiques, regardless of whether they are incoming or outgoing.

On the other hand, we expect the patient who is suffering *only* from aphasia to be relatively unimpaired with respect to propositions in *ostensive* forms, that is, expressive processes such as gestures,* facial expressions, or acts that do not in any way depend on symbolic codes. In short, the aphasic should exhibit nearly normal competence for expressing his intentions or understanding those of others, so long as they are presented in the form of signal communiques. (For some related research, see Goodglass and Kaplan, 1963; and De Renzi, *et al.*, 1966.)

Our view is that the patient is giving an accurate report when he says, "I know what I want to say, but I can't say it." The patient has no fundamental thought disorder; he comprehends the figural aspects of the situation; he knows what he wants and intends; but he cannot formulate propositions in the symbolic mode. As Jackson said (1874):

> Speaking is not simply the utterance of words. The utterance of any number of words would not constitute speech. Speaking is "propositionizing." To this meaning of the term, speech must be rigidly kept. That the speechless patient cannot propositionalize *aloud* is obvious— he never does. But this is only the superficial part of the truth. He cannot propositionalize internally. He can neither say, "Gold is yellow" aloud nor to himself. The proof that he does not speak internally is that he cannot express himself in writing. He may write in the sense of copying writing, and can usually copy print in writing characters. Now, if he can speak internally, why does he not write what he says to himself? He can say nothing to himself, and therefore has nothing to write." (p. 130)

While we believe that writing is more difficult than speaking for most patients, for a variety of reasons that will be examined later, the force of Jackson's argument is clear. The symbolic deficit that impairs speech is similarly fundamental in writing.

---

*Gestures, of course, fall into two categories: those that signal a proposition such as a threatening gesture (e.g., a raised closed fist) or a come-hither gesture (e.g., the crooking of a finger), and those that symbolize a proposition such as finger spelling or the victory or peace gestures. The signal gestures are capable of pure figural processing since they simulate in part or abbreviate an action that can be carried out, while symbolic gestures derive their meaning solely from learned conventions.

From this point on, however, our view differs from Jackson's and from the entire classical treatment of aphasia. Jackson thought that aphasia was a deficit of production but not of reception. This was in accord with his view that the right hemisphere was concerned with the reception of propositions and that reception was automatic rather than voluntary. For both of these reasons he believed that aphasia, being due to left-hemisphere damage, affected only the voluntary act of formulating propositions.

As we will argue in detail below, the best interpretation of the evidence seems to be that both production and perception in *all* language modalities exhibit the aphasic deficit. For the present we offer the following definition of this primary disorder of the symbolic mode: Aphasia is a general language deficit that crosses all language modalities. The primary symptoms exhibited by the aphasic are: reduction of available vocabulary, impaired verbal retention span, impaired perception of symbolic communiques, and impaired production of symbolic communiques.

DISORDERS OF INSTANTIATION

Fairbanks (1954) has described a communication model as a servosystem in which part of the output is returned to the place of input for purposes of comparison and control. Something akin to this is what we envision as the major dual functions of the planner–interpreter component. The dual functions of this component are, first, that of *selecting* and *coordinating* commands for synergisms which are then *assembled* and *enacted* by the two subordinate components, respectively, and, second, *monitoring* the enacted communique through feedback control and using the interpreted results to *modify* the planning, assembly, and enactment of later portions of the communique.

The production of communiques is the result of many converging processes under the control of a multiply determined intentional proposition. The intentional proposition can be considered a plan which evolves as it passes from the higher-order components, through the lower-order ones, into ever finer-grained means–end analysis. Finally it emerges as a sufficiently differentiated command signal, which triggers an assembly of appropriately organized effector synergisms, which finally make it a public enactment.

Comprehension of the proposition afforded by a perceived communique is no less complex than production. It is presumed that perception of a communique involves the activity of appropriate receptor synergisms. These synergisms achieve an analysis of the lower-order phonic, graphic, or action structures available in the communique. The resultant analyzer signal patterns are assimilated by interpreter plans which satisfy certain means–end analyses in an appropriate cognitive mode. The means–end analysis pattern is presumed to be a propositional form which agrees in intent with some propositional form the person himself might have formulated. For this reason no person can truly understand a communique which expresses a proposition foreign to him.

It is no wonder that a faulty command signal due to a dysfunction of any single component may have multiple effects throughout the whole system. Undoubtedly, because of these elaborate patterns of interaction among so many diverse components, the symptoms usually exhibited by aphasics are a mixture of primary and secondary symptoms, accompanied by those due to a variety of complicating conditions such as visual, auditory, or sensorimotor impairments.

We will now proceed to discuss the impairments in instantiation. Dysfunctions of these components obviously affect the enactment of propositions, on the one hand, and the decoding of propositions, on the other. Deficits here provide the complicating symptoms that we wish to separate from the primary symptoms of aphasia. In addition, as we will see later, these complicating symptoms have real importance for the classification of aphasic patients, as well as implications for treatment and prognosis.

Disorders of the planner–interpreter.

As we have already remarked, accurate speech production requires extremely high reliability of the central nervous system. In a single minute of discourse as many as 10,000 to 15,000 neuromuscular events must be enacted with appropriate continuous control of the manner and precision of articulation. Because at least part of that control may be exercised through feedback from the speech signal, we have chosen to combine the planner and interpreter functions. A disorder of this function, then, should show itself in joint disorders of both speech production and speech reception. We have called this a *sensorimotor* involvement. As we will see later, this involvement tends to correlate with the severity of the accompanying aphasia, as well as with indices of severity of neurological involvement.

Patients with disorders of the planner–interpreter show articulation errors as a function of the complexity of the productions required and as a function of the length of the utterance to be produced. They fail to correct their utterances by ear and show a loss of auditory discrimination of speech sounds. In reception as in production, they perform better on short units than on long or complicated ones.

Disorders of effector synergisms.

Impairment at this level differs from the impairment described above in that it is not necessarily accompanied by impairment of auditory discrimination, and the patient shows considerable ability to correct his errors by ear. The kinds of production errors are also characteristically different. The production is not due to failure to produce phonemes; the patient's problem seems to lie in the appropriate initiation of the correct bundle of synergisms. Thus, he may substitute unrelated phonemes for the one desired and is likely to articulate more difficult productions for simpler ones, as well as the reverse.

This disorder appears to us to be similar to what Alajouanine *et al.* (1939) called "phonetic disintegration," Bay (1962) called "cortical dysarthria," and Nathan (1947) called "apraxic dysarthria." In a study of what we think to be the same disorder, Shankweiler and Harris (1966) write:

> Phonetic disintegration can occur in combination with widespread disorders of expression or, less frequently, in remarkably "pure" form. In the latter case, in spite of difficulties in emitting speech sounds, expressive abilities (e.g., as shown in writing) may be well preserved, indicating

continued access to vocabulary and continued adherence to the rules of syntax. Thus, speech may be selectively impaired at the phonetic level.

The patients they studied made highly variable errors which had little relation to the similarity of phonemes. They made most errors in initial position on monosyllables and most errors on difficult consonants (fricatives) and consonant clusters. The errors their patients made indicated that they had difficulty in coordinated sequencing of the several articulators and that they frequently produced unintended phonemes differing in both manner and place from the target phoneme.

We suspect that patients with this symptom cannot utilize (or are not receiving) proprioceptive feedback. Such a patient often does not know where his tongue is in his mouth and tends to control his productions by false starts that he can monitor by ear. In listening to aphasic patients who demonstrate this kind of symptomatology, we have been impressed with the degree to which their speech resembles the speech of subjects who have been orally anesthetized (Gammon et al., 1971; Scott and Ringel, 1971).

Disorders of the effectors.

It is well known that disorders of the effectors form a large family of overlapping disturbances in the production of speech. It is also well known that such disorders are relatively independent of aphasia. Darley, et al. (1969) have given a clear and concise definition of this class of disorders:

> Dysarthria is a collective name for the group of speech disorders resulting from disturbances in muscular control over the speech mechanism due to damage of the central or peripheral nervous system. It designates problems in oral communication due to paralysis, weakness or incoordination of the speech musculature. It differentiates such problems from disorders of higher centers related to faulty programming of movements and sequences of movements (apraxia of speech) and to the inefficient processing of linguistic units (aphasia). (p. 246) [It encompasses] . . . coexisting motor disorders of respiration, phonation, articulation, resonance and prosody (those variations in time, pitch and loudness that summate to produce emphasis and interest in speech) . . . (p. 247)

Darley et al. have related the various aspects of dysarthric symptoms to particular disorders of the nervous system and have further performed a cluster analysis of the kinds of disturbances that appear together both within and across disease entities.

Disorders of receptor synergisms.

Little is known about disorders of central auditory processes. It is clear, however, that a patient with essentially normal hearing, as evaluated by pure tone audiometry, may fail simple auditory discrimination tasks when speech stimuli are employed. In aphasic patients we have seen a phenomenon that we have called *intermittent auditory imperception*. These patients were sometimes referred to the clinic as deaf even when testing revealed no hearing loss. Usually, repeated or redundant messages can eventually be perceived, and generally such utterances are better understood than single words or short units that are not redundant. Sometimes slowing the rate of the message helps.

Some patients report recognizing speech patterns as familiar word patterns that they should comprehend, but say that the words all seem to run together. The same patient may not exhibit difficulty in using those words at another time in spontaneously produced sentences.

We assume that a comprehensible pattern is not being delivered to the planner–interpreter. These patients could sometimes match printed words to pictures but still made errors matching printed words to spoken words. Yet, in general, they had difficulty in reading and writing even single words. Luria (1966) has suggested a tapping pattern repetition task which we sometimes used with these patients. Ordinarily they found it quite difficult. It would be interesting to know whether these patients have trouble discriminating musical compositions, rhythms, and other nonspeech sound patterns. Unfortunately, we have no such data.

Disorders of receptors.

Here, of course, we would place the communication disorders that flow in an obvious fashion from deafness, blindness, and all other impairment of the sensory systems that convey information to the higher levels for analysis.

Comment.

It must be obvious that some of our distinctions are speculative and weak. To the best of our knowledge, for example, no one knows, or even has any very good guesses about, the boundaries between the sensory organs and the perceptual analyzing systems that yield information about the world to the normal individual. In the case we are considering here, the problem is confounded by the problems of intermodality transfer. At some point (or points) the written symbols for language must make contact with the phonetic system which we believe must be primary and basic for language. We do not know how this is accomplished. It is similarly a problem to give a detailed account of writing and its simultaneous dependence on the visual, motor, and language systems. It is likewise a problem to say how information is transferred between the symbolic and figural systems and the extent to which information can be multiply coded in each, etc.

Clearly the schema we have presented is just the very beginning. It does give us a way to discuss what we know and a framework in which to consider the evidence from the various disciplines; but, importantly, it also points up the severe limits of our information and indicates the great need we have for further systematic study of communication disorders.

APHASIA: A COALITION OF SYMPTOMS

In the final section of this chapter, we wish to characterize aphasia as the clinician is most apt to encounter it, namely, as a complex coalition of symptoms. Some of the symptoms of the patient are directly due to the patient's aphasia. Others are a result of complicating conditions that affect the communication processes independent of the aphasia itself. Still others are due to a host of variables such as how the patient is reacting to his disorders and what he has learned to do to cope with his problems.

THE PRIMARY SYMPTOMS OF APHASIA

As we argued earlier, we believe that the primary symptoms of aphasia are due to an impairment of the ability to formulate psychological propositions in the symbolic mode. This means that the aphasic patient will show deficits both in perceiving and in producing symbolic communiques. The observed communication deficit is not modality specific and exhibits a rather impressive regularity of symptomatic errors. This regularity is shown both in the kinds of errors that occur and in the level of impairment observed. There is inconsistency of individual responses, but kinds of errors and percentage of errors on given tasks remain remarkably stable from day to day, and from week to week. Improvement, when it occurs, is orderly and predictable.

Two prominent primary symptoms consistently observed in all aphasics are a reduction of available vocabulary and an impaired verbal retention span. Qualitatively speaking, these symptoms consist of errors that nonaphasic speakers make under conditions of fatigue, duress, or inattention. Aphasics in general make the same kinds of errors, but with far greater frequency. In other words, there seems to be evidence that the same cognitive system is involved but is working with much less efficiency.

Difficulty in perceiving and structuring verbal propositions seems dependent on both the ability to retrieve the required vocabulary from the symbolic mode and the ability to retain simultaneously the lexical items retrieved in some kind of store until they can be wedded into a well-formed proposition. However, this process of synthesis must satisfy the whole descriptor index if the proposition is to be properly formulated.

The values for descriptor index in turn must satisfy the matrix of intent laid down by the executive control component. In this sense, then, the verbal retrieval and retention mechanisms seem dependent on the control of the executor of intent. It is because of the mutual interdependence of these subprocesses supporting the formulation of symbolic propositions that we are led to characterize the primary symptoms of aphasia as a coalition rather than a hierarchy or aggregate of symptoms.

In this decision we find ourselves in substantial agreement with Brain (1961) when he argues that the "two factors in meaning, which we may call the syntactical and semantic, must be very intimately related at the physiological level, because the serial order of words and their syntactical relationships influence their meaning, and, conversely, meaning is reflected in serial order and syntax." To separate these aspects of language into distinct levels would be extremely arbitrary.

If we consider how language must be learned, we must come to the same conclusion that language processing is indivisible. The discrete elements and the rules of the code are both mediated through the auditory channel. The child at one and the same time is learning phonology, morphology, syntax, and semantics in all of their functional interdependence. There is surely no basis for postulating unrelated mechanisms for learning elements and learning combinatorial rules at separate levels. The complex interaction between meaning and structure and their simultaneous acquisition would lead one to predict a high correlation between retrieval of words and retrieval of rules in aphasia at all levels of severity, and this seems to be the case. It follows that the dichotomy assumed in categorizing aphasia as amnesic versus syntactical, or grammatic versus agrammatic, is artificial.

This kind of categorization implies that aphasic subjects who have difficulty finding words operate with the rules for combining words intact. Conversely, it implies that aphasic subjects who have difficulty combining words do not have difficulty finding them. It is possible that this dichotomy reflects the old error of observing only the most obvious symptoms, symptoms that fit some a priori assumption, or symptoms prominent at one point in time.

When an "amnesic" patient, asked what you pound with, replies, "You pound with —we know that thing—what it is. We have him back down there—we go down there —the pound bench," it is obvious he could not readily retrieve the word hammer. Presumably he is trying to tell us he knows what you pound with, and that he has a hammer downstairs on his workbench. Isn't it obvious that he is also having a little trouble discriminating gender of pronouns, and structuring and sequencing a message, as well as, or perhaps because of, trouble finding words?

On the other hand, when a "syntactical" patient, asked what he did today, responds, "Eat—doctor—go—I can't say it—you know?—haircut," it is obvious that he has difficulty generating sentences. It may be less obvious that he can't think of the word *breakfast*, his doctor's name, or a label for *barber shop*, that his retrievable vocabulary is confined to common words of high immediate utility, and that he uses common grammatical combinations on occasion.

The following are three protocols of an aphasic subject who had no speech 3 weeks after onset of aphasia, but gradually began to recover language. The first was recorded 5 months, the second 10 months, and the third 11 months after occlusion of the left middle cerebral artery.

1. Picture description, January 16, 1962 (5 months)

   This. This. Kite. God (dog), Bailbox. House. Vone (smoke). Timming (chimney). Gor (door). Windows. A. Smith (name on mailbox). Dog. Tree. Dills (hills).

2. Retelling paragraph, June 14, 1962 (10 months)

   The park—Yell Park—Yellowstone Park in Wyoming. The pots are on the rock bubbling over. Bright red, blue, and white are the—bubbling over. Bubble over, red, blue, orange— (Clinician: What did you see when you were in Yellowstone?) Old Faithful. (Clinician: Tell me about Old Faithful.) Goes off every hour. 40 feet—under 40 feet. (Clinician: Did you see any animals?) Bears, elk, bears, goats, chipmunks, squirrels. (Clinician: Tell me about the bears.) The bears come up to the car. (Clinician: What for?) Rob, eat. (Clinician: Did you feed them?) No, no, no. Dangerous. (Clinician: Why?) Because you can't tell what might happen. (Clinician: What might happen?) The bear is—shakes the children.

3. Picture description, July 13, 1962 (11 months)

   The children being led by the boat. Two carrying the boat. The oars are carried. The boat —a string attached to it—a rope. The field—corn—grain—a field of grain. The girl has on tennis shoes. The boy has on a straw hat—cap. Two houses are visible. Two houses across the bay. The dock is floating. The rock was across the bay. By the rock is—sticking up. Two boys are in the boat. A mast—the boat has a mast. Two children is following the boat. The car is a Ford. Two pines. The weather is fall. They dock the boats.

These protocols are presented in support of the previous statement that there is a relatively high correlation between retrieval of words and retrieval of rules at various levels of severity of aphasia. As available vocabulary increases, the beginnings of structure appear. The percentage of well-structured responses increases slowly but steadily, although impairment of vocabulary as well as impairment of structural usage continues to be evident. This is illustrated in the last sentence of protocol 2, where a structural break occurred when the patient could not retrieve the word he wanted, and substituted an example accompanied by a vivid gesture. We suggest that loss of structural forms represents a more severe disruption of language processes than difficulty finding words, which occurs in normal speakers and in mild as well as in severe aphasia.

Zipf (1935) pointed out that naming is more than an imitative process and that it involves continuous categorization of experiential data. For example, *"bow-wow* 'animal' may be split into *bow-wow* 'small animal,' and *moo-cow* 'large animal'; *bow-wow* 'small animal' is later split into *bow-wow* 'small quadruped' and *kluck-kluck* 'bird.' " Thus the semantic as well as the syntactical aspects of language involve abstraction, generalization, and learning of rules. A single word may in fact represent an extremely complex category of experience.

The point at which we have most often been challenged, however, is in the insistence that the language deficit in aphasia is "all of one piece." Defense of this view against the older compartmentalized theories is called for again and again. We did not begin with this position, but arrived at it by consideration of the data that we collected. As we came to know better what we were looking for, we saw that the language deficit that we observed across patients differing in severity of aphasia could also be seen in a single uncomplicated case as the patient regained "access" to his previous linguistic competence.

As we have argued earlier, there is no easy way to "prove" the hypothesis of a unitary dimension of language deficit. Rather, it is a strong inference from data from a wide variety of observations and many different kinds of experiments. In our case, the network of evidence began to grow when Schuell (1950) made a careful study of the errors of aphasic patients and discovered that the vast majority of them were identical with responses made by normal speakers when they are asked on a word association test to "respond with the first word this makes you think of." The patient trying to identify a table calls it a "chair"—the same response a normal speaker makes to the word "table" on the free association test. Furthermore, these same kinds of errors are made when the aphasic is trying to read the word "table," name a picture of a table, write the word "table," or tell you what his plate sits on when he eats dinner. Nor is it just that this particular word is unavailable to him. When asked a few moments later to name a chair, the patient is highly likely to call it "table" as he searches for the correct word.

Two salient aspects of these findings impressed us. First, the aphasic still had (in some form) the semantic and grammatical relations that must be supposed to account for the normal speaker's behavior on the association test. Second, the form of error and the patient's difficulties extended across the traditional modalities of input and output and the several sensory or motor systems involved.

As our comprehensive test battery developed and we had an opportunity to see the patients behave in a wide variety of situations, we came to recognize that each specific task involved a mixture of skills and knowledge and made different demands on the sensory and motor systems, as well as on the extent to which the symbolic system was involved. In general, however (Schuell, 1953), it became apparent that level of the patient's comprehension of spoken and written language paralleled his level of effectiveness in formulating speech and writing.

By 1959 (Schuell and Jenkins) we had enough data on our major categories of patients to attempt a statistical test of the hypothesis of a single major dimension of language deficit. The hypothesis was not original with us, of course, since the major studies of Head (1926), Weisenburg and McBride (1935), and Wepman (1951) had already implied a relatedness among the seemingly different aspects of language by failing to find the isolated disorders postulated in the old literature. Ours was the first attempt to perform an explicit psychometric test of the hypothesis, however.

The study employed the Guttman scaling technique (1950) to examine the scores of 100 patients on 18 tests from the aphasia battery. The patients were consecutive admissions to the aphasia clinic. The tests were selected as tests that involved the symbolic domain but that varied widely across the modalities of presentation, materials required, and responses needed (for example, pointing to objects and letters, following directions, listening to sentences and paragraphs and answering questions, matching printed words with pictures, repeating words, naming months of the year, naming objects and pictures, answering questions, giving biographical information, rhyming, telling three things the patient had done that day, describing a pictured situation, stating similarities between words, and writing letters and sentences to dictation).

The tests turned out to be scalable. This simply means that when we arranged subjects in order of severity of aphasia (defined by number of tests passed) and arranged the tests in order of difficulty (defined by the number of subjects passing each test), we formed a matrix that was highly predictable from one axis to the other. That is, if one knew how many tests a patient passed, it was possible to say which they were. Conversely, if one knew what proportion of patients failed a test, it was possible to say which patients they were with high accuracy. Such scalability is usually considered as evidence of a single hierarchy in the universe being explored, in this case, aphasic language behavior.

In other words, we identified a continuum of language deficit that crossed all the usual language modalities and was present in patients who showed simple aphasic impairment, as well as in patients who had additional problems that interferred with communication. This scale was found to apply adequately to an independent sample of 23 patients not included in the original analysis. Later Jenkins and Schuell (1964) demonstrated that the scale applied satisfactorily to a sample of 157 patients used in the next study reported below.

A different statistical technique was employed by Schuell et al. (1962) in a factor analysis of the Minnesota battery. The sample consisted of 157 aphasic patients. Here, the intercorrelations of 69 tests were examined by several factor analytic techniques in an attempt to discover the major dimensions which could account for the pattern of relationships. Five major factors were identified:

Factor 1. Language behavior

Factor 2. Visual discrimination, recognition, and recall

Factor 3. Visuospatial behavior

Factor 4. Gross movements of the speech musculature

Factor 5. Recognition of stimulus equivalence

Because of the general importance of the results, a complete table of the factor loadings for all the tests in the battery is given in Appendix 2, Table 1.

Factor 1 clearly represented a general dimension of language behavior that crossed all language modalities. Of the 69 tests, 45 had meaningful loadings on this factor, and it accounted for 41% of the estimated common factor variance. The tests used in the previous scaling study had very high loadings on the first factor (median loading 0.83) and, in general, only small loadings on the other factors.

Tests from every section of the test battery were heavily dependent on this primary factor. Tests for speech and language, auditory comprehension tests, visual and reading tests, visuomotor and writing tests, numerical tests, and tests that involved naming or recognition of body parts were all represented with substantial loadings. In short, when a test involved comprehension, retention, or manipulation of symbols, it appeared on this factor regardless of its surface form or its input or output modality.

The tests that did *not* appear on this factor were also informative. Exclusively visual tests, such as matching forms and matching letters, did not appear. Neither did tests which involved copying forms and pictures or drawing a man or assembling a mannequin. Tests which involved the gross movements of the speech apparatus (phonation, movements of the tongue, jaw, palate, and pharynx) did not load appreciably on this factor. This latter finding, of course, substantiates the view that impairment of the speech musculature is not an essential component of reduction of language in aphasia.

Factor 2 involved visual discrimination and recognition and recall of learned visual patterns. It was moderately correlated with Factor 1 and was interpreted as reflecting the integration of learned visual discriminations and previously acquired language patterns. Both reading and writing tests had high loadings on Factor 2. We found no evidence for "pure alexia" or "pure agraphia" existing independently of language.

Factor 3 was interpreted as a visuospatial factor, dependent on proprioceptive as well as visual information. Tests with high loadings on Factor 3 included all matching, copying, drawing, and object assembly tasks in the battery.

Factor 4 involved gross movements of the speech musculature. It is related to paralysis or paresis of these structures, and does not correlate with overall language deficit.

Factor 5 was the most weakly determined of our factors, but we consider it to involve recognition of stimulus equivalence. Tests included on this factor involved matching letters and forms, matching printed words to pictures, matching spoken words to pictures, and explaining proverbs. Our best guess at this time is that bilateral neurological damage is implicated, but the data are far too fragile to warrant much interpretation.

All in all, the factor analysis served to confirm our view that the core of aphasia was a deficit in symbolic processing that extended over vocabulary, auditory retention span, and ability to deal with language formulations at various levels of complexity in all the modalities tested. Further findings by other investigators and ourselves have continued to strengthen our conviction.

At the time of this writing we have just received a brief report from our Japanese colleagues concerning a factor analysis for a group of aphasic patients similar to our sample. Sasanuma administered the Schuell–Sasanuma Differential Diagnostic Test of Aphasia, Form 2, to 269 consecutively admitted aphasic patients at a large rehabilitation center. Scores of 68 subtests were used as the basis for factor analysis. Ten principle axes accounted for 95.5 % of the common factor variance. Orthogonal rotation resulted in the following factors:

Factor 1. Language behavior

Factor 2. Visuospatial and/or visuomotor processes

Factor 3. Programming of articulatory movements

Factor 4. Auditory discrimination and recognition

Factor 5. Movements of the speech musculature

It should be noted that the findings reinforce important interpretations made above. First, the most salient factor is again the general language factor. Second, the visuospatial factor and the factor dealing with gross movements of the speech musculature are both confirmed and found to be relatively independent of the language factor. Our earlier Factor 2 was not confirmed (reading and writing), but it is not clear whether this is due to differences in the subject population or due to the fact that two very different orthographies are available to the Japanese patient, one a *syllabary* and the other a *logographic* system, while Americans have a single *alphabetic* system. The Japanese Factors 3 and 4 (programming articulatory movements and auditory discrimination) were missing from our analysis (presumably swallowed up in the general language factor). The factors are welcome additions, however, and fit appropriately with the classification system we will present later.

Reduction of vocabulary is the most adequately studied aspect of language deficit. In normal adults, it is well known that the ability to read a word on short exposure or to hear it correctly in the midst of noise is a function of the frequency of usage of that word. Highly frequent words are most easily read and heard, and infrequent or rare words are the most difficult. In parallel fashion, the reduction of vocabulary in aphasia is a function of frequency of word usage. Frequent words are most likely to be available to the aphasic, and rare words are least likely to be understood or employed. Wepman, *et al.* (1956) first confirmed this phenomenon. Howes and Geschwind (1960) showed it to be true of the free speech of aphasics. Schuell *et al.* (1961) found the relationship in auditory-word-to-picture matching, and Bricker *et al.* (1964) demonstrated the same relationship in written spelling to dictation.

Finally, in a study that takes this section to full cycle, Schuell and Jenkins (1961) studied the reduction in vocabulary and the errors made by aphasic patients in a variety of tasks. These tasks were specially designed where necessary to make the form of the errors clear. In pointing to pictures, for example, cards were constructed which displayed: (1) the desired test object, (2) an object whose name rhymed with the test word, (3) an object associated with the test word (as determined from the Russell and Jenkins, 1954, norms for word association), and (4) an unrelated object. An example is a card containing the four pictures: chair, stair, table, and apple. When a test word was spoken, the subject had an opportunity to show a correct response, a phonetic error, an associative error, or a random error. With phonetic stimulus alone, 59% of the patients' errors were association errors, 21% were phonetic errors, 10% were unrelated words, and 10% were "don't know" responses. The percentage of associative errors was negatively related to overall errors; that is, if a patient made only one error, it was certain to be an associative error. As he made more and more errors, first phonetic errors increased, and then, finally, his errors were evenly distributed across all types.

The same patterns of errors were found in naming pictures, reading printed words, and writing to dictation. We concluded that as precision of vocabulary breaks down in aphasia, the symbolic association processes still intact serve to mediate the errors that appear. At more severe levels of vocabulary deficit, these processes become faulty, and errors of more remote origin appear. At the most severe levels of deficit, the errors become even more irrelevant, finally becoming random or "no response" errors.

Another aspect of language deficit on which we have extensive data is auditory retention span. While we have published no special analyses of this phenomenon, it is apparent from the test data themselves that reduction of span is a pervasive characteristic of aphasia. Repetition of sentences, repetition of digits, pointing to items named serially, following directions, and writing sentences to dictation all rely on retention span. All these tests show parallel limitations in a patient and vary directly across patients with the severity of the overall language deficit. And as in the case of vocabulary, improvement in span in the case of the individual patient is an important concomitant of the recovery process.

SECONDARY SYMPTOMS OF APHASIA

Secondary symptoms are due to disturbances of language-related processes that occur as reactions to the primary symptoms of aphasia. For instance, the moderately impaired aphasic patient may develop a pathological retardation of the intent to speak due to depression over his inability to continue the pursuit of his chosen profession, or due to the disruption of his life with his family. Such reduction of intent to speak usually passes as a result of supportive therapy.

Another secondary symptom of aphasia may be manifested as a change in attitude toward communication. The aphasic patient may fail to function cognitively at the maximum level his competence actually allows, due to the lack of communication demanded by the clinical environment. The patient may find that his new circumstance neither requires, permits, or socially rewards his attempts to communicate. He finds himself in a caretaker environment which both understands and anticipates his needs and whose routinized social patterns preclude most of the natural, day-by-day requirements and opportunities for spontaneous verbal interaction with family, co-workers, and peers. To the extent that such conditions prevail, or the patient perceives them as prevailing, his competence for communication may appear more impaired than it actually is.

COMPLICATING CONDITIONS IN APHASIA

Specific auditory impairment.

Probably because of the great dependence of language on the auditory system, there is almost always demonstrable impairment of auditory processes in aphasia. Even subjects with mild aphasia usually show initial loss of auditory discrimination on tasks such as pointing to letters of the alphabet named in random order, tending to confuse letters whose names sound alike, such as *bcdegptvz*, or *ahjk*, or *iy*. They also show reduction of auditory retention span observable on repetition of digits, and on sentences containing series of words or phrases, such as "Benjamin Franklin was a printer, an editor, and an inventor." Patients with moderate aphasia usually have difficulty in rhyming or associating by sound, as do children who are partially deaf.

Some aphasic patients show more severe and persisting auditory impairment than others. Instead of being able to correct a defective response readily by ear, they require many stimulations to be able to repeat a common word. Sometimes it is necessary to increase intensity, reduce rate, or use combined auditory and visual stimulation to enable the patient to repeat. Auditory retention span is often reduced to two or three digits, or to meaningful units of three or four words. With intensive auditory stimulation there is slow, gradual improvement.

A small percentage of aphasic patients show such severe auditory impairment that they are sometimes considered deaf, although it can be demonstrated that they hear. This condition usually improves. Patients begin to respond to parts of messages, then to perceive short messages in entirety. However, there continue to be occasions when the patient fails to perceive a common word. He may or may not recognize the word when it is repeated several times. When recognition occurs it appears to be an all-or-none event. The patient is completely bewildered or responds unhesitatingly, unlike patients who vacillate between a knife and a fork, or a lock and key, and make a tentative response. Patients with severe auditory impairment often have persisting difficulty discriminating between words such as *fish* and *dish*, *rake* and *lake*, *lock* and *clock*, *rain* and *train*, and so on, and in responding to long messages.

Specific visual impairment.

Although all aphasic patients have difficulty in reading and writing because language is not intact, some aphasic patients, and not others, show persisting impairment of visual discrimination. These patients tend to confuse letters with similar visual configurations, such as *E–F, C–G, J–L, A–N–H, M–W,* and *B–P–R* in upper case type; *b–d–p–q, h–n–r–u, f–t, w–m,* and *m–n,* in lower case type, and *f–b, h–k, g–q, y–j,* and u–w in script. Such confusions appear in both reading and writing. The patient may read or write *dark* for *park*, *match* for *watch*, *house* for *horse*, *store* for *stone*, and so on. Patients frequently perceive the beginning of a word and guess at the ending. *Housewife* may be read as *household*, *blackboard* as *blackbird*, or *Minneapolis* as *Minnesota*. In writing, reversals and distortions of letter forms occur. There is special difficulty with double letters and silent letters to which sound offers no clue. Patients frequently spell words aloud correctly, but make errors in writing them, and oral spelling generally exceeds written.

When visual impairment is severe, matching, copying, and drawing are also defective. Sometimes all letter forms have to be relearned individually before reading and writing are possible. Impaired discrimination and recall of learned visual forms may or may not be combined with impaired spatial discrimination.

Specific sensorimotor impairment.

Some aphasic patients, and not others, have persisting difficulty performing the intricate and rapid sequences of movements required for normal speech. They sometimes seem not to know where the tongue is in the mouth, or how to move it in a given direction or to a given position. One of the phenomena of such impairment is confusion of phonemes with similar articulatory characteristics, such as *p–b–m, t–d–n–l, k–g, r–l*, and *f–v*. This impairment is sometimes difficult to observe, because it may be obscured initially by grosser impairment, and by impaired recall of auditory patterns. Usually the gross errors disappear first, then this striking pattern characteristic of sensorimotor deficit is revealed, until it, in turn, begins to give way to normal articulation, at least of common words and phrases.

That sensorimotor impairment is secondary to reduced proprioceptive and auditory discrimination is demonstrated by the fact that the same kinds of errors appear when patients are asked to point to letters or words named by the examiner and to write letters or words to dictation, as well as when they are asked to read aloud, repeat, or produce words beginning with a given sound.

Specific articulatory impairment.

Sometimes, with aphasia, there is demonstrable paralysis or paresis of some of the speech musculature, although this is relatively infrequent. Mild general weakness results in slurred speech, characterized by loss of precise movements and firm contacts. Marked weakness of the tongue or palate each produces a recognizable pattern of articulatory impairment. Sometimes there is a reduction of kinesthetic or proprioceptive feedback (without reduction of auditory feedback) which is characterized by placement errors of articulatory movements. These inconsistent errors can be corrected by ear, which results in a pattern somewhat like primary stuttering. These deficits do not correlate with the amount of language reduction present and should be considered dysarthria or dysfluency rather than aphasia, since they may exist when no aphasic disorders are present.

Perhaps at this point it would be helpful to specify some of the things we think aphasia is not. It is not loss of memory for recent or past events. It is not even loss of memory for words. As Hughlings Jackson pointed out, aphasic patients have words, and most good clinicians know tricks to elicit them. The patient, however, cannot retrieve his words readily to serve him in communication. Good clinicians know, too, that they do not teach the aphasic patient words, although they use words (and phrases and sentences) to stimulate language processes. If the clinician is successful, what comes out is happily more than he put in.

Finally, aphasia is not general confusion, disorientation, instability, or psychosis. When these manifestations are present, one is dealing with more than aphasia, and with deterioration that includes more than the language system. Most aphasic patients are reasonable, responsive, and well-oriented. They are stable, highly motivated, able to work persistently and hard, and to withstand more than ordinary amounts of frustration and discouragement in a manner that commands respect and admiration.

part three

DIAGNOSIS AND PROGNOSIS

chapter 7

THE RESEARCH PROGRAM AND
THE PATIENTS

THE EVOLUTION OF A TEST BATTERY

Schuell constructed Form I of the Minnesota Test in April, 1948 (Brown and Schuell, 1950). She knew that she needed uniform test procedures in order to compare performances between patients and performances of the same patients from one time to another. She hoped to find out which symptoms were reversible and which were not, and what changed in relation to what. For this, a comprehensive battery of tests graduated in difficulty was needed.

She asked what she could observe in the behavior of aphasic patients that distinguished them from nonaphasics. The obvious thing that was different was language behavior. The next question was what could be observed about language behavior.

It is possible to observe when subjects understand or fail to understand spoken language under controlled conditions. It is possible to observe similar behavior with reading materials. It is possible to make observations about the way people talk, the way they write, and about their ability to manipulate other common symbol systems such as numbers. Some of this behavior can be evaluated by conventional achievement-type tests.

Schuell asked, also, to what extent aphasic and nonaphasic subjects differed in nonverbal behavior. To answer this she explored responses to various kinds of perfor-

113

mance tests, such as the Goldstein—Scheerer Color–Form and Stick Tests, block-tapping, block-design, object-assembly tests, Raven's Progressive Matrices, the Bender Gestalt, and other projective tests.

The third question asked was why aphasic subjects could not perform specific tasks, when they could not. The procedure here was to observe the behavior in question until she was able to make some sort of hypothesis about what was operating and then to construct tests to evaluate the hypothesis.

Schuell continued to use new tests experimentally, tabulating and studying responses obtained from both aphasic and nonaphasic subjects. For example, she wondered if patients failed to identify body parts because of the somatic or because of the part–whole relationship, and added a test requiring identification of parts of a bicycle. She found no evidence of specific difficulty with parts of objects. On all recognition and naming tests errors increased when less common words were used. She found occasional patients, however, who showed evidence of impaired perception of body schema.

To test the concept of *anomia,* and the inference that aphasic patients have more difficulty recalling nouns than other parts of speech, Schuell constructed a test requiring various parts of speech in response to simple questions, such as *What do you shave with? What do you do with a razor?* Patients who answered the first question with a statement such as, "I have it back there," usually said something like, "Well, on your face," in response to the latter. She concluded the difficulty lay in producing a specific rather than a general response, regardless of grammatical form.

Patients responded better to some tests than to others. They tended not to like unusual tasks, such as those involving nonsense syllables, for example, and generally responded negatively to them. On other tests, responses tended to be equivocal and uninformative. Sometimes Schuell could revise test items or test instructions to secure less ambiguous responses. When she could not, she dropped the tests.

Schuell used pass–fail scoring whenever possible. When qualitative judgments were necessary, she collected responses made by a diversified group of patients, analyzed and rated them, and established empirical scoring criteria.

At the end of each year Schuell tabulated and studied the test score distributions, and revised the test battery. In general she revised to simplify administration and instructions, to eliminate tests that were duplicated by other tests or seemed not to yield meaningful information, and to add other tests that might be useful or promising.

Eventually Schuell eliminated most performance tests, because, although they discriminated between brain-injured populations and those without brain injuries, they either contributed little to our knowledge of aphasia, or gave the same kind of information as other tests. Some tests tended to be failed initially, but passed on retest when patients were better able to grasp and retain instructions. This was particularly true of many of the tests for "abstract attitude."

In 1954, the test battery was administered to a population of 40 hospitalized patients with no history of neurological involvement. While nonaphasics made scattered inconsistent errors, there was only one record that resembled an aphasic pattern. This was the test of an older patient. Obviously, any population including 50- and 60-year-old subjects might contain individuals with previously undetected brain damage, resulting from arteriosclerotic changes, subclinical strokes, or other causes. Resultant mental changes were often interpreted as forgetfulness, and attributed to age rather than to brain damage. These patients showed mild aphasia, as well as other mild neurophysiological symptoms.

In 1955, Schuell completed the sixth overall revision of the test, and made it available to hospitals and universities for experimental use. The 1955 research edition, form 6, was used for material in the first edition of this book.

PARAPHASIC RESPONSES

Schuell recorded all the paraphasic responses, word changes, and word substitutions patients made on naming and reading tasks during treatment periods. She was struck by the similarity of these responses to those normals produced on word association tests. In general the word-finding errors of aphasic patients fell into the categories of word associations defined by Jung (Schuell, 1950). This is the first clearcut indication we had that the language behavior of aphasic patients, bizarre as individual responses sometimes appeared, was predictable and orderly and related to general laws governing language behavior.

IMPAIRMENT OF AUDITORY COMPREHENSION

Another early observation was that there appeared to be a relationship between difficulty understanding spoken language and available speech. Schuell tried to document this, to see if the evidence supported the clinical impression (Schuell, 1953). She had test and retest records for 138 aphasic patients who had been studied throughout a period of treatment. Using preestablished criteria, the clinic staff divided the subjects into four groups determined by the amount of speech present at discharge. The groups were essentially as follows:

Group A, excellent speech (35 patients), defined as ability to discuss previous interests, without obvious impairment.

Group B, good speech (47 patients), defined as speech that usually sounded normal in everyday situations, but broke down when subjects tried to express long or complicated ideas.

Group C, limited speech (25 patients), defined as ability to communicate needs and wishes through intelligible but limited or defective speech.

Group D, no functional speech (31 patients), defined as inability to express needs and wishes voluntarily, although some kinds of language responses occurred.

Schuell tabulated errors on tests for auditory comprehension on initial examinations. All subjects made errors on tests ordinarily passed by nonaphasics. More than twice as many subjects in Groups C and D as in Groups A and B made errors on all tests except one. This was the most difficult test, paragraph comprehension, on which 99 % of subjects made some errors.

The easiest test required pointing to common objects named by the examiner. No subjects in Groups A and B and only four subjects in Group C made any errors on this test. However, all 31 subjects in Group D failed some items. This meant that out of 107 aphasic patients with functional speech, less than 4 % made errors on this test. In contrast, 100% of subjects who regained no functional speech with intensive therapy failed some items. Thus Schuell had not only confirmed the original hypothesis but had also found a simple test with high predictive value.

She recorded the complete initial and final test scores of these 31 subjects. All of them had been considered neurologically stable at the time of initial examination. The data yielded a consistent picture of severe damage, amounting to almost complete loss of function in all language modalities on both initial and final testing. Thus the study led to identification of a test profile for which prognosis for recovery from aphasia was clearly negative.

It was puzzling to find patients who scored above the 90th percentile for normal adults on the Ammons (Ammons and Ammons, 1948) test for auditory recognition of words but made errors following simple directions. One day, however, Schuell found a patient who could not write sentences like *The grass is green*, or *We have a new car* to dictation, although spelling tested at Grade 6 level. On a hunch she repeated the sentences, but dictated them in two- or three- rather than four- or five-word units. This time the patient wrote the sentences easily and correctly.

This clearly pointed to a retention span difficulty. Schuell constructed tests to explore this probability. She found patients who could point to items in a picture when they were named singly, but not when they were named in series of two or three. Some patients could follow simple directions, but not two or three of the same directions combined. For patients who could talk, repetition of sentences equated for word frequency but progressive in length showed the same difficulty dramatically. The cutoff points were sharp. The same effect appeared on repetition of digits.

This turned out to be a highly reversible phenomenon. Moreover, performance tended to improve in all language modalities as retention span increased.

CLASSIFICATION OF PATIENTS

Schuell had studied several hundred patients before she began to see clearcut evidence of recurring patterns of impairment.

Error patterns can be dramatic. Not only does the same patient make the same kinds of errors every day over periods of weeks or months, but new patients come along and repeat the same errors day after day.

Schuell had identified the test pattern of severely impaired patients with no functional language skills in any modality. She had worked with these patients enough to know what happened with intensive treatment. She knew they could learn to repeat and to copy, to count, and to recite the alphabet, the days of the week, or even the Lord's Prayer, if someone started them. They learned to produce reactive responses to high strength associations or other strong stimuli. They could usually match simple printed words to pictures. But no matter how much practice she provided, language never became voluntary or functional in any modality.

The next time she analyzed test data she extracted the records of these patients and copied them on separate data sheets. She found the expected homogeneous set of error distributions. It seemed a good idea to contrast these with the records of patients who showed no gross visual or motor disturbances. The results looked highly consistent, in spite of differences in severity between subjects, and between initial and final tests. In general, patients in this group made no errors on easy tests, but errors increased in all modalities as length of stimuli or length of required responses increased.

There were other records that looked much the same on tests for auditory comprehension and tests for speech and language, but differed markedly on tests involving matching, copying, reading, and writing. She studied these profiles. The records clearly reflected aphasia with additional involvement of visual processes.

Next she looked for records that showed motor involvement without specific visual signs, and detached this group.

The remaining records showed evidence of both visual and motor impairment. This analysis identified a group of subjects previously not recognized as clinically homogeneous. All of them had some residual language in one modality or another. Some had severe motor impairment, but only mild visual involvement. Others showed only mild slurring of speech, but visual involvement was severe. One patient showed mild involvement of both processes.

When Schuell looked at the background data she found this was the most homogeneous of all the groups identified. There were only five patients in this first sample, but they were all over 60, they were all hypertensive, and all of them had had more than one cerebrovascular accident. Later we found that although these details differed in other subjects, the neurological findings were always compatible with scattered or generalized brain damage.

For several months the clinic staff reviewed all new test records, seeing the patients to verify the findings, and classifying them independently. Agreement was remarkably high.

The system made sense to the neurologists. The clinic had a file of test–retest records as well as clinical experience from which to determine prognosis. This enabled us to make predictions on completion of initial testing, if patients were neurologically stable. We included classification and prognosis in the initial case summaries, which were placed in the medical charts. The results began to be impressive, and we gradually acquired confidence in them.

We continued to work with severely impaired patients. We developed new techniques for intensive stimulation to try to penetrate the barrier that seems to exist between reactive responses, on the one hand, and voluntary control of language, on the other. The intensive methods produced accelerated results for patients in all the other categories, but we were forced to conclude that there is a level of language deficit at which functional recovery is not possible.

Further data, to be presented later, have confirmed the original patterns of deficit identified here and the prognoses attending these classifications. Additional patterns have been recognized from time to time, and two of them have appeared consistently enough that we have included them in our major categories (aphasia with persisting dysfluency and aphasia with intermittent auditory imperception). Other patterns have occurred rarely, at least in the population of some 1200 aphasic patients whom we have studied. In view of the infinite complexity of the brain, of cerebral processes in general, and language processes in particular, we consider it probable that aphasic patients will continue to be found who do not fit the major patterns of impairment identified. Any classification system would be suspect if this were not true. A simplification of complex behavior so gross as to be all-inclusive would have little clinical or theoretical value.

SUBJECTS AND METHODS

The best way to present diagnosis and prognosis is to consider data from patients we have examined and (for the most part) treated and followed for a substantial period of time. In the remainder of the chapter, therefore, we shall describe the patients who are the subjects of our study and the nonaphasic patients who agreed to be tested to provide matched controls. In addition we shall mention the kinds of data we collected and some general findings that define the patient population more precisely.

The date were derived from 157 aphasic and 50 nonaphasic subjects, tested on the 1955 research form of the Minnesota Test for the Differential Diagnosis of Aphasia, and 23 aphasic subjects tested on the 1965 published form of the examination. The first group of aphasics includes 155 patients admitted to the Minneapolis Veterans Administration Hospital between June 1955 and June 1958, and two patients examined by Dr. Schuell at Syracuse University through the courtesy of Dr. Louis M. di Carlo. (These two test records were added to increase the number of subjects in one diagnostic category.) The second group of aphasics was selected from admissions to the Minneapolis VA Hospital between June 1965 and January 1970. Unlike the first group, these do not consist of all admissions during the period, but rather were selected to illustrate the two diagnostic groups which were previously considered minor syndromes: Persisting Dysfluency and Intermittent Auditory Imperception.

PATIENTS EXCLUDED FROM THE STUDY

First, we excluded patients from the research series when extensive testing revealed no evidence of aphasia. Some had a history of transient aphasia. Others had suspected organic involvement or major hemisphere lesions. In addition, a few patients referred for problems not related to brain damage, such as stuttering present since childhood, a hearing loss of long duration, or a voice disorder were excluded.

Second, we excluded patients who were unresponsive to any test materials. Untestable patients were often acutely ill, and inability to respond appeared related to this factor. It was established clinical practice to request that these patients be referred again when overall physiological conditions improved. Death often intervened, which supported the initial impression.

Third, we excluded records of patients who were not neurologically stable, because we did not consider test results reliable.

Finally, we excluded patients with psychiatrically confirmed diagnoses of psychosis or regressive behavior, because test responses reflected more than aphasic impairment.

We studied patients in the last two categories, and treated them for aphasia when indicated, but did not include them in the research series.

TEST DATA

Patients were tested on the research edition and the published form of the Minnesota Test for Differential Diagnosis of Aphasia, which is described in the next chapter. Examiners were nine trained speech pathologists who were members of the clinical staff of the Aphasia Section of the Neurology Service during some period of the study. Subjects were assigned to clinicians in random order, determined by the size of individual case loads when a new patient was referred. Patients were classified in diagnostic categories on completion of testing, and findings were reviewed in staff conferences.

MEDICAL DATA

Patients received neurological examinations on admission to the Neurology Service. These findings were usually reviewed in medical conferences, and there was always a free interchange of information between speech pathologists and staff neurologists. We recorded the final diagnosis in every case.

THE TEST–RETEST SERIES

Retests on termination of treatment were available for 91 of the 178 Minneapolis subjects. This included all the patients in the series for whom two tests that met criteria were obtained. Loss of subjects resulted chiefly from the nature of the sample of aphasic subjects. The veterans population is aging, and about half of the Minneapolis patients were classified in diagnostic groups characterized by massive or generalized brain damage, often with a history of successive episodes or progressive changes. Since patients with massive brain damage tend not to respond to treatment for aphasia, and patients with generalized brain damage usually make only limited gains, most of these patients received only a short period of patient and family counseling or of therapy directed towards limited goals, and retests were not administered.

In addition, some patients with mild aphasia also received short-term therapy, because they were anxious to return to work, and were not retested. Treatment in these cases consisted of helping patients to understand and to predict difficulties they could expect to encounter, and demonstrating what they could do at home to insure continued improvement.

Some patients were not retested because treatment was discontinued abruptly by sudden onset of illness, or by a personal or family emergency. In some cases, also, initial examinations had to be discarded because patients were not neurologically stable or because an older test form had been used when the first test was administered. In these cases, final tests were used in the single-test, but not in the test–retest, series. We adopted this procedure because the only criterion for the single-test series was a diagnosis of aphasia in a neurologically stable patient. Subjects were heterogeneous in age, in educational and vocational levels, in time elapsed since onset of aphasia, in etiology, and in locus and extent of brain damage.

For the test–retest series the requirements were two reliable tests separated by a reasonable interval of time. The test–retest interval ranged from 1 to 13 months, with a mean interval of 3 months. Practice effects from test to retest must certainly be negligible for aphasic subjects, who require intensive reinforcement to hold language acquisitions from one day to another.

The clinician who treated the patient administered both the initial and final test. This procedure is subject to criticism, but it was the only practical plan when we were operating a clinical service with patients admitted and discharged each week, and all clinicians carried full case loads. This method is defensible on some grounds. All examiners were trained in making objective observations, not only during testing but also throughout the course of therapy. Final test performances tended to fall below clinical performances in almost all cases. This was predictable, since recently acquired skills hold up less well in stress situations than skills reinforced over longer periods. Changing examiners, had this been feasible, would probably have increased tension during testing and have made results less reliable.

NONAPHASIC SUBJECTS

Fifty patients on the Medical Wards of the Minneapolis VA Hospital were also tested on the research edition of the Minnesota Test for comparison with the aphasic patients tested on that edition. The examiner was a research associate, Barbara Stansell Street, a former member of the clinical staff of the Aphasia Section of the Neurology Service. Mrs. Street obtained medical clearance for available subjects each week and then screened them by review of medical charts and personal interviews. She eliminated patients who were unwilling to cooperate, patients with visual or hearing problems severe enough to interfere with testing, patients who had never learned to read or write, and patients with a history of neurological or psychiatric problems. In addition, she selected subjects to match the age distribution of the aphasic population, as far as possible. Thirty-eight percent of subjects in both series were under 50 years old and 62% were over 50. Age distributions were as follow:

Age	Nonaphasic subjects	Aphasic subjects
19-29	8%	10%
30-39	14%	8%
40-49	16%	20%
50-59	12%	14%
60+	50%	48%
TOTAL UNDER 50	38%	38%
TOTAL OVER 50	62%	62%

Thirty-four percent of the nonaphasic subjects were high-school graduates, and 2% were college graduates. This was a lower educational level than was found in the aphasia series, in which 32% of subjects were high-school graduates, and 14% were graduated from college.

Ten percent of the nonaphasic subjects compared with 20% of the aphasic series followed occupations listed as professional or semiprofessional on the Minnesota Scale for Parental Occupations. Fifty-four percent of the nonaphasic subjects and 53% of the aphasic subjects were classified as semiskilled or unskilled laborers, and the remainder of subjects in both groups were clerical or skilled workers. The Minnesota Scale differs from the United States Census Classification of Occupations in that it discriminates levels within general types of services.

The Minneapolis VA Hospital does not provide custodial care. Both aphasic and nonaphasic subjects were admitted for medical treatment, rehabilitation, or both. Most aphasic subjects were admitted to the Neurology Service, where they were on the acute ward until diagnostic procedures and treatment for conditions requiring intensive care were completed, then transferred to the neurological rehabilitation ward. The difference between the two wards is in the kind of nursing care provided. On the rehabilitation ward, personnnel are trained to encourage patients to do as much as they can independently and to give assistance only when patients are unable to help themselves.

Some patients were admitted specifically for treatment of aphasia. This undoubtedly operated as a selection factor and probably accounts for the slightly higher educational–vocational level in the aphasia series.

In general, nonaphasic subjects made occasional random errors on testing, such as would be expected to result from carelessness or inattention, or sometimes from educational deficit. We did not find the recurring patterns of impairment that characterize the performances of aphasic subjects. However, nonaphasic subjects over 50 averaged significantly more errors on tests for reading, writing, and arithmetic, and significantly more total test errors than subjects under 50. Differences between means for the two age groups were not significant on tests for auditory comprehension, tests for speech and language, or tests for body scheme. This would seem to indicate that the older and younger subjects did not differ in functional use of language, although they differed in specific educational skills.

It is probable that observed differences were attributable in part to differences in educational level, since 40% of subjects under 50 were high-school graduates, compared with 13% of subjects over 50. But this was not the whole story. Mrs. Street reported that older nonaphasic patients tended to comment that they did not remember as well as they used to or that their eyes bothered them when they tried to read or write. She noted that all performances seemed to be slowed down a little in the older subjects. She recorded overall testing time for 43 subjects. The average time for all nonaphasic subjects was one hour and 22 minutes. For 16 subjects under 50, the average testing time was an hour and five minutes, compared with an hour and 32 minutes for subjects over 50. These findings emphasize the danger of using college or graduate students as controls for aphasic subjects, as some studies have done.

TEST PERFORMANCE OF APHASIC AND NONAPHASIC PATIENTS

The range of total errors on the 73 tests was 1–29 for nonaphasic subjects, and 7–602 for the aphasics. The median number of errors was 8, and the average 10.4 for nonaphasic subjects, compared with 170 and 213.1 for the aphasics. Means and standard deviations for each section of the test and for total scores are shown in Table 7–1.

It is obvious on inspection that the two distributions of scores are drawn from different populations. No nonaphasic subject performed as poorly as 92% of the aphasics, and only one aphasic performed as well as the average nonaphasic. Thirteen aphasics made between 7 and 29 errors, which means that 8% of the aphasic subjects scored within the normal range. These patients were classified as aphasic because of discrepancies between test performance and educational and vocational achievement, and because the pattern of errors was characteristic of aphasia.

Table 3 in Appendix 2 shows that correlations between test sections were high for the aphasic subjects, reflecting a general language deficit present in all modalities. For the nonaphasic subjects, correlations were generally low, indicating that errors resulted from diverse factors. The highest correlations tended to be between areas where scores might reasonably be expected to reflect educational deficits.

Because the nonaphasic subjects were well-screened for neurological involvement and other conditions that would invalidate test results, there were no nonaphasic subjects who showed obvious signs of brain damage. In former studies, however, such subjects have occasionally been found, and this is to be expected. There are undoubtedly individuals in the general population with no known history of neurological trauma or disease who are brain-injured to some extent. Concussions sometimes occur without being recognized as such, and people have "little strokes" that are never diagnosed. Adequate testing would be expected to reveal such damage. The pertinent questions are whether a patient has difficulty with tasks he once performed easily, what this difficulty stems from, how disturbing it is, and what can be done to ameliorate it.

TABLE 7-1. Means* and Standard Deviations of Errors for 154 Aphasic and 50 Nonaphasic Subjects Over All Sections of the Minnesota Test for Differential Diagnosis of Aphasia

Test section	Aphasic subjects		Nonaphasic subjects	
	M	SD	M	SD
Auditory	29.94	27.18	1.80	1.65
Visual and reading	25.88	21.84	1.96	1.70
Speech and language	69.82	60.89	10.08	1.48
Visuomotor and writing	58.85	41.71	4.12	3.89
Numerical and arithmetic processes	8.65	6.65	1.10	1.17
Body scheme	20.00	19.71	.36	.84
All tests	213.10	162.02	10.42	7.32

* Means over test sections have no significance except for comparisons between groups of subjects, since number of tests and test items vary from one section to another.

GENERAL FINDINGS FOR THE APHASIC POPULATION

AGE, EDUCATION, AND OCCUPATIONAL LEVEL

Aphasic subjects ranged in age from 19 to 72 years old, with a mean age of 52. Of the subjects: 8% were in their twenties, 14% in their thirties, 16% in their forties, 12% in their fifties, and 50% were over 60. Eighty-two percent of subjects over 60 were classified in diagnostic groups characterized by massive or generalized brain damage or both.

Information on education was available for 136 subjects. The range of schooling was from less than six years to professional degrees in law and medicine. Fifty-four percent of subjects were not graduated from high school, 32% were graduated from high school but not from college, and 14% were college graduates. The average number of school years completed was more than 10 but less than 12. All subjects with less than six years of schooling were over 50, but, on the other hand, all patients with professional degrees were over 60.

Occupational data was obtained for 147 subjects. These data necessarily refer to the occupation the patient followed before the onset of the condition for which he was admitted to the hospital. Occupations ranged from day labor to professional positions of major responsibility. Twenty percent of subjects were in occupations rated as professional or semiprofessional, 26% in occupations rated as clerical or skilled, and 54% were skilled or unskilled laborers. Patients over 50 had a slightly higher vocational level than patients under 50, although this difference was not statistically significant.

HANDEDNESS

Information on handedness was obtained by questioning the patient or an informant, who was usually the patient's wife. We asked which hand the patient generally used before his illness, how strong this preference was, and if there were any activities for which he frequently used the nonpreferred hand. In addition, we asked which hand he normally used for eating, writing, using tools, and playing games.

The preferences expressed were conclusive enough for us to combine the initial categories of right and chiefly right, and left and chiefly left, when we analyzed the data. The most ambiguous case was a man who considered himself left-handed, but reported

TABLE 7-2. Handedness and Hemisphere Involvement

Handedness	Left Hemisphere Lesions		Right Hemisphere Lesions		Bilateral Involvement		Total
	N	Percent	N	Percent	N	Percent	
Right-handed	102	76%	5	4%	27	20%	134
Left-handed	5	50%	3	30%	2	20%	10
Ambidextrous	2		0		0		2

he had been forced to write with his right hand in school, and continued to do so. Only one subject reported he could and did use either hand interchangeably for almost all activities, although he wrote and ate with the right hand because he found it more convenient. The first patient was classified as left-handed, and the second as ambidextrous. It is undoubtedly true that there are individual differences in degree of handedness dominance, but we were unable to discriminate them by questioning, and testing was impossible because a large number of subjects had neurological involvement affecting one hand or the other.

Table 7–2 summarizes the handedness data in relation to cerebral hemisphere lesions for 146 aphasic patients. The judgment of right or left hemisphere damage was made on the basis of contralateral involvement of extremities, with no observed signs of bilateral impairment. Bilateral damage was determined by bilateral weakness of extremities found on neurological examination, or by positive neurological findings on both sides of the body. The latter included such things as unilateral weakness of extremities, with facial paralysis, reduction of sensation, a positive Babinski, or a homonymous visual field defect on the side opposite the weakness. Subjects with no paralysis or paresis were excluded from consideration, since determination of the hemisphere involvement was less conclusive for these patients.

If we exclude subjects with known bilateral damage, we can say that 95% of the right-handed aphasic patients, and 70% of the left-handed and ambidextrous subjects had left-hemisphere lesions. However, the number of left-handed and ambidextrous subjects is too small to permit conclusions to be drawn from these date. Furthermore, it is not always possible to rule out bilateral involvement conclusively, even when there are no obvious clinical signs.

ETIOLOGY AND TIME SINCE ONSET

In 83% of subjects, aphasia was the result of a cerebrovascular accident (CVA). Age, of course, was important; 61% of subjects under 50 and 94% over 50 had incurred a cerebrovascular accident.

Unless there was clearcut evidence to indicate the nature of the CVA incurred, we attempted no further classification. We present the following breakdown of the incidence of kinds of CVAs in our population merely as a matter of interest:

Embolism	8%
Hemorrhage	11%
Thrombosis	22%
CVA involving distribution of the middle cerebral artery	59%

The diagnosis of a CVA involving the distribution of the middle cerebral artery was made on the basis of clinical and not laboratory findings. This means that cause was undetermined. The category reflects two general policies of the Neurology Service. The first is not to subject patients to what are essentially surgical procedures when it is not critical to do so. The second is not to make more precise diagnoses than the evidence permits.

The period that elapsed between onset of aphasia and initial testing of subjects in the research series ranged from just under three months to 10 years. The average period was between three and six months. The patient who was treated 10 years after the onset of aphasia stayed nine months, and learned to speak and write in sentences and to read with enjoyment for the first time in 10 years.

ELECTROENCEPHALOGRAMS

Electroencephalograms were obtained for 106 of the 155 Minneapolis subjects. It is necessary to interpret these data cautiously, since some of the records were made during the period of acute illness, and others were obtained a year or more after onset. Seventy-eight percent of the records were abnormal. Fifty-two percent showed focal findings in the left hemisphere, and 8% in the right. The most significant finding was that 85% of the EEG's with focal findings in the left hemisphere, and all the EEG's with focal findings in the right, showed temporal lobe involvement.

HEARING LOSS

Audiometric tests were available for 142 aphasic subjects. Overall, 83% showed some hearing loss, and 43% showed loss in speech frequencies. However, when the better ear was used as a criterion, 12% of subjects were judged to have mild, 3% moderate, and 2% severe hearing loss in the speech range. Most of the speech frequency losses were found in patients over 50, and were of long standing.

As in previous analyses performed, there was no indication of a relationship between hearing loss measured by pure-tone audiometry and aphasic difficulty understanding spoken language. Six out of 10 subjects with severe auditory imperception showed no hearing loss in either ear. Subjects with moderate or severe hearing loss were scattered through all diagnostic groups and performed like other subjects in their diagnostic categories on language tasks when tested under conditions in which they could hear. The only conclusion we can draw from these data is that pure-tone audiometry is not sensitive enough to reveal alterations of auditory perception in aphasic subjects.

CONCLUSION

Our sample of aphasic patients differed from the young war-injured populations reported in many of the earlier studies. In general, it was an older group of patients, with aphasia usually resulting from cerebrovascular lesions.

It was also a different population from the patients Penfield and Roberts studied postoperatively in Montreal, since our patients were all neurologically stable when tested.

It was a slightly older group of patients than we had seen before. In 1954, we analyzed data obtained from 65 subjects. Forty-two percent of these subjects were over 50, compared with 62% of the present sample, and 55%, as compared with the present 83% had incurred cerebrovascular accidents.

However, subjects covered the entire age range and included all etiologies found in earlier studies. The same patterns of test errors were obtained. As we worked with these patients, the only difference we were aware of was the increasing number of patients found in the group characterized by findings compatible with scattered brain damage.

It is important to make it clear that since we analyzed data by diagnostic categories determined by recurring test patterns, what we have to say about aphasia cannot be considered to be about patients with massive or generalized brain damage only. Previous studies had in fact made it possible to recognize these patients on admission, and to compare their performance on testing and throughout the course of treatment with the behavior of patients with less extensive involvement.

chapter 8

EXAMINING APHASIC PATIENTS

TO TEST OR NOT TO TEST

Objections have always been made to systematic testing of aphasic patients. A common argument is that aphasic responses are inconsistent, and consequently test results are unreliable. Criticisms have been directed at plus–minus scoring and quantification of data. Some clinicians consider test procedures traumatic to patients. Perhaps the most frequent complaint is that comprehensive testing is economically unfeasible because it requires so much time.

There is partial truth in all these statements. Some aphasic responses are inconsistent in some ways. Plus–minus scoring and quantification of data can obscure important information. Some examinations are traumatic, and all searching and thorough explorations take time. Instead of tilting at these traditional windmills, however, let us try to look at them critically.

INCONSISTENCY OF RESPONSES

Performance of aphasic patients fluctuates with transient physiological states during the first few days and sometimes the first few weeks after brain damage is incurred. Penfield and Roberts (1959) described a condition of neuroparalytic edema, characterized by transient symptoms that usually occur a day or so after brain surgery, and then subside. Less dramatic fluctuations during convalescence are a familiar occurrence.

127

In addition to fluctuating states, progressive changes take place. The immediate and remote effects of physiological recovery are reflected in functional improvement that may go on for considerable time. In addition to healing taking place in the brain, pulse, temperature, and blood pressure tend to stabilize, as the organism recovers from shock. The patient responds increasingly to what is going on about him. He attempts more activity from day to day and fatigues less readily. As a result of all these factors there may be marked improvement from one day to another.

This is the period of spontaneous recovery. It is impossible to predict its rate or limits, and no one can distinguish between transient and persisting symptoms while these processes are going on. Sometimes an adverse condition is present, such as infection, recurrent bleeding, or a chronic disease process, and then regression rather than recovery may occur. If the condition is arrested, recovery may begin at some unknown point.

Eventually most patients become neurophysiologically stable, and the residual damage in the brain is irreversible. The only further changes to be expected are slow gradual ones resulting from stimulation, practice, and exercise. At this time performance becomes predictable.

There is general agreement in the literature that test findings are unreliable if aphasic patients are examined before they are neurologically stable. An arbitrary limit of three months after onset is the common clinical rule, although it is recognized that significant spontaneous recovery occurs after three months in some patients. In others with ongoing destructive processes, test performances may continue to fluctuate indefinitely. A series of initial tests within a month of onset, followed by retests obtained eight months or more later, provided an opportunity to document the reliability or unreliability of early findings (Schuell and Nagae, 1969). Although diagnosis was unchanged for 19 (63%) of 30 aphasic patients retested, the converse of this is that one would be wrong, and sometimes grossly wrong, 37% of the time in predicting outcome for aphasic patients who were diagnosed before they were neurologically stable. For clinical purposes, it is wise to withhold differential diagnosis and prognosis for recovery from aphasia until patients are neurologically stable. (This statement does *not* imply that treatment should necessarily be deferred until this time.)

However, even stable aphasic patients show inconsistency on individual responses, and this persists. On one occasion, a patient may call a *man* a *woman*, a *knife* a *fork*, and designate a *telephone* correctly as a *telephone*. The next day he may label a *man* a *man*, a *knife* a *cutter*, and produce *talk* uncertainly for *telephone*. The early localizationists, thinking in terms of destruction of word images, could not explain these inconsistencies. There is no difficulty, however, if one thinks in terms of processes operating with reduced efficiency.

But even these variable responses show two remarkable kinds of consistency. First, the percentage of errors is remarkably stable from day to day, not only on identical but also on similar tasks. For example, on naming pictures, different pictures may be used to elicit different words without altering the level of performance, if words of the same general frequency are used.

The pattern of recovery is one of gradual improvement, more apparent from week to week than from day to day, and from month to month than from week to week. These gains result from persistent practice, and accrue slowly.

The second kind of consistency is in individual error patterns. If three patients are asked to name a set of pictures, one patient may usually produce jargon, another intelligible though defective approximations of words, while a third frequently misnames the pictures, though the words he produces sound normal. Patients usually make more than one type of error, and error patterns change gradually along predictable lines. However, a patient whose responses are 90% jargon one day does not change suddenly and show an altogether different response pattern the next day.

The speech of aphasic patients varies under different conditions in reasonable ways. In general aphasic patients talk more readily when they are rested and relaxed than when they are tired or tense. It is easier for most aphasic patients to talk to one person at a time than to enter into a group conversation. Like most of us, aphasic patients find some people easier to talk to than others. It is difficult for aphasic patients to talk to anyone who seems busy or hurried. The patient knows it takes him longer than most people to say what he wants to say and that, if he reacts to real or imagined impatience on the part of the listener, his speech may break down altogether.

Aphasic patients differ also in individual reactions to situations, probably much as they differed before they were aphasic. One patient with a good deal of speech hesitates to talk to anyone because he is afraid he will make a mistake. Another, with a repertory of three or four stereotyped phrases, grins and greets everyone he encounters with "How are you doing, pretty good?"

Most aphasic patients, understandably, do not talk as easily in medical conferences as they do on the hospital ward or in the clinic. Some patients, however, are stimulated by a friendly audience and almost forget they are aphasic. However, even in such circumstances, differences are in total verbal output and not in altered speech or language patterns.

In contrast to fluctuating environmental conditions, testing is a controlled situation. If the patient is neurologically stable, and if a relationship of confidence is established, maximal responses can usually be obtained. It is a maxim of psychometric testing that while scores may be depressed for many reasons, it is not possible for a subject to perform better than he can. As Goldstein (1948) has pointed out, aphasic patients are highly motivated to perform well, and experienced examiners rarely have trouble finding out what the patient is able to do.

In the course of treatment, daily performances are so predictable that consistent failure on tasks previously performed well should be reported to a physician. Performances may suffer if the patient did not get enough sleep, has a cold, or didn't get a letter from his girl, but in these circumstances fluctuation remains within characteristic individual ranges. Even patients subject to emotional disturbances can usually be quieted and work as well as usual. However, language is such a sensitive indicator of brain damage that the first symptom of progression or recurrence of a destructive process may be unexpected changes in language performances, and it is irresponsible not to report them.

We have obtained the following correlations between initial and final test scores of 73 aphasic patients who were tested on the *Minnesota Test for Differential Diagnosis of Aphasia* (1955 research form) and 22 aphasic patients who were tested on the 1965 published form before and after treatment for aphasia.

	1955 Research Form	1965 Published Form
Tests for auditory comprehension	0.89	0.77
Visual and reading tests	0.83	0.80
Speech and language tests	0.79	0.60
Visuomotor and writing tests	0.82	0.78
Numerical and arithmetic tests	0.76	0.78
Tests for body image	0.73	—

These correlations indicate good test–retest reliability, particularly considering that subjects were heterogeneous in age, education, and etiology of brain damage, as well as in pattern and severity of aphasia. To the extent that some age, educational, etiological, or diagnostic categories favor or inhibit recovery, such heterogeneity should reduce pre- and post-therapy correlations. In addition, there were subjects with moderately severe aphasia who made good recovery, and subjects with mild aphasia who made little improvement because of generalized brain damage, or some other limiting condition. This would also be expected to depress test–retest correlations.

PLUS–MINUS SCORING AND QUANTIFICATION OF DATA

Goldstein (1948) and others have rightfully held that plus–minus scores do not give meaningful information about the nature of aphasic disabilities. A minus score does not tell why a patient failed, or discriminate one failure from another. A plus score does not tell whether a patient performed a task in a normal manner or used some compensatory method.

This is a problem of test construction. Any complex behavior must be explored by more than one type of test. Consider an aphasic patient who has trouble following oral directions. He might fail because he can not discriminate enough words to receive the message. Perhaps he hears something that sounds like *pen*, sees a penny and a pencil, and guesses one or the other. Perhaps another patient hears, "Show me the lock," sees a key, and responds to the association between the two words. A third patient hears, "Put the spoon, the penny, and the key in the box," and picks up the penny and the key, but can not remember what else the examiner said. More tests are needed to determine why the patient fails. This is just another way of saying that it is necessary to observe a variety of specific behaviors.

Suppose, on the other hand, a patient, asked to multiply 21 by 6, produces the correct answer by writing 21 six times, and adding. His method would be impractical if he were consequently asked to multiply a three-digit number by another three-digit number. Failure on the second task would indicate difficulty multiplying. When method of performance or type of error is considered important information, different scoring categories can be assigned to different methods or types of errors. Identifying the significant dimensions to be explored is one of the tasks of test construction. In Loevinger's (1957) words, the problem is "one of finding items which are sensitive signs of those areas of behavior which are significant for practical and theoretical purposes," and a good test will provide such signs.

Additional information is obtained from the overall pattern of test errors. Taking account of the general pattern of test performance is part of all good psychometric procedure. For simplicity, let us suppose an examiner, using the Binet, finds a five-year-old child who passes all tests at the three-year- level and fails all tests at the four-year level. The examiner will probably write in his report that the tests indicates mental retardation of about two years.

If another five-year-old child fails one or two tests at the three-, four-, and five-year levels, but passes some tests at six and seven years, it is necessary to look for another kind of explanation. The examiner will then study the tests that were missed and the tests that were passed to try to find a reasonable explanation for the discrepancies. He will look for evidence of specific disabilities that interfere with the performance of some tests but not of others.

Aphasic patients frequently have specific disabilities of this kind. For example, both aphasic and nonaphasic subjects frequently show dysarthria and various degrees of visual and spatial imperception. The frequency of these sequelae of brain damage in both groups tends to support the validity of the principle of differential diagnosis in aphasia based on identification of the nature of the underlying processes that are involved. Identification of these disabilities is essential to differential diagnosis. This is far more important than counting pluses and minuses. It does not by any means imply, however, that test scores have no value. They can be used to compare the performance of a patient at various stages of recovery, and this is often useful information. They can be used to compare the performance of an aphasic subject with that of nonaphasic subjects, to estimate how handicapped a patient is vocationally. Finally, it is often informative to study distributions of errors of large populations of aphasic subjects for similarities or differences that occur in segments of the population studied.

But there is a further justification for objective testing, which Loevinger (1957) summarized as follows: "There are no natural units for the study of behavior. The problem of discrete, unambiguously identifiable units of behavior can be solved by the use of objective test items. Because tests are samples, what we know about behavior in general applies to test behavior. Because tests are signs, what we learn from tests can help structure and interpret knowledge of other, more amorphous behavior."

Certainly we need quantified data for precise description of any complex behavior. It constitutes all the evidence there is for what we talk about when we talk about aphasia. Both systematic exploration and repeated observations are necessary for understanding the complexities of the problem with which we are dealing.

TRAUMA TO PATIENTS

Aphasic patients are vulnerable, and sometimes become disturbed without obvious cause, although not generally without reason. Goldstein (1948) has shown that transference develops with organic as well as with neurotic patients, and that when transference exists, the patient is able to do whatever the physician asks him to do without fear, because he trusts the physician.

This confidence is a critical factor in all clinical relationships. It is as essential in testing as in therapy. In psychological literature, the term *rapport* is sometimes used instead of transference. This is acceptable, if one gives rapport a deeper meaning than casual bonhomie. A clinical relationship must include supportiveness on the part of the clinician, and confidence on the part of the patient. It is not easy to write the rules for establishing this confidence.

Probably the first requirement for the clinician is an awareness of what has happened to the patient, and what his illness means to him. This involves knowing something about the kind of person the patient was before his illness, and what he is like outside the hospital or clinic. In order to build effective clinical relationships, we must somehow counteract the institutional tendency to depersonalize patients or clients.

It is particularly important to help aphasic patients bridge the present and the past. We ought, for example, to talk about *Hamlet* or *Macbeth* or the *Furness Variorum* to a Shakespearian scholar, a new bridge or highway to a civil engineer, and crops and farm machinery to a farmer, whether he can discuss them or not, because these are the things he cares about. They are also apt to be the kinds of patterns that are best organized in his brain and to which he responds most readily.

Often we are so afraid of causing a "catastrophic reaction" that we deal too much with trivialities and are superficial in consequence. The patient rejects our false bright reassurances, and no meaningful communication takes place. He feels that we do not understand, or are avoiding his problems because there is no hope for him.

The examiner should understand that aphasic patients know something has happened to them, and that they want him, in his professional capacity, to know this, too. They react as anyone does who goes to a doctor because something is wrong. If the doctor makes a thorough examination and explains what he finds to the patient, the patient usually experiences relief, although the symptoms have not changed. Relief occurs even when serious conditions are present, because the patient no longer faces nameless fears alone. The physician's attitude has told him that other people have adjusted to similar conditions, that this is possible, and that he can do it, also.

This kind of supportiveness is essential in all clinical relationships. The physician alone accepts responsibility for life and death and for maintaining optimal physiological conditions. Every aphasic patient should be under the care of a physician, who sees him as often as necessary to maintain an adequate medical regime. The speech pathologist has no responsibility for survival of the organism, for medication, or for physiological care. He is, however, responsible for establishing communication with the human personality, which may also be struggling for survival. If this seems of lesser importance, it is instructive to meditate upon the number of aphasic patients who have gone through a period when they would have chosen death if a choice had been offered. There are no statistics on attempted suicides among aphasic patients, but such attempts have been made, sometimes repeatedly, and many aphasics have expressed a death wish at one time or another:

"When I woke up and found I couldn't talk, I'd have shot myself if there'd been a revolver under my pillow. I wished there was."

"I might as well go out in a field and shoot myself. What else can I do? I'm not good for anything."

"I wish I could die, but I don't know how. Well, I know how, but I don't suppose I would do it."

"I don't know what is to become of me. I'd be better dead."

"I wish I had died when I had the stroke. It would be better for everyone."

These statements were made by men who could communicate reasonably well, but could not resume their work.

One point of all this is that under such circumstances, confidence cannot be won by evasion. Another is that when confidence exists there is no need for evasion on the part of the clinician or the patient. The job for both is to assess disabilities honestly, to clear the way for potential resources and strength to emerge.

It seems sensible to start with the reality that something is wrong, that the patient knows it, and wants us to know it, too. There can be no confidence unless we deal seriously and honestly with existing problems.

The interview usually works best if the examiner begins with the assumption that the patient is concerned about the trouble he is having with his speech. If the patient can talk, it is constructive to ask him to tell you about it from the beginning. When he has told all he can, the examiner should ask questions. Searching questions often elicit a surprised how-did-you-know expression, which may signal the beginning of acceptance of the examiner in his clinical role.

When the patient cannot talk, the examiner can ask questions the patient can answer with an appropriate sign or gesture. He can ask, for example, if the patient is comfortable, if he tires easily, if he stays up all day, if he understands what the examiner is saying, if he has trouble understanding what people say, if he can say any words at all.

Then, with a patient like this, it is usually a good idea to proceed directly to a peripheral examination of the speech musculature, and go on to show the patient that it will work, at least to some extent. The examiner can try, in this order, for phonation, singing, counting to 5 , then to 10, saying the alphabet, and naming the days of the week. Each task should be tried several times, and the examiner and patient should perform it in unison. Sometimes it is possible to go on to repetition of common words, and to elicit words by supplying common associations, such as *a cup of*—, *bread and* —, *read the*—, or *go to*—. One should not go on to a new task unless some success has been achieved on an easier one. The level or quality of obtained responses is immaterial. The important thing is that the patient should do something he did not know he could do, even if it is as simple as opening his mouth and saying *ah*, then opening and closing his mouth or moving his tongue around while he is saying it. The idea is to get the musculature in motion, preferably while phonation is going on.

Next, the idea of testing should be presented directly. The simplest method is to tell the patient that you want to give him some tests, that some will be easy for him and some will be hard, but that you want to find everything that gives him trouble.

If the examiner maintains this interested but objective attitude throughout the examination, patients do not usually find tests threatening, because they feel the supportiveness of the examiner. It is a good idea to comment casually on what the patient does well, but it is even more important to acknowledge his failures, reminding him that this is what you want to know about. It is a good idea to prepare the patient for a difficult task by telling him it will be hard, but that you want to find out where the trouble lies.

This procedure is supportive because a failure is not regarded as a failure, but rather as a way to help the examiner find out what is wrong. Patients often ask if the examiner has seen other people with similar problems. This question is asked so often that it would appear to be an important kind of reassurance to give to all patients. The known is always less frightening than the unknown, and panic begins to recede when the patient no longer feels isolated with his disability or afraid he is losing his mind because he cannot do things he once did easily.

It is startling how many people equate aphasia with insanity, perhaps because they never heard of aphasia. One of the therapeutic effects of examination is probably that it corrects this misapprehension more convincingly than words. This insight can not occur, however, unless the examiner treats the patient as a reasonable and responsible adult who is justifiably concerned about what has happened to him.

Defensiveness almost always decreases during the course of examination. Instead of trying to cover up disabilities, patients become anxious for the examiner to observe them. They begin to show the examiner things they cannot do, as though they were afraid something might be overlooked. Patients who can talk frequently ask about problems unrelated to aphasia, such as fear of seizures, fear of another episode, fear that they will die or that they won't, or anxieties about family, money, work, or the general loss of confidence they have experienced.

Such communications should be regarded seriously, and something should be done about them when possible, to justify the confidence of the patient. Professional ethics require recognition of the limits of the field in which one is trained, and the domains and competencies of others. This should present no problem. It is always possible to say, "This is something you should talk to your doctor about. Would you like to have me explain what you have told me, and ask him to talk to you about it?" It may be the doctor, the social worker, the vocational counselor, physical therapist, rabbi, priest, or minister. Referral is not only responsible professional procedure, but it enables the aphasic patient to form significant relationships with more people. These relationships have the effect of making the patient's world a little wider, and this tends to increase confidence and reduce anxiety. Aphasic patients are often necessarily dependent upon the clinician, who not only spends a good deal of time with them, but is frequently the person with whom they can communicate most easily. The clinician accepts this responsibility, but also that of gradually decreasing dependency needs. Encouraging other rewarding relationships from the beginning works in this direction.

The examiner must be sensitive to signs of tension and fatigue in the patient. He should stop procedures as soon as these appear, either for an interval of relaxation or to continue in another session. As Goldstein (1948) has observed with such deep insight, fatigue is usually a reaction to stress. Almost all aphasic patients can work for an hour, and patients who are physiologically stable can go on much longer, provided that there are changes of activity and that they do not feel threatened. If, however, the examiner attempts to force procedures upon a patient who is uncomfortable or disturbed, the results are an indication of tolerance level and not of ability to perform a set of tasks.

In conclusion, searching exploration of aphasic disabilities can be a therapeutic rather than a traumatic procedure. This is true because the process of testing establishes communication on a level that is highly meaningful to the patient. As a result, he feels less isolated and less anxious. By means of the tests, the examiner leads the patient toward objectivity by helping him understand the nature of his problems and their limits. The patient discovers things he is able to do, which tends to restore confidence and alleviate depression. Patients become less and less defensive as confidence in the clinician increases.

TEST REQUIREMENTS

Any testing methods that enable the examiner to observe adequate samples of language behavior may be used. No tests or test methods are sacrosanct. There are some advantages to using tests standardized on aphasic populations. For one reason, test instructions are usually better because they have been revised to anticipate and reduce difficulties of presentation. Clinically tested materials tend to be more effective because common sources of error have been eliminated.

There is probably no such thing as a pure test. All tests administered to aphasic subjects are influenced by the ability of the patient to understand or to remember test instructions. They are probably also influenced by the patient's ability to explain the task to himself, retain the sequences of his plan, and tell himself what to do next. However, some tests do better than others in screening irrelevant variables and in revealing specific disabilities.

Much of the earlier literature shows the tendency of observers to find what they were looking for and to ignore other dimensions of deficit. The only correction for this kind of subjectivity seems to be to develop as much sophistication as possible about what to look for. A good test may serve to increase sophistication by extending insights into what is operating to alter language behavior. On the other hand, it may limit insights by discouraging further exploration. Probably the best answer to this dilemma is to make use of the best instruments available, to investigate new ones as they appear, and to continue to study the daily performances of aphasic patients searchingly from an open-minded and eclectic point of view.

Uniform test procedures are necessary to compare performances between patients and to compare performances of the same patients over intervals of time.

Pierre Marie pointed out in 1906 that it was necessary to have tests of graduated difficulty in order that mild forms of aphasic disorders should not be overlooked. It is necessary to have easy tests to obtain samples of language behavior from subjects with severe aphasia. Tests of intermediate difficulty are required for subjects who make no errors on easy tests but cannot perform on hard ones. As we pointed out earlier, "easy" and "hard" must be defined by the percentage of aphasic subjects who make errors on a given test. As Goldstein contended, it is not safe to assume that a test easy for nonaphasics is also easy for aphasics. It is instructive to study test difficulty empirically. Results often differ from those most of us would have predicted naïvely. When we understand why, we have increased our knowledge of aphasia. This is one of the reasons it is necessary for a test to sample diverse kinds of language behavior.

There is always some overlap on language tests between errors resulting from aphasia and errors resulting from low intelligence or low educational level. Borderline intelligence or below, as well as illiteracy, is found in aphasic as in normal populations. A patient with mild aphasia will perform better than an illiterate on some language tests, and less well on others. It is not possible to eliminate this overlap completely. It can be minimized, however, to a considerable extent, since aphasic deficits usually appear on language tests below fifth- or sixth-grade achievement level, even in patients with considerable intelligence and intellectual attainment.

Only rarely is a patient found with a mild aphasic disability that is not revealed by a comprehensive battery of language tests held to grade-school level. Then it is necessary to use supplementary tests with higher ceilings. Results can be compared with educational level, but the pattern of deficit is more discriminating than obtained score. If, for example, the patient scored at college level on tests for reading vocabulary, at the eighth-grade level on tests for sentence comprehension, and at fourth- or fifth-grade level on tests for paragraph comprehension, one would infer reduction of verbal retention span, which is a characteristic aphasic deficit. One would predict that the same pattern would appear in other language modalities if tests of equivalent difficulty were used. For such subjects, the discrepancy between performance on verbal and nonverbal tests is often discriminatory, also, if "verbal" is given a sufficiently broad interpretation. For this purpose, tests that involve any kind of symbolic behavior must be considered verbal tests.

PROBLEMS TO BE INVESTIGATED

Briefly, the examiner needs to find out what abilities are retained, what disabilities are present, and how to account for them. Another way of saying this is that the examiner needs to know the level of performance in all language modalities, and why performance breaks down when it does.

We observe language behavior in the usual modalities, listening, speaking, reading, and writing, because this is what there is to observe about language. Perhaps this accounts for the traditional tendency to talk about sensory or motor, or reading and writing disturbances. *But while we observe behavior, we think in terms of processes that underlie behavior.* This is harder, because processes cannot be observed but must be inferred.

We have seen that some language disabilities, such as reduction of vocabulary and reduction of verbal retension span, cross language modalities. This must be because the same processes operate in retrieval of words and retention of sequences of words, regardless of the use to be made of them. We once had a patient who had learned sign language to communicate with deaf parents. When he could think of the word he wanted, he could say it, write it, and sign it. When he could not say it, he could neither write it nor produce the manual sign.

Impairment of auditory processes is usually reflected in all language modalities, also. The patient may mispronounce, misread, or miswrite words because of impaired auditory feedback, or impaired recall of learned auditory patterns. If he calls a *house* a *fouse,* he may write it *fouse,* and it may or may not look wrong to him. He may repeat, read, or write *necessity* as *necesty,* because he cannot recall learned sequences of sounds or letters.

Impairment of visual processes, on the other hand, is reflected only in reading or writing. The patient may read or write *match* for *watch,* but if you ask him what he tells time with, he will probably never say *match.*

Dysarthrias affect only speech. We can be less sure of this with sensorimotor impairment. Studies of auditory perception (Liberman *et al.,* 1967) indicate that discrimination of phonemes is probably dependent upon articulatory as well as auditory, information. It is therefore reasonable to suppose that impairment of proprioceptive processes may affect auditory discrimination, as well as articulation, to some extent.

In summary, we observe language behavior in the usual modalities, because this is what discriminates aphasic from nonaphasic patients. We infer disturbances of processes underlying various kinds of language behavior and look for evidence to support our inferences. Testing involves asking questions and making observations. If testing is done under controlled conditions, observations can be repeated and compared from one patient to another, and from one time to another.

THE MINNESOTA TEST

Because it represents our most refined application of the principles just discussed and because it is the basis for the work reported in this book, we have listed below a brief description of each of the tests in the Minnesota battery. The reader will notice that the tests are grouped under five main headings: Auditory Comprehension, Visual and Reading Tests, Speech and Language Tests, Visuomotor and Writing Tests, and Numerical Relations and Arithmetic. Under each heading the tests proceed from easy to difficult; thus, the tests for Auditory Comprehension begin with the simplest task (pointing to an object or picture named by the examiner) and end with more complex and taxing tasks (repetition of sentences and digit strings of progressive length).

The research form of the Minnesota Test which provided the basis for the first edition of this book differed slightly from the published form used here. The research form included a section on Body Parts (now omitted since it contributed little new information relative to aphasia) and a few different subtests. The major categories of tests were identical.

DESCRIPTION OF TESTS IN THE 1965 PUBLISHED EDITION OF THE MINNESOTA TEST FOR DIFFERENTIAL DIAGNOSIS OF APHASIA

The figures in parentheses indicate the number of items on the test.

TESTS FOR AUDITORY COMPREHENSION

1. *Recognition of words* (18). Patients are required to point to 6 objects and 12 pictures of common objects named by examiner.

2. *Discriminating between paired words* (24). Cards with two pictures representing words that sound alike are presented. Patients point to the picture named by the examiner (for auditory discrimination).

3. *Recognition of letters* (26). Cards containing five or six large printed letters are presented serially. Patients are required to point to the letter named by examiner.

4. *Items serially* (6). Patients are required to point to objects in a picture, named in series of two, and series of three.

5. *Understanding sentences* (15). Sentences are read aloud to patient who is required to answer *yes* or *no*.

6. *Directions* (10). Items are equated for vocabulary difficulty but are progressive in length. Examples: *Ring the bell; Put the spoon in the cup; Put the bell between the pencil and the spoon.*

7. *Understanding a paragraph* (6). A short narrative paragraph is read to the patient, and he is asked questions about content, which are answered *yes* or *no*.

8. *Repetition of sentences* (6). Patients are required to repeat sentences equated for vocabulary difficulty, but progressive in length (test for auditory retention span).

9. *Repetition of digits* (6). Patients are required to repeat series of four, five, and six digits forward, and four digits backwards. Binet procedures are followed (for auditory retention span).

VISUAL AND READING TESTS

1. *Matching forms* (5). A card is presented containing six large clear geometric forms. Single forms for matching are presented on individual cards.

2. *Matching letters* (20). A series of cards is presented, each containing five or six large upper- or lower-case printed letters. Individual letters are presented for matching.

3. *Matching words to pictures* (32). Cards are presented containing pictures of six common objects. Cards containing single words are presented individually for matching.

4. *Matching printed to spoken words* (32). A card is presented containing the 12 printed words used in Test 3. Patients are required to point to words spoken by examiner.

5. *Reading comprehension, sentences* (12). Patients are required to check printed questions *yes* or *no*. Example: *Does everyone put money in the bank? Yes (   ) No (   ).*

6. *Reading Rate* (6). It was ascertained that most nonaphasics completed Test 5 in less than 60 seconds, and few aphasics required more than three minutes. A seven-point scale was constructed ranging from 60 seconds or less, to more than three and a half minutes, and performance on Test 5 was timed and rated.

7. *Reading comprehension, paragraph* (8). Patients are required to read a short

narrative paragraph (approximately Grade 6 level), and check questions on content *yes* or *no*.

8. *Oral reading, words* (15). Patients are required to read 15 words aloud, ranging from one to four syllables in length. Any mispronunciation is scored wrong.

9. *Oral reading, sentences* (30). Patients are required to read six sentences aloud, ranging from Grade levels 1 through 6. A sentence is scored wrong if it contains an error in pronunciation or wording.

SPEECH AND LANGUAGE TESTS

1. *Imitating gross movements* (10). Patients are asked to produce phonation, and to protrude and move tongue laterally. Palatal movements are observed on phonation. Pharyngeal movements are checked by questioning patients are nurses regarding difficulty swallowing liquids and solids.

2. *Rapid alternating movements* (8). Patients are asked to pronounce a given syllable, then repeat it as rapidly as possible, after demonstration. Error scored if patient cannot repeat syllable 15 times in five seconds.

3. *Repetition of monosyllabic words* (32). Patients are required to repeat phonetically edited list of common monosyllabic words.

4. *Repeating phrases* (20). Patients are required to repeat a phonetically edited list of phrases.

5. *Counting to 20* (20). Patients are asked to count aloud to 20. Numbers are supplied when necessary, but scored as errors.

6. *Days of week* (7). Procedure as in Test 5.

7. *Sentence completion* (8). Sentences are read to patients, who are required to supply last word. Example: *I want a cup of—*.

8. *Answering simple questions* (8). Patients are asked questions requiring single-word responses. Example: *What do you do with a hammer?*

9. *Information* (15). Patients are asked for factual biographical information. Examples: *Where do you live? Where were you born?*

10. *Expressing ideas* (6). Patients are asked to tell three things they have done during the day, and three things a good citizen should do.

11. *Producing sentences* (6). Patients are asked to produce a sentence using a specific word.

12. *Picture description* (6). Patients are asked to describe a picture, and tell what is happening. Scale was developed by classifying responses of aphasic subjects.

13. *Naming pictures* (20). Patients are required to name 20 pictures of common objects.

14. *Defining words* (10). Patients are asked to tell in their own words, what given words mean *(robin, apple, return, opinion, etc.)*. Scale was developed by classifying responses made by aphasic subjects.

15. *Retelling paragraph* (6). Patients are asked to retell a paragraph read to them by the examiner.

VISUOMOTOR AND WRITING TESTS

1. *Copying Greek letters* (5). Patients are asked to copy Greek *pi, psi, theta, lambda,* and *phi.*
2. *Numerals to 20* (20). Patients are asked to write numerals from 1 to 20.
3. *Reproducing wheel* (6). Picture of a wheel is presented for 10 seconds, then withdrawn. Patients are asked to draw it as well as possible.
4. *Reproducing letters* (18). Upper- and lower-case printed letters are exposed individually for two seconds, then withdrawn. Patients are asked to copy letters as they were on the cards.
5. *Writing letters to dictation* (26). Patients are required to write letters of alphabet dictated in random order.
6. *Written spelling* (10). Words from graded spelling lists 3 through 6 written to dictation.
7. *Oral spelling* (10). Patients are required to spell aloud words written on Test 6.
8. *Producing written sentences* (6). Patients are required to write sentences using words such as *door, want,* and *became.*
9. *Sentences to dictation* (7). Sentences equated for vocabulary difficulty, but progressive in length, are written to dictation.
10. *Writing paragraph* (6). Patients are asked to write a paragraph describing a picture, and telling what is happening in it. Scale was developed by evaluating responses of aphasic patients.

NUMERICAL RELATIONS AND ARITHMETIC PROCESSES

1. *Change* (8). Coins are presented, and patients asked to indicate correct change for nickel, dime, quarter, and simple transactions.
2. *Setting clock* (5). Patients are asked to set hands of clock to show when they get up, eat supper, go to bed, and to specified times.
3. *Simple arithmetic combinations* (12). Patients are required to select correct response to common numerical combinations, e.g., addition, subtraction, multiplication, and division (combined visual and auditory presentation, with verbal, written, or gesture response permitted).
4. *Written problems* (6). Patients are required to work two each of addition, subtraction, multiplication, and division problems at the Grade 5 level.

THE DIAGNOSTIC SCALE

In keeping with our earlier discussion of test scores, it is obvious that neither the total number of errors on the test battery nor the total number of errors on a subset of tests are the most meaningful information for differential diagnosis. The problem at this point is to go from specific evidence provided by the patient's performance on the battery to an assessment of the kinds of difficulties the patient is having with respect to symbolic communication. For this purpose we have developed a Diagnostic Scale which summarizes the critical information obtained from each test section and presents an overall view of the pattern of impairment observed in each patient.

The Diagnostic Scale also provides a method of comparing diagnostic findings over a series of patients examined with different subsets of tests determined by obtained baselines and ceilings, and has been used to compare diagnostic findings across two languages.

Diagnostic ratings are completed after testing. It is essential that positive findings be documented by test evidence, since agreement between examiners is contingent upon clear operational definition of what is rated. The scale includes observations of auditory functions, visual and visuospatial functions, motor and sensorimotor functions, and use of language. The last deals with ability to use the words and rules of an acquired language for communication, and is not specific to any modality. In other words, you must know a word to understand it in a lecture or on the printed page, or to use it in speech or in writing. Probably all of us have had the experience of having to look up a rarely encountered word more than once. In general the aphasic patient retains best and recovers first the words that are most common in the language. In addition to vocabulary, we learn the rules of a language. We must know the rules of German, for example, before we know whether to use *das, der,* or *die* before a given German noun. Most English speakers know, consciously or unconsciously, that we can say *a man,* but not *a men,* and that we say *you are,* but not *you is.* The ability of the aphasic patient to use the rules of his language usually correlates with the amount of language that is available to him. In other words, the ability to combine words appropriately is related, to some extent at least, to size of vocabulary and length of verbal retention span.

Most investigators agree that the term aphasia should not be used unless some reduction of language can be demonstrated. If we accept this definition, it becomes meaningful to talk about simple aphasia, when no complicating conditions are present, and aphasia complicated by involvement of visual processes, sensorimotor processes, or by dysfluency, and so on. The advantages of this method of diagnosis are, first, that it makes it possible to describe any form of aphasia in a simple empirical manner; and second, that it is possible to demonstrate the interferences that are present with considerable precision, which facilitates agreement between examiners. This is the rationale of the Diagnostic Scale, which is presented below.

Essentially the task of the examiner is to review under general functional headings all of the specific behavior that he has obtained in response to the examination. For each kind of function he must appraise the evidence and rate the performance of the patient on the following four-point scale:

0   No impairment: performance within normal limits for age and educational level
1   Mild impairment: occasional difficulties that do not disrupt performance
2   Moderate impairment: consistent difficulties; performance possible but limited or defective
3   Severe impairment: almost complete disruption of performance

The functional categories that we use are the following:

		Rating
1.	Auditory discrimination	( )
2.	Auditory recognition	( )
3.	Auditory retention span	( )
4.	Visual discrimination	( )
5.	Visual recognition	( )
6.	Visual recall	( )
7.	Spatial orientation	( )
8.	Involvement of speech musculature	( )
9.	Sensorimotor involvement	( )
10.	Word finding	( )
11.	Functional speech	( )
12.	Functional writing	( )

The first three items on the scale refer to observable impairment of the auditory system. Relevant observations are as follows:

1. *Auditory discrimination* refers to ability to discriminate sounds and sound patterns used in speech. Does the patient frequently confuse the names of letters, or words, that sound alike, on appropriate tests?
2. *Auditory recognition* refers to ability to understand spoken words. Does the patient make errors pointing to objects or pictures named by the examiner? Can he demonstrate understanding of less common words appropriate to his educational level, on suitable tests? For example, some patients may be able to identify *window* but not *illumination, car* but not *transportation, recreation* but not *isolation,* which is a somewhat less common although not a rare word.
3. *Auditory retention span* refers to ability to retain a series of words that are heard. Repetition of random series of digits is the most precise test for this. The examiner begins with two digits, pronounced at a rate of one per second, and proceeds to series of three, four, and so on, until the patient fails two series of any given length. Seven digits is usually considered normal for adults, although six is probably average for subjects over 50. Patients unable to repeat can be tested by being asked to point to common objects in a picture in series of gradually increasing length. Aphasic subjects who cannot repeat often have difficulty pointing to two or three objects named in a series.

The next four items refer to observations of visual or visuospatial disturbances. Relevant observations are as follows:

4. *Visual discrimination* refers to ability to discriminate learned visual patterns and is tested by matching. Does the patient make errors matching geometric forms, or matching letters of the alphabet? Does he tend to confuse letters that look alike, in isolation, or in words?
5. *Visual recognition* refers to reading vocabulary. Can the patient match words to pictures? Does he frequently confuse words that look alike? Is reading vocabulary significantly below the vocabulary level observed in speech, or on tests for auditory comprehension, for no apparent reason (such as educational deficit, foreign back-

ground, or reduction of visual acuity)? Visual recognition is not labeled defective on the diagnostic scale when reading impairment results from vocabulary deficit common to all modalities, in the absence of specific visual signs, such as confusion of letters and words with similar visual configurations.

6. *Visual recall* refers to retention of learned visual patterns. Does the patient have difficulty recalling letter forms? Does he produce reversals and distortions of letters? Does he often substitute one letter for another that looks somewhat similar? Does he tend to spell phonetically? Is spelling significantly below general vocabulary level for no apparent reason (educational deficit, etc.)? *Visual recall* is not labeled defective when writing reflects a language deficit common to all modalities, in the absence of specific visual signs, such as reversals, distortions, and substitutions of letters with similar visual configurations.

7. *Spatial disorientation* refers to impaired perception of relationships in space. On testing, impairment is shown by gross distortions on drawing and copying, by confusion of directionality on writing, and by difficulty on object assembly tests.

The next two items on the scale are related to production of speech sounds. It is important to remember that mispronunciations and even initial jargon may appear as a result of defective recall of auditory patterns. In the latter case errors are inconsistent, can usually be readily corrected by ear, and some connected speech is usually present that sounds normal.

8. *Speech musculature* includes relevant observations of gross movements of the speech musculature, usually in imitation of the examiner. Is phonation present? Is there evidence of difficulty swallowing? Is the palate elevated on phonation? Are palatal movements equal bilaterally? Can the patient protrude and retract the tongue? Can he elevate the tongue tip? Are lateral tongue movements equal?

9. *Sensorimotor involvement* refers to disruption of learned phonemic patterns in the absence of weakness of the musculature. The patient sometimes behaves as though he did not know where the tongue was in the mouth, or what to do to move it in a given direction or to a given position. Both auditory and proprioceptive feedback and control appear defective. Appropriate tests include repetition of phonetically edited monosyllabic words and repetition of phrases. Diadochokinetic movements are usually impaired initially but often improve as voluntary control is regained. Sensorimotor impairment is correlated with reduction of language throughout the course of recovery. Impairment that can be accounted for by weakness of the musculature is not designated as sensorimotor.

The last three items on the diagnostic scale refer to ability to use language for communication. They are concerned with the patient's ability to use the words and conventional rules that are learned as language is acquired. Occasionally a patient is found who has so much paralysis of the musculature that speech is almost unintelligible, but writing shows language to be intact. Such a patient is dysarthric rather than aphasic.

10. *Word finding* refers to ability to retrieve words from the memory store. Is the patient able to name common objects? Does he confuse words that are related in meaning? Does he frequently grope for words? Is language limited, or generally

vague and imprecise, because vocabulary is limited? With mild word finding difficulty the patient may be able to name common objects, since common words are most resistant to aphasic breakdown, but may not have enough language to explain the use of an object or the meaning of a familiar term.

11. *Functional speech* refers to the ability to communicate in phrases and sentences according to the established conventions of the language. Normal speech contains many abbreviated utterances. The question is, can the patient use connected units of language in spontaneous speech, or does communication repeatedly break down because utterances are fragmentary and incomplete? Are sentences coherent, or does the patient get lost before he has succeeded in communicating the information he intended? One useful test is to ask the patient to produce sentences using given words, since this is something nonaphasic adults are able to do easily (Schuell, 1965).

12. *Functional writing* refers to spontaneous writing and is evaluated in terms of meaningfulness of content and use of acceptable linguistic patterns. The patient may be asked to write sentences using given words, and then to write a short paragraph describing a picture. Can the patient produce sentences in writing? Are sentences usually fragmentary and incomplete? Are sentences coherent? Does the paragraph consist almost exclusively of enumeration of objects? Is writing consistent with the educational or vocational level of the patient?

In using the diagnostic scale, the examiner must make allowances for nonaphasic conditions that may affect performance and, in some cases, make reliable diagnosis impossible. The patient may be too ill to respond. Scores may be depressed by hearing loss, reduction of visual acuity, absence of glasses, or educational deficit. *It should be emphasized that the diagnostic scale designates the nature of the impairment that is observed. A diagnostic rating does not necessarily reflect the level of function in a given language modality.* It is possible, for example, for the diagnostic scale to show no involvement of visual processes, at the same time that reading and writing are almost nonfunctional because of severe reduction of language. The diagnostic scale is an attempt to specify the underlying processes that are impaired, and to document this impairment by appropriate observations.

THE SEVERITY SCALE

Obviously it will also be useful to us to have a way of describing the patient's level of functioning in each common language situation. This descriptive task can be accomplished through the Severity Scale. The Severity Scale presented in this section was initially developed to interpret test findings to individuals to whom scores on the various specific tests were not meaningful. It has since been used to evaluate changes in patients when their pre- and post-tests were not strictly comparable and has been used to compare patients tested in different languages.

The Severity Scale and the Diagnostic Scale complement one another. The Severity Scale estimates the residual function in each common language modality, and the level at which performance breaks down. It indicates what can be expected of the patient at a given time in some natural situation, as well as the functional limitations imposed by aphasia. It is sensitive to differences that occur over time and can be used to report and evaluate progress in therapy. On test–retest rating of 75 aphasic patients (pre- and post-therapy) highly significant differences were observed in each modality rated—auditory comprehension, speech, reading, and writing.

It may be argued that clinical rating scales are notoriously unreliable. This is true when ratings are based on unstructured impressions or intuitions, because these are not reproducable by other examiners who may have different frames of reference. If, however, a scale is used to summarize specifiable test results, and is documented by test findings, a high degree of reliability can be achieved.

Correlations between severity ratings and number of errors made by 157 aphasic patients on corresponding sections of the Minnesota Test were all significantly high (0.86 for auditory ratings, 0.80 for reading, 0.84 for spoken language, and 0.79 for writing). (The scale for dysarthria was not included in the computations, since it was developed later.) These findings indicate that the Severity Scale is a reliable tool for comparing aphasic involvement between subjects and for indicating test–retest differences, when it is used in conjunction with a test that permits adequate documentation of the behavior rated.

It should be emphasized that the Severity Scale designates level of impairment of common language behaviors, but does *not* specify the nature of the observed impairment. It is in no sense diagnostic.

In contrast to the Severity Scale, the Diagnostic Scale indicates the nature and the overall pattern of deficit that underlies the communication impairment observed in an aphasic patient. The Diagnostic Scale remains stable, even with statistically significant changes in severity of aphasia, as indicated by the consistent pattern of errors obtained on each test section on test and retest.

The Severity Scale uses the following categories of communicative behaviors:

	Rating
Auditory comprehension	( )
Reading	( )
Spoken language	( )
Written language	( )
Dysarthria	( )

We have found it possible to use a scale from 0 to 6 within each of the categories except Dysarthria, where we have used cruder groupings. Zero always indicates no observable impairment, and higher numbers indicate progressively more severe disabilities, as indicated by the descriptive statements given below. It is assumed that the statements are scalable, that is, that a patient rated at a particular level can perform the tasks at the higher numbered levels but cannot perform the tasks at levels with lower numbers.

Auditory Comprehension
0   No observable impairment
1   Follows radio program or general discussion with only minimal difficulty

2   Follows ordinary conversation with little difficulty
3   Follows most conversation but sometimes fails to grasp essentials
4   Follows simple conversations but requires repetition
5   Follows brief statements with considerable repetition
6   Usually responds inappropriately because he did not understand

Reading
0   No observable impairment
1   Reads average adult materials with only minimal difficulty
2   Reads paper and short magazine articles
3   Reads simple sentences and simple paragraph materials
4   Reading vocabulary of 100 or more words: reads some phrases and sentences
5   Matches words to pictures and some spoken to printed words
6   No functional reading

Spoken language
0   No observable impairment
1   Converses easily with only occasional difficulty
2   Conversational speech, with mild impairment of formulation or fluency
3   Some conversational speech but marked difficulty expressing long or complex ideas
4   Ready communication with single words and short phrases
5   Expresses needs and wishes in limited or defective manner
6   No functional speech

Written language
0   No observable impairment
1   Can write acceptable letter with only minimal errors
2   Spontaneous writing present with mild impairment of spelling and formulation
3   Can write short, easy sentences spontaneously and to dictation
4   Spelling vocabulary of 100 or more words: can write some phrases and sentences
5   Can write name and a few words to dictation
6   No functional writing

Dysarthria
0   Normal articulation and fluency
1   Minimal impairment: occasional or very mild slurring
2   Mild impairment: mild slurring that does not interfere significantly with intelligibility
3   Moderate impairment: speech is usually intelligible but listener has to follow closely to understand
4   Severe impairment: speech is usually unintelligible

It is readily apparent that the clinician can fill out the Severity Scale without difficulty after observing the patient through the course of the examination. It should also be apparent that such a scale makes a firm base for reports to physicians, nurses, personnel of other medical services, and family with regard to what the patient can and cannot be expected to do at that time. Again, however, it must be emphasized that its major value is just this description; it is not adequate for diagnosis *precisely because* it deals with the surface level of the communication behaviors. If the diagnosis is fortunate and the treatment adequate, the Severity Scale is further convenient in reporting progress and evaluating gains.

SHORT TESTS FOR APPRAISING APHASIA

In our experience there has always been a steady pressure to develop a short examination for aphasia. Some years ago we yielded to the demand and published such an examination by selecting test items from the test battery then being developed for the complete examination (Schuell, 1957). We are now convinced, however, that the development of the short form was a mistake and that arguments for brief examinations are far outweighed by arguments against them.

We argue first that it is irresponsible to try to work with a problem as complex as aphasia without as much information and understanding of what has happened to the patient as can be obtained. The examiner learns a good deal about the patient during the course of the examination. He learns what the patient can do and what he cannot do, what processes are intact and what processes are impaired. He not only learns the maximal level of performance in all language modalities, but a good deal about the underlying sources of the difficulties the patient experiences. He also acquires insight into the patient's feelings, interests, and needs. As a result, he knows what to do, where to begin, and how to work with direction and purpose. This means the patient will make gains from the beginning, and frustration and discouragement will be avoided. The clinician will not waste time on trial-and-error forays that accomplish nothing, perhaps, except alienation of the patient.

The patient is also ready to work after a thorough examination. He has become less anxious and has lost his initial defensiveness. He has found there are some things he can do and others he cannot do. He has learned that this has happened to other people, that something is known about it, that something can be done about it. He has begun to face his limitations and discover his resources. He has confidence in the clinician and is eager and ready to work. Upon conclusion of a successful examination, the patient's attitude tends to be, "Tell me what to do, and I'll do it."

Complete examination also leads to identification of patients who will not recover functional language skills. This prevents fruitless expenditure of resources, of time, and of effort. We shall discuss counseling in such cases in a later chapter.

There is still the objection that patients who are paying for treatment by the hour will object to several sessions spent in testing. Actually they do not, if the reasons for it are explained first, and if they are told there is a set fee for the examination, which is not affected by the amount of time it takes. If the speech pathologist is convinced of the importance of the information to be obtained, it is not difficult to explain its importance to others. In practice, this procedure tends to make clients feel the clinician knows what he is doing and understands the problems. It builds confidence and prepares the way for acceptance of limitations that may have to be accepted.

There are good reasons why a short test for aphasia cannot be completely satisfactory. In the first place, an adequate test must evaluate behavior in all language modalities lest important aspects of aphasic disability be overlooked. If any dimension of aphasic impairment is neglected, misdiagnosis and corresponding errors of prediction may result.

The ability of many aphasic patients to respond appropriately to people, to situations, to visual cues, and to occasional words or phrases often obscures relatively severe impairment of auditory comprehension. If a patient has difficulty producing speech sounds, it is important to know if he can perceive differences between various sound patterns, and this is not usually obvious. Reading and writing may reveal impairment not observable in speech.

In the second place, as we have argued repeatedly, an adequate examination must do more than specify major areas of disability. It must explore aphasic behavior within each language modality to determine why performance breaks down when it does. Reading is often disrupted simply because the patient does not have enough language. One cannot read Sartre, for example, with tourist French. Or reading may break down because verbal retention span is reduced, and the patient cannot hold on to a long-enough string of words to perceive the meaning of a sentence or a paragraph. These are both language disabilities reflected in reading and have nothing to do with the visual system, which is an important diagnostic consideration.

To other aphasic patients, however, the printed page may appear as an array of random ink marks, one indistinguishable from another. Some patients may perceive letters and words, but often fail to discriminate between *b* and *d*, *m* and *w*, or *E* and *F*, for example. Still others have little or no difficulty discriminating letters in isolation, but tend to confuse words in context with words of similar appearance. *Store* may be read as *stone*, *mouth* as *month*, or *house* as *horse*, for example, even when the substitution results in a meaningless sentence. The nature of the impairment underlying a functional deficit, whether in listening, speaking, reading, or writing, is important diagnostic information.

Finally, aphasic impairment covers a wide range of severity in all language modalities. This range necessitates easy tests that make it possible to observe specific behaviors in patients who cannot perform on more difficult tests, and difficult tests for patients who make no errors on easy tests. Between these extremes are patients who pass the easy tests and cannot perform on the difficult tests, but require tests at some intermediate level.

A short examination may cover all language modalities and ask discriminating questions about the nature of observed deficits, and still fail to elicit an adequate sample of aphasic behavior from many patients for whom most of the tests on an abbreviated scale may be too easy or too difficult. To the extent that this occurs, test results will be unreliable.

In summary, an adequate diagnostic test must sample relevant kinds of behavior in all language modalities over the entire range of aphasic deficit. Test reliability is always to some extent a function of test length. Length becomes particularly important when fine differential diagnosis is desired.

These considerations led to the decision not to include a short form on the current revision of the Minnesota Test, but to adopt a different strategy to reduce testing time when it is essential to do so. As an alternative, the use of scaled tests, which permits the examiner to select appropriate items for each patient, is proposed.

As we have seen in the 1965 edition of the *Minnesota Test for Differential Diagnosis of Aphasia,* tests in each language modality have been arranged in order of difficulty determined by the percentage of aphasic subjects failing each test. In other words, tests in each section were scaled for difficulty. The use of scaled tests enables the examiner to shorten testing time by obtaining a baseline and a ceiling for each subject on each test section. This principle has been used in Binet testing for some 60 years, and today many standardized tests employ a similar method.

The procedure we recommend for the Minnesota Test is as follows. Before administering any test section the examiner estimates performance level in the language modality to be explored. He then selects the highest test he thinks the patient can pass and begins with this test. If the patient makes more than one error, the examiner goes back to an easier test until the criterion of not more than one error is met. This is the baseline for the given test section. The examiner than proceeds to administer more difficult tests until the patient has failed 90% of the items on a given test. This is considered the ceiling in the modality tested.

A reasonable estimate of performance level in auditory comprehension and in spoken language can usually be derived from a preliminary interview with the patient. The best guess for performance in reading and writing is that it will approximate the level of speech. When this prediction does not prove true, the discrepancy serves to alert the examiner to begin searching for sources of interference that may affect language modalities differentially.

The method of obtaining a baseline and a ceiling for each patient in each language modality selects the best tests for each patient. Each patient is given only the tests on which he can perform and upon which aphasic disabilities can be observed. A short test is thus obtained without the constraints imposed by arbitrary selection of a limited number of tests, of which only a fraction may be appropriate for any individual patient.

SUMMARY

Reliable tests cannot be obtained from aphasic patients until they are neurophysiologically stable. Aphasic patients make inconsistent responses on individual test items, but percentages of errors and types of errors are remarkable constant.

Tests are not given simply to obtain numerical scores that summarize total errors or even errors grouped by subtests. Tests are employed because they are standarized situations in which we may discover what the patient can and cannot do in a controlled environment, which permits us to discover where and why the patients fail.

Testing need not be traumatic if the examiner is supportive and if the patient knows that the examiner's purpose is to find out what is giving him trouble in order to help him.

An adequate test battery must use tests that cover a wide range of language behavior and a wide range of difficulty in each modality tested. Differential diagnosis is based on observations of performances in the usual language modalities and inferences about the underlying processes involved.

The Diagnostic Scale requires the clinician to review the test performances and record the degree of impairment present in each of 12 functional areas. This requires careful appraisal of comparative performances and inferences about the source of the patient's difficulties.

The Severity Scale summarizes the patient's level of functioning in each common language situation. While it is not diagnostic, it has considerable practical value in describing the patient's current level of linguistic functioning to nonspecialists.

Although the clinician may be urged to dispense with an extensive examination, he should resist such pressures. Time required for comprehensive testing is justified by time saved in treatment. Better results are secured when the clinician knows what he is dealing with and can work with direction and purpose from the beginning. Patients are able to work better because they have become less anxious and have confidence in the examiner. If examinations must be shortened, the Binet method of establishing baselines and ceilings is recommended.

The process of testing is essentially that of asking significant questions under controlled conditions and making pertinent observations. A good test battery helps the examiner to make systematic and thorough observations. It is always good procedure, however, to extend observations beyond the limits imposed by any conventional test. There is no substitute for a thoughtful and insightful examiner.

chapter 9

CLASSIFICATION OF APHASIC PATIENTS

There are several important things to say about classification systems in general. First, there is no right or wrong way to classify phenomena, in the sense that one way is right and all other ways are wrong. A classification system is only a sorting system. On the *Weigl–Goldstein–Scheerer Color–Form Test,* (Goldstein and Scheerer, 1941) for example, it is correct to sort the figures by color, and it is equally correct to sort them by form. Nothing makes one way better than the other. All that is necessary for sorting is a set of rules or identifying criteria that can be applied to all the figures.

Second, a classification system is an abstraction. It does not tell everything about the entities it categorizes. Sorting by color gives no information about form. Cow_1 is not cow_2, but if we had to take full account of individual uniqueness we could not talk about cows at all.

A classification system is an attempt to abstract dimensions that are meaningful and useful in dealing with complex processes or events. It is valid to classify aphasic patients according to criteria based on age, etiology, total test scores, linguistic characteristics of their speech, or any other observable differences between subjects. Indeed, at some times, and for some purposes, we might select any one of these methods. The choice of method depends on what we want to know, and what we want to be able to say about aphasia.

It would seem that two important things to know about any aphasic patient are first, what is interfering with communication, and second, what the outcome is going to be. In other words, the most useful kind of a classification system would be descriptive and predictive. Theoretically it would provide classes for all the aphasic disorders that have been observed or may be observed in the future. In this sense it would constitute a very complete and precise description of aphasia.

We have rejected the three-way relay systems for classification of aphasia because they are incompatible with what is known about cerebral function and with clinical data. We have also rejected systems based on an expressive–receptive dichotomy, because we believe that no such dichotomy exists. If there is always some expressive and some receptive component in aphasia, as our data indicate, these are wastebasket terms. A similar objection can be made for classes such as amnesic and syntactical aphasia. These are not mutually exclusive categories, and so do not offer a meaningful basis for classification.

We hold the view that a general classification system for aphasia must be based on comprehensive observations of large numbers of aphasic subjects over long periods of time. Longitudinal studies are needed to determine which symptoms are transient, which are persistent, and which are interrelated. The most obvious presenting symptom is not a good basis for classification, because symptoms change. There can be no stable classification system without long-term studies of large numbers of individual patients.

SEVEN DIAGNOSTIC CATEGORIES OF APHASIA

The classification system we have evolved is an empirical one, based on test and retest findings obtained from a large series of aphasic subjects studied intensively throughout the recovery period. Essentially we followed Hughlings Jackson's (1888) dictum that the clinical observations must come first and generalizations afterwards.

The categories themselves are based on recurring patterns of impairment identified by successive analyses of test data obtained on various experimental forms of Schuell's *Minnesota Test*. Since classification is determined by overall pattern of deficit rather than by severity alone, this has proved to be a remarkably constant system. The same general patterns appear on final as on initial testing, if patients are neurologically stable when examined. If one tests to limits, the same elements can be detected as long as residual impairment remains.

The classification system has predictive value. The patterns have been studied systematically enough to make it possible to see the end in the beginning. We know how patients in all the major categories looked when they were acutely ill, and we know that only limited predictions can be made from such behaviors. Sometimes the only hopeful thing one could say about a patient was that time was in his favor, and sometimes, though not always, time was enough. We know what changes came about day by day and week by week when patients were receiving intensive treatment in the clinic. We know what some patients in each category were like five or even 10 years later when they returned to the hospital as patients or visitors, or we looked them up in other parts of the country.

As long as we have classified aphasic patients we have included prognosis in the initial

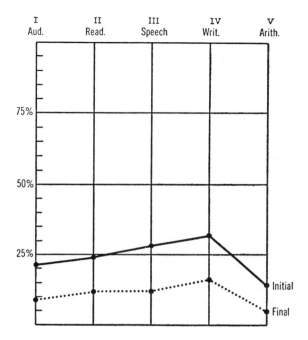

Fig. 9–1. Mean percentage of test-retest errors over modalities: Simple Aphasia (N 17).

case summary, and placed this in the medical record on completion of the admission examination. At first, this was frankly experimental procedure, but gradually we have come to have confidence in initial test results. We are still using the five diagnostic categories we reported in 1955, although we have changed the ordering of the groups to effect a more logical structure and have added two categories that have recurred from time to time in the population we have studied.

The seven major categories are as follows:

Simple aphasia.

Available language is reduced in all modalities, with no specific perceptual or sensorimotor involvement and no dysarthria. Prognosis for recovery from aphasia is excellent. Most simple aphasic subjects resume former occupations.

Aphasia with visual involvement.

Reduction of language is complicated by impaired discrimination, recognition, and recall of visual patterns used in reading and writing. The prognosis for recovery of language is excellent, as in Simple Aphasia. Reading and writing recover more slowly. Patients approximate former performance level, but rate tends to remain retarded and occasional inconsistent errors tend to persist.

Aphasia with persisting dysfluency.

These patients have only a mild language impairment, except for the presence of dysfluency. The prognosis for recovery from aphasia is excellent. Excellent articulation may be achieved, but conscious control must be exercised. Articulation continues to disintegrate whenever control is relaxed. The extent to which control is exercised after it is achieved varies from patient to patient and appears to be related to personality traits.

Aphasia with scattered findings.

These patients show moderate aphasia with additional impairment which is compatible with generalized or scattered brain damage. Some functional language is retained in speech or writing or both. Some visual findings and some dysarthria are usually present, although one system is often more severely involved than the other. Spatial perception may or may not be disturbed. Emotional lability is often present. Aphasics with scattered findings tend to have many physiological complaints, and personality changes sometimes occur. Patients sometimes work well when the clinician is present, and achieve more language or improved intelligibility, but tend to be incapable of consistent effort. Prognosis for recovery tends to be limited more by physiological and psychological status than by severity of aphasia.

Aphasia with sensorimotor (somatosensory) involvement.

Sensorimotor patients show severe reduction of vocabulary and verbal retention span in all language modalities, complicated by impaired perception and production of phonemic patterns. The prognosis is for limited but functional recovery of language. Patients learn to communicate through intellible speech, usually common words and phrases, and later short sentences, but language continues to break down when longer or more complex responses are required. Normal articulation is usually achieved for common words and short language units, but continues to break down when longer sequences are attempted.

Aphasia with intermittent auditory imperception.

This syndrome is characterized by severe involvement of auditory processes, usually with some functional, normal speech present or recovered early. Patients frequently behave as though they were deaf. Early attempts at repetition may result in jargon. Although appropriate utterances may occur, patients have difficulty naming objects and expressing specific ideas. Reading and writing mirror language impairment. Patients often improve remarkably but do not achieve normal language functions.

Irreversible aphasia syndrome.

Irreversible aphasic subjects show almost complete loss of functional language skills in all modalities. They have difficulty pointing to common words named by the examiner and following simple directions. They cannot name common objects or give simple biographical information. They can sometimes match common words to pictures, but reading is nonfunctional. They sometimes learn to copy and to write their names, but are unable to write simple words to dictation. They sometimes learn to repeat and to count. Some reactive speech usually emerges, but it does not become voluntary or functional.

It should be emphasized that neither the classification of subjects nor the prediction of outcome is reliable unless patients are neurologically stable when examined. The first three diagnostic categories usually show "mild" aphasia. Patients in these groups are more successful on language tests *on the average* than a nonselected group of aphasic patients. Individuals may display aphasia that is so slight that it is found only on the most difficult tests in the battery, or they may show aphasia that is so severe that the patient can do little more than cope with single words. In general, however, patients in these groups demonstrate their characteristic patterns with a mild aphasia. Patients in the remaining categories show "moderate" to "severe" aphasia. Their scores on language tests cluster around or fall below the mean for a nonselected group of aphasic patients. Table 9–1 summarizes the various classification system in use. It should be obvious from the table that different classifications are used for different purposes and change radically with different approaches to aphasia.

TABLE 9-1. Classification Systems

Schuell	*Wepman (1951)*	*Popular Eclectic Terminology*	*Luria (1966)*
Based on patterns of impairment. (Stable over time)	**Based on verbal output at a given point in recovery. (Changes over time)**	**Based on classical localization**	**Based on cortical divisions and functional systems or analyzers.**
Simple aphasia	Semantic or syntactic (depends on severity)	Anomic aphasia	Semantic aphasia
Aphasia with visual processes impairment	Semantic or syntactic (depends on severity)	Anomic aphasia	Amnestic aphasia with optic alexia
Aphasia with persisting dysfluency	Expressive apraxia	Broca's aphasia	Efferent (kinetic) motor aphasia
Aphasia with scattered findings		Conduction aphasia	Generalized organic defects
Aphasia with intermittent auditory imperception	Jargon	Wernicke's aphasia	Sensory (acoustic) aphasia
Aphasia with sensorimotor (somatosensory) impairment	Expressive apraxia	Broca's aphasia	Afferent (kinesthetic) motor aphasia
Irreversible aphasia	Global	Global	

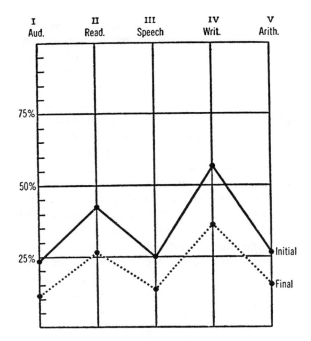

Fig. 9–2. Mean percentage of test-retest errors over modalities: Aphasia with Visual Involvement (N 16).

While aphasic populations drawn in any clinic constitute specially restricted groups and it is difficult to generalize results, the classification system presented here seems to be nearly exhaustive. In 1961 Schuell and Jenkins estimated that 90% of their aphasic patients could be classified in one of the five major diagnostic categories then in use. In the study presented in the first edition of this book, 96% of the patients were reliably classified. Using the published form of Schuell's *Minnesota Test* with seven diagnostic groups, 73 out of 75 patients were classified in our most recent analysis.

In 1969 the results of a study comparing Japanese and Minnesota subjects was reported (Schuell and Nagae, 1969). Using the Diagnostic Scale, 15 Minnesota and 15 Japanese subjects were independently classified into the seven categories by the two investigators. There was only one case of disagreement in classification for the 30 subjects.

Figures 9–1 through 9–7 show test–retest profiles for each of the diagnostic categories. The curves represent the mean percentage of errors for each group of subjects over five sections of the *Minnesota Test*, before and after treatment for aphasia. Table 8–2 shows test–retest correlations. Table 4 in Appendix 2 shows the means and standard deviations for each test section by diagnostic groups, and Table 5 in Appendix 2 presents the data shown graphically in the figures. Here mean percentages of error were calculated to make it possible to compare performances over test sections.

The most important observations to be made about the figures are the distinctiveness of each of the seven patterns, and the general consistency of test–retest results. The

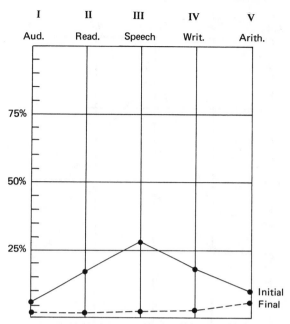

Fig. 9–3. Mean percentage of test-retest errors over modalities: Aphasia with Persisting Dysfluency (N 4).

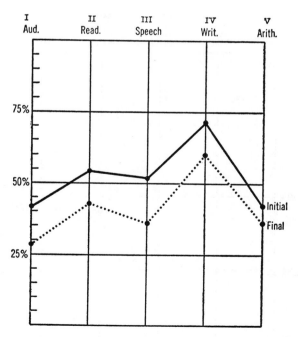

Fig. 9–4. Mean percentage of test-retest errors over modalities: Aphasia with Scattered Findings (N 22).

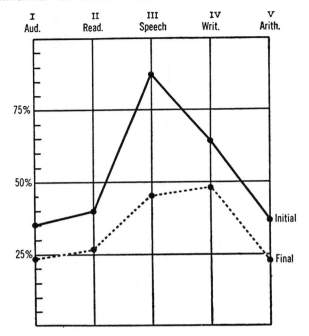

Fig. 9–5. Mean percentage of test-retest errors over modalities: Aphasia with Sensorimotor Involvement (N 10).

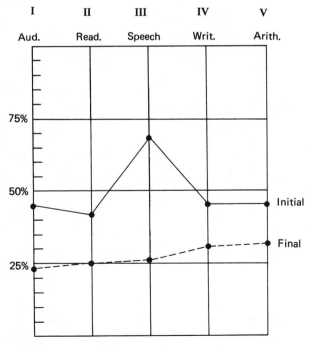

Fig. 9–6. Mean percentage of test-retest errors over modalities: Aphasia with Intermittent Auditory Imperception (N 12).

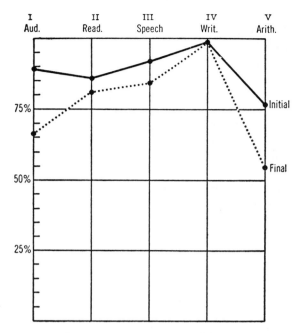

Fig. 9–7. Mean percentage of test-retest errors over modalities: Irreversible Aphasia (N 4).

distinctiveness of the curves is evidence that pattern of impairment, and not severity alone, is operating. The general consistency of test–retest results indicates the stability of patterns over periods of time, in spite of statistically significant changes in severity of symptoms.

TEST–RETEST DIFFERENCES

As the test–retest profiles suggest, there was significant improvement on almost all tests during the course of therapy. Statistical tests confirmed the reliability of such changes over the entire group of patients. Given this general improvement, it is especially interesting and instructive to look at the tests that did *not* show improvement.

Among the tests for auditory comprehension, only the test for recognition of common words failed to show improvement. This confirms our earlier finding that language deficit at this level tends to be irreversible. Most aphasic patients pass all of the items on this test even when first tested. Failure of items, therefore, is of considerable diagnostic importance and is not ordinarily correctible (except in the case of some patients with intermittent auditory imperception).

Patients showed significant improvement on most visual and reading tests. The exceptions were patients who reported subjective visual complaints and patients who made errors in matching forms and letters. Errors at this level were characteristic of patients with irreversible impairment of visual processes.

Improvement was significant on all speech and language tests except those involving gross movements of the tongue, jaw, palate, and pharynx. Errors on these tests reflected irreversible weakness of the musculature.

Patients showed significant improvement on all writing tests except copying forms and Greek letters. Similarly, there was improvement on all arithmetic tests except for simple numerical combinations (specifically multiplication). Failure of these simple tests probably reflects spatial disorientation found in a small proportion of the population. Patients with even mild impairment of perception of spatial relations usually have difficulty multiplying by more than one digit. They set the products down in such an inconsistent manner that it is impossible to deal with the array in the final addition.

We have indicated that aphasic patients failed to show improvement on a small number of tests because of severe impairment that was modality specific. These were tests that were easy for a majority of patients; thus, failure indicated either very severe aphasia or specific impairment in the modality examined. In either case, improvement is unlikely.

While we have here stressed the differences that result with therapy for specific

TABLE 9-2
Diagnostic Scale Values for Categories of Aphasia*

Functional Category	Simple Aphasia	Visual	Dys-fluency	Scattered Findings	Sensori-motor	Auditory	Irrever-sible
Auditory discrimination	0	0	0	1	1	2−3	3
Auditory recognition	0	0	0	1	2	2−3	3
Auditory retention span	2	2	1	2	3	2−3	3
Visual discrimination	0	1−3	0	1−3	0	0	0−3
Visual recognition	0	1−3	0	1−3	0	0	0−3
Visual recall	0	1−3	0	1−3	0	0	0−3
Spatial orientation	0	0−3	0	1−3	0	0	0−3
Motor involvement of speech musculature	0	0	0	1−3	0	0	0−3
Sensorimotor involvement of speech musculature	0	0	2	0	3	0	0−3
Word finding*	1−2	1−2	1	1−2	3	2−3	3
Functional speech*	1−2	1−2	1−2	1−3	3	2−3	3
Functional Writing*	1−2	1−2	1	1−3	3	2−3	3

* All aphasic patients
Note: 0 means no impairment; 1 means mild impairment; 2 means moderate impairment; 3 means severe impairment.

groups, we must again emphasize the fact that the *patterns* of test performance are stable from beginning to end of therapy, as demonstrated by the test–retest correlations for the various sections of the test battery given in Chapter 8. The test–retest correlations are highly satisfactory, especially considering that differences as a result of therapy occur in the interval between testings. The relatively low correlation between test and retest scores on the speech section of the test for the small sample of patients can be explained on the basis of the remarkable recovery in many speech and language tasks for Auditory patients and those with Dysfluency (the two categories that make up this sample). Although Auditory patients continue to make errors based on inadequate auditory information, they usually recover to a point where repetition is easy for them. The Dysfluency patients continue to have difficulty in spontaneous speech and must exert conscious control, but their performance on speech tests is nearly without error after treatment.

DIAGNOSTIC SCALE

It must be realized that while the test profiles for the group are both impressively different and impressively stable, they are not in themselves the most powerful form of arranging the data. As we argued in the previous chapter, the clinician can get even more impressive separation and consistency by using the Diagnostic Scale. In making the diagnostic ratings, the clinician uses all the data from the testing situation to make inferences about the disruption of processes. It is these inferences, then, that are arrayed in the Diagnostic Scale.

For ease in assigning patients to categories, the typical patterns seen in each category are given in Table 9–2. You will notice that this simply gives in tabular form the material which we are elaborating in the text. The Diagnostic Scale makes a convenient and powerful way to summarize the relevant data for classification and comparison of cases. This scale is put forth with the caution that no figures are absolute. There will be exceptions in diagnosing patients. All aphasics have a reduction of auditory retention span and word finding. All aphasics have some reduction of functional speech and writing. Complicating conditions vary in severity. Aphasia alone will depress function in all modalities; the Diagnostic Scale is used to identify impairment of processes in a particular way, over and above the aphasia involved. Ratings should be well documented by evidence from specific subtests.

SIMPLE APHASIA

Figure 9–1 shows that these subjects presented relatively mild aphasia in comparison with subjects in other diagnostic categories. The percentage of error was slightly higher on tests for speech and writing, which required generation of language, than on tests for auditory comprehension and reading, which required analysis of stimuli presented to the patient. One could reasonably ask if this pattern resulted from differences in the difficulty of items on the major test sections. We do not think this is the explanation. Profiles for Simple Aphasic and Dysfluent patients tended to flatten a little on retest, making the pattern a little less marked as recovery occurred. Visual and Scattered Findings patients and nonaphasic subjects all made a larger percentage of error on reading and writing tests than on tests for auditory comprehension or speech. The more tenable hypothesis seems to be that the principal sources of variance reflected in the profiles were in the population rather than in the tests.

On the other hand, the relatively low percentage of errors on tests of numerical relations and arithmetic processes was found in all diagnostic groups, and probably does indicate that these were relatively easy tests. Tests were confined to basic operations in addition, subtraction, multiplication, and division to avoid overlap with performance of nonaphasic subjects. Problems involved carrying, borrowing, multiplying by three digits, and long division, however. We included fractions and decimals on earlier test forms, but found such a high correlation with educational level that we dropped these items, preferring to use supplementary tests when necessary.

We have observed that aphasic patients often improve in arithmetic skills without specific training, as more language becomes available. Initially they tend to confuse names of numbers, as well as names of things. The most common confusions are between words with strong associational linkages, which numbers present. In addition, aphasic patients frequently have difficulty recalling learned combinations, such as $6 + 7 = 13$, or $8 \times 9 = 72$.

It is obvious that retests profiles, even for Simple Aphasic subjects, do not show complete recovery from aphasia. Patients in all diagnostic groups were usually discharged from the hospital when we felt they had acquired a solid basis of language skills on which to build. This will be discussed further in later chapters.

APHASIA WITH VISUAL INVOLVEMENT

Figure 9–2 shows that these patients could not be distinguished from subjects in the Simple Aphasic group by performance on tests for auditory comprehension or tests for speech and language. Differences between means were not significant, nor was there anything clinically observable that would enable a listener to discriminate patients in one group from patients in the other.

Profiles for Visual patients are distinguished by sharp error peaks on reading and writing tests. These peaks reflect the difficulties Visual subjects had with discrimination, recognition, and recall of learned visual symbols.

On reading and writing tests, differences between means obtained by Simple Aphasic and Visual subjects were significant on both initial and final testing. We surmise that writing tests are more discriminating than reading tests for two reasons: First, there seems to be a tendency for aphasic patients to make more errors on tests that require subjects to generate responses, and this provides a larger sample of differential behavior to observe and analyze. Second, all writing errors are observable. On tests for reading comprehension, on the other hand, it is possible to misread occasional letters and words and still grasp the general meaning and respond correctly, because of the redundancy of language.

Both Simple Aphasic and Visual subjects improved in arithmetic between initial and final testing. However, Visual subjects continued to misread and miswrite numbers. They tended to omit digits, and to confuse numerals such as *6* and *9*, *3* and *5*, or *3* and *8*. Since this type of error was rarely found in the Simple Aphasic group, it is understandable that the two groups should separate more widely as linguistic errors decreased.

APHASIA WITH PERSISTING DYSFLUENCY

The profiles for the Dysfluency group in Fig. 9–3 show an aphasia which is extremely mild. When first examined, these patients appeared much like the Simple Aphasics, except that speech was hesitant and labored and there were many articulatory errors. We have never been able to demonstrate any unequivocal weakness of the speech musculature in these patients. Of the seven studied intensively, one had mild weakness of the tongue initially, one had slight deviation to the right on protrusion, and none of the remaining five had any weakness of the tongue. Two had reduced gag reflex, while one showed assymetry of the palate while vocalizing. These findings do not account for the extreme difficulty in articulation these patients encountered. As recovery takes place, these patients learn to control articulation and learn to repeat short units as well. This accounts for the reduction of speech errors in the retest profile. Dysfluent patients usually recover almost completely from the reduction of language they show initially. Brief utterances often sound normal, but articulation continues to disintegrate in connected speech, unless they speak slowly and exert conscious control. Some of these patients are unwilling to make the continuous effort required for clear articulation when it fails to become automatic. Without continuous effort, these patients tend to talk fluently but much less intelligibly.

In our early studies, Dysfluent patients were considered mild Sensorimotor patients, but further study makes this untenable. For one thing, auditory stimulation helps the Dysfluent patient to increase vocabulary and retention span, but does not improve articulation as it does with Sensorimotor patients. Phoneme discrimination is good in these patients. When one listens carefully to the pattern of speech, it often appears that the patients are self-correcting by ear as they speak. This causes some of them to sound much like stutterers, with hesitations and easy repetitions as they continually test articulatory placement. If Sensorimotor patients lack proprioceptive and auditory feedback, Dysfluent patients seem only to lack the proprioceptive feedback which enables them continually to correct by ear.

What helps the Dysfluents most is facilitation by means of strong rhythmic drill on consonants and consonant blends, first in nonsense syllables, then in various positions and combinations, then in words, phrases, and sentences. These patients never sound completely normal, and must always exert control of the speech musculature.

Schuell surmised earlier that this pattern of impairment may result from lesions in the frontal area that involved descending tracts. All seven patients studied in this series had frontal lesions. This evidence indicates that the syndrome of Persisting Dysfluency, rather than the one presented by the unhappy Tan, should be considered Broca's Aphasia.

APHASIA WITH SCATTERED FINDINGS, USUALLY INCLUDING BOTH VISUAL INVOLVEMENT AND DYSARTHRIA

These profiles show error peaks on reading and writing tests, reflecting cerebral involvement of visual processes. Sometimes the error patterns found on these tests were indistinguishable from those found in the Visual group. Sometimes performances showed only a general blunting of visual discrimination, rather than the specific confusions characteristic of Visual patients' performances. The overall effect was one of carelessness or, more precisely, inattentiveness to visual detail. Sometimes spatial disorientation was present, also, and patients had trouble keeping the place and following the line in reading, and produced gross distortions on copying and drawing tests. Such symptoms are often accompaniments of right-hemisphere brain damage.

Profiles for these patients differed from Visual profiles in showing an elevated percentage of errors on speech and language, as well as on reading and writing tests. Sometimes there was general slurring of speech, resulting perhaps from mild weakness that prevented precise movements and firm contacts. Sometimes there was paralysis of the tongue or soft palate, usually accompanied by weakness of the pharyngeal musculature with attendant difficulty swallowing. In severe cases, the larynx was also involved, as well as the muscles of respiration. In traumatic cases, particularly, we sometimes found speech similar to that observed in spastic paralysis, and occasionally we found other forms of dysarthria as well.

Sometimes the visual involvement was mild and the motor involvement severe, and sometimes the opposite was true. Thus, these subjects frequently presented clinical pictures with little resemblance to one another. The differentiating criteria are, first, the presence of some residual functional language in one modality or another, and second, scattered test findings compatible with bilateral or generalized brain damage.

Both visual and motor processes were almost always involved. Involvement of both processes was, in fact, the initial differentiating criterion, and it is still a sound one. However, we have occasionally classified an aphasic patient in this group when involvement of one process or the other might appear questionable, if test behavior clearly indicated generalized brain damage. Among such signs are impairment of recent memory, differentiated from aphasic reduction of language, generalized confusion, and persistent and severe emotional lability. These signs were not, however, found in all Scattered Findings subjects.

APHASIA WITH SENSORIMOTOR INVOLVEMENT

The profiles for Sensorimotor patients are shown in Figure 9–5. Initially, this group was contaminated by inclusion of patients with mild, as well as patients with severe, reduction of language. In the test–retest series, 10 patients showed the severe reduction of language we usually associate with sensorimotor involvement. Four patients showed mild though clearcut aphasic impairment, together with persisting disturbance in control of movement patterns required for speech, with no demonstrable weakness of the musculature.

It seemed reasonable at first to regard these four subjects as milder examples of the basic syndrome, representing perhaps the lower end of a continuum of severity. We have now seen enough of these patients to accumulate a reliable body of data, and further study of individual subjects has led to a revision of the earlier concept. We now consider this to be the Persisting Dysfluency syndrome. We have redefined the Sensorimotor group to include only those patients with severe reduction of language in all modalities, as well as a sensorimotor deficit. Figure 9–5 is the profile obtained from the 10 patients considered to form a homogeneous group.

For subjects in the Sensorimotor group, as redefined, auditory comprehension was generally good within the limits of observed retention span, but this span was very short. Reading and writing were severely impaired by reduction of language, but subjects utilized visual cues effectively. Visual discrimination, visual recognition, and recall of learned visual symbols were more intact than similar auditory processes. For example, these subjects made fewer errors matching printed words to pictures than matching printed to spoken words. They usually learned to write a list of words to dictation, with all the silent letters intact, before they could evoke the same words to name pictures.

The discrepancy between test–retest profiles for the Sensorimotor group is more apparent than real. The sharp peak of errors on speech and language tests found on initial examination tended to flatten somewhat, as soon as the speech mechanism began to function. On initial testing, these subjects frequently had great difficulty repeating single monosyllabic words. This was in fact one of the most discriminating tests for this group. On final testing, difficulty producing speech tended to appear only on longer responses, although reduction of available language continued to be reflected on both speech and language tests.

APHASIA WITH INTERMITTENT AUDITORY IMPERCEPTION

The profiles for intermittent auditory imperception in Figure 9–6 show a very severe aphasia. The peaks in errors in initial testing are evident in the auditory tests and in the speech and language tests. Our factor analysis did not show an auditory factor, but the Japanese factor analysis did. In our sample, auditory tests showed a meaningful loading on the language factor. This is further supported by the high error percentage in speech tests in this group. These patients have difficulty finding the auditory pattern for the words they want to say. Because language itself is so highly dependent on auditory integrations, impairment in the auditory system is usually not confined to one modality.

Some of these patients are able to read aloud without error, but when asked if they know what they read, admit that the words had no meaning for them. One patient, when asked if he knew what "paper" was after he had read the sentence *The paper is here*, said, "No, I don't believe I do." After a long explanation, he said, "Oh, yes, we have a boy who fetches that up to our house every night!" Most Auditory patients do not speak as well as that patient did, but most have flowing jargon or overlearned phrases which sound almost normal. The retest profile shows that the errors in auditory comprehension are fewer as the patients learn to listen again.

The difference between Auditory patients and the group of patients who show a simple reduction of language is more than one of severity. These patients have an auditory imperception that is intermittent. When asked to respond to spoken words by pointing to pictures, these patients clearly demonstrate an on–off phenomenon. They will correctly point to two, three, or four pictures, then will miss three to five in a row, then begin to respond correctly again. It is almost as if a switch is being turned on and off.

Auditory patients often show severe aphasic impairment, together with apparent disturbance in control of movement patterns required for speech, with no demonstrable weakness of the musculature. These patients were at first considered to be Sensorimotor patients because of the struggle pattern of speech movements. When connected speech appeared early, together with jargon, these patients were no longer considered to have sensorimotor impairment, and it became apparent that the struggle was due to the difficulty the patient was having with auditory patterns. As available language increases, the labored speech, articulatory inaccuracies, and jargon responses gradually decrease and disappear. In intermediate stages of recovery, utterances tend to show restricted vocabulary and little variety of syntactic structure, but usually sound normal. At no time in the course of recovery is spontaneous speech limited to single-word utterances; nor do "telegraphic" utterances, in which words without referents are characteristically omitted, occur in spontaneous speech.

The aphasia, or reduction of available vocabulary and verbal retention span, is reversible, but these patients will always need to have words and sentences repeated to them.

AN IRREVERSIBLE APHASIC SYNDROME

Profiles for Irreversible aphasics reflected severe impairment, amounting to almost complete loss of functional language skills in all modalities. The profiles in Figure 9–7 represent test–retest profiles for four subjects who received intensive treatment, because in each case some aspect of language appeared a little more intact on initial examination than is usual in this syndrome. Although the signs that led us to question the diagnosis were minimal, we followed the clinical practice of giving the patient the benefit of the flicker of doubt they engendered. In this sense these are not typical profiles.

Final testing showed a significant reduction of errors on tests for auditory comprehension, although an average of 67% of items were still missed. Our experience has been that these patients tend to lose these gains when intensive auditory stimulation is discontinued. On reading tests there was no performance beyond chance except on matching printed words to pictures, and matching a few printed to spoken words. On speech and language tests, all four patients passed some items on final testing that involved repetition, counting, and naming the days of the week in serial order and produced some high-frequency associative responses. On writing tests, patients succeeded in writing a few numerals and letters, and one patient wrote the word *boy* to dictation. This was the highest performance obtained. No patient achieved functional speech, reading, or writing. This is a consistent finding. We are therefore forced to the conclusion that there is a degree of cerebral damage that is incompatible with recovery of functional language skills.

MEDICAL FINDINGS, HOSPITAL COURSE, AND OUTCOME

Tables 2 through 5 in the Appendix summarize data obtained from analysis of medical records of aphasic subjects initially classified in the seven diagnostic groups we have just described. We shall review these findings briefly in this chapter, and discuss them in more detail when we talk about the subjects in individual diagnostic groups in ensuing chapters.

Neurological findings for subjects with Simple and Visual Aphasia were generally mild, as predicted, and are considered compatible with limited and circumscribed brain damage. Simple Aphasics diverged from Visual Aphasics in only two respects: The incidence of visual field defects was significantly higher in the Visual subjects, and there was a higher incidence of sensory reduction. More data are needed to determine whether or not the latter is a true difference. Neurological findings for Simple Aphasic and Visual groups were consistent with the observed language deficit and with the additional visual involvement found in Visual patients, which can only be accounted for by a difference in locus or extent of the lesion.

It should be noted that the presence of visual field defects does not necessarily result in impairment of perceptual discrimination. The two findings frequently, but not invariably, coexisted.

Dysfluency patients also had neurological findings compatible with limited and circumscribed brain damage, but these patients diverged from the Simple and Visual Aphasics on four neurological findings. They had a significantly lower incidence of cerebrovascular accidents as etiology, and of sensory reduction, and they had a significantly higher incidence of facial paralysis and focal EEG findings.

Results for Scattered Findings patients confirmed previous impressions of generalized or bilateral brain damage and the presence of many adverse physiological and psychological conditions that imposed limitations upon recovery. Neurological findings were compatible with the generally scattered aphasic findings. Involvement of language, as well as involvement of extremities, was frequently much milder than in Sensorimotor patients, but drive toward recovery and capacity for intensive and persistent effort was always diminished to some extent, and this was usually a limiting factor.

Sensorimotor patients showed almost as severe neurological damage as the Irreversible subjects, but without the high incidence of complicating neurophysiological conditions found in the Scattered Findings and Irreversible groups. The authors postulate a sizable lesion with the remainder of the brain relatively intact and overall physiological conditions generally favorable. This would account for the excellent response to rehabilitation, within the limits of the irreversible damage incurred, which characterized Sensorimotor subjects. With the use of the left hand, and a brace on the right leg, Sensorimotor subjects achieved physical independence. With limited and effortful speech, they became communicating and useful individuals, and some of them achieved gainful employment. It is important to note that without examination, many Sensorimotor subjects were initially indistinguishable from Irreversible subjects.

Auditory patients had a significantly higher incidence of complete thrombosis of the internal carotid or middle cerebral artery than any group except the Sensorimotor or Irreversible subjects. On the other hand, these patients had a significantly lower incidence of paralysis or paresis of the extremities and of sensory reduction. With the exception of the Visual group, they had a significantly higher incidence of visual field defects than any other classification. In spite of the fact that Auditory patients had a low incidence of paralysis or paresis, they showed, along with the Scattered Findings group, a significantly higher incidence of bilateral neurological signs.

Irreversible subjects showed the most severe neurological damage of all diagnostic groups and a significantly high incidence of neurophysiological complications. In general these findings are compatible with large focal lesions, although further brain damage is by no means ruled out.

We conclude that these data support the hypothesis that differences between aphasic subjects in the major diagnostic categories reported are true differences, related to locus and extent of brain damage and incidence of complicating neurophysiological conditions, as well as to obtained patterns of aphasic impairment.

Finally, we should like to point out that the classification system described is a relatively simple and logical one from the viewpoint of language behavior and functional cerebral systems. Most investigators who are aware of the infinite complexity of language and the hypothetical nature of theory related to cerebral mechanisms subserving complex behaviors are advisedly cautious about relating clinical data to localization. Although aphasia is an extremely sensitive indicator of brain damage, probably at present the chief value of aphasic findings to the neurosurgeon is that positive findings indicating the presence or extension of a lesion often appear before other neurological signs are present. To the clinical neurologist, however, knowledge of aphasic syndromes and the expected course of recovery is of considerable importance in the management of brain-injured patients. Language is a unique human attribute, and one should neither assume that nothing can be done when communication processes are disturbed, or that all aphasic patients can recover normal language skills.

CATEGORIES OF APHASIA

PREFACE TO PART IV

In Chapters 5 and 6 we saw how the process of communication could be represented in terms of a functional schema which specified the complex interaction of various cognitive, effector, and receptor components. We argued that the primary symptoms for a wide range of communication disorders might be explained as the failure of specific functional components to provide necessary support for the normal communication process. We sketched the way the schema could be used to distinguish the primary symptoms of aphasia from those of other communication disorders which sometimes resemble aphasia due to overlapping symptomatologies.

A further test of the heuristic value of the schema is the extent to which it can be used to differentiate among the different types of aphasia. In other words, in order for the schema to be descriptively adequate for diagnostic purposes, it must be sufficiently precise not only to distinguish aphasia from other communication disorders but also to capture the often subtle distinctions among the seven categories of aphasia discussed above. With reference to the functional schema, we defined aphasia as an impairment of the ability to formulate propositions in the symbolic mode, rather than as a disorder of need states, intents, intellectual competence, or the processes effecting the instantiation of communiques. This means that each of the seven categories of aphasia shares a set of primary symptoms as indicated in Fig. 10–0 below.

Since the primary symptoms of aphasia arise due to impairment of the ability to formulate propositions in the symbolic mode of cognition, this component is designated as the source of fault propagation. In the following chapters each of the seven categories

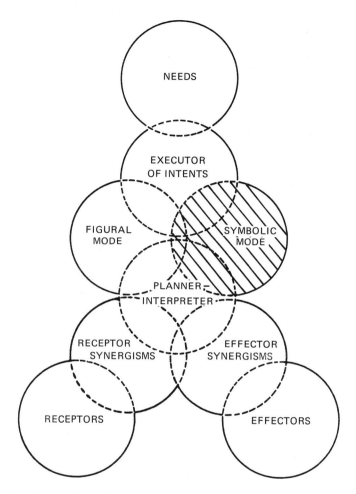

Fig. 10–0. Functional schema for aphasia.

of aphasia will be represented similarly by designating those components of the functional schema for communication which are most likely involved in producing the symptoms of the disorder. The root designation for each of the categories of aphasia is the same as that for simple aphasia, since this constellation of symptoms represents the primary characteristics of the disorder.

In addition to this root designation, each category of aphasia, beyond the simple type, possesses its own unique configuration of dysfunctioning components in the schema.

Part IV of this book devotes a full chapter to the detailed discussion of the symptomatology of each of the seven categories of aphasia. The fact that each of the seven types of aphasic disorders consists of a complex cluster of symptoms with a common core lends credence to the claim made earlier in Chapter 5 that aphasia, although not at all simple, is a unitary disorder.

chapter 10

SIMPLE APHASIA

Bill Masterson, a young man of superior intelligence, left college to enlist after Pearl Harbor, and spent the last years of the war in the European Theater. Within three years after the war he had completed a course in business administration and was selected for the executive training program of a large corporation. By this time Bill was married, had a young son, and was buying a house in a pleasant suburban community.

A few days before his second son was born, Bill complained of a headache and a stiff neck that grew progressively worse for several days. Bill finally went to the hospital for diagnostic tests, which showed evidence of cerebral bleeding. An angiogram revealed an arteriovenus malformation in the left posterior parietal region. During the subsequent surgery two ruptured vessels were seen in the malformation. The large vessels seen by angiography were not exposed, but four lesser vessels were clipped. After the operation Bill was aphasic, and the right side of his body was paralyzed. The aphasia subsided in the course of a few weeks, and the paralysis improved to the extent that Bill could walk with a brace and a cane. Nine months later he went back to work.

Fourteen months after the initial onset Bill incurred a second subarachnoid hemorrhage. It began with a nagging headache, followed several hours later by abrupt occurrence of aphasia. Bill knew what was happening and dialed the clinic. By the time a doctor reached the telephone, Bill could not talk. Fortunately, one of his colleagues completed the call, and Bill went back to the hospital. This time studies showed that an aneurysm had ruptured. The neurosurgeon decided to ligate the left common carotid artery to reduce the probability of further bleeding.

A few months later, when Bill was having a routine medical examination, well-advanced pulmonary tuberculosis was found. Bill spent the next 18 months in a hospital that specialized in treatment of pulmonary disease. He was still hemiplegic and aphasic. He had further surgery, this time a partial pneumectomy involving removal of four ribs and the lingular and part of the superior division of the superior lobe of the left lung.

By this time Bill's third son had been born, and since the material resources of the family were nearly exhausted, Bill's wife was forced to sell their house and move back to her parents' home with the three children.

Eighteen months later, when the tuberculosis was arrested, Bill was transferred to the Minneapolis VA Hospital for treatment of aphasia. Though he was almost 34 years old, and tired of hospitals, he was unwilling to settle for the limited amount of language that had returned in 22 months.

INITIAL FINDINGS

On auditory tests, word recognition was superior, but verbal retention span was seriously impaired. Bill scored at the 95th percentile for adults on the Ammons *Full-Range Picture Vocabulary Test.* This reassured and encouraged him. He could follow oral directions, but could not answer questions about a simple paragraph read aloud by the examiner. He could repeat a series of four digits, but not five. He could repeat sentences of four or five words, but not of six or seven.

Bill read sentences and simple paragraphs with good comprehension, but reading rate was slow. He averaged 160 words per minute on easy narrative material, but could recall little that he read. Bill read slowly because he constantly had to go back to reread. He explained that unless he did this he lost the continuity, and did not know what he was reading. Although he had always loved to read, it was no longer any pleasure to him.

Bill had usable speech. Articulation was normal. Occasionally, however, he mispronounced a word because he could not recall sound sequences accurately. On testing, for example, he wanted to say *utensils.* He said, "uten . . . uten . . . utensils."

Sometimes Bill could not think of the word he wanted at all. He talked in hesitant and disjointed fragments, and he found it impossible to express ideas of any length. Asked to tell three things a good citizen should do, he replied, "Pay taxes—the law—abide the law—just can't."

He had trouble expressing ideas precisely. When he tried to define a familiar word, he could usually produce associations and give examples, but he did not have enough language at his command to give a synonym or a clear explanation. For example:

bargain: Where the . . . something that you . . . if you buy a merchandise . . . and they have a sale on it . . . it might be called a bargain.

repair: Something is broken . . . you repair it.

method: Method means . . . surgeon . . . repairs a broken leg . . . he has a method . . . of fixing it.

Spelling tested close to seventh-grade level. Bill wrote much the way he talked. He had trouble recalling sequences of letters, as well as sequences of sounds and words. For example, he wrote *responsible, responable,* and *institution, instition.* Written spelling was better than oral. Bill could write short sentences to dictation, although he sometimes omitted words. Errors increased as sentences increased in length. He wrote a well-formulated paragraph, but produced only 10 words in five minutes.

Bill could not remember the multiplication tables and tried to compensate by adding digits the desired number of times.

There was no evidence of impairment of perceptual discrimination or of dysfunction of the speech musculature. Bill showed simple aphasia, characterized by reduction of available vocabulary and verbal retention span, reflected in all language modalities.

THE COURSE OF RECOVERY

We subjected Bill to a barrage of intensive controlled auditory stimulation. The instructions were always, "Listen. Try to hear it. Try to think it. Then say it." Bill repeated hundreds of words, phrases, and sentences of gradually increasing length, every day. He spelled words aloud, used them in sentences, and tried to define them. He read hundreds of paragraphs aloud, first in unison with the clinician, then alone. First he answered questions on content, and later retold the paragraph unassisted. He progressed from isolated paragraphs to magazine articles and chapters in books. He wrote words and sentences to dictation every day, short easy ones first, then longer and more difficult ones. For homework, he studied spelling, and moved from writing sentences to writing paragraphs and clever original essays.

Bill was a highly literate person. He felt oddly lost because aphasia was like a wall between him and many things he cared about. The clinician spent part of each period giving him words to evoke his own associations. One day, using place names in Europe, which Bill knew well, she said, "Dardenelles." Bill was tremendously excited, but he could not explain why. He had never been in the Aegean. He said, "Man—wrote." Not Lord Byron. Bill added, "Died there—England—April." He was thinking of Rupert Brooke (1915), and the sonnet that begins:

> If I should die, think only this of me:
> That there's some corner of a foreign field
> That is forever England.

"April" was a tangential association to English poetry, apparently. We traced it to the lines from Robert Browning's poem (1845), "Home Thoughts, from Abroad," that begin:

> Oh, to be in England,
> Now that April's there.

But this was not all. That night Bill remembered a pocket book of modern poetry he had carried all through the war. His wife found it and mailed it to him. Bill tried to express what this meant to him. He said: "Will you wait—wait just a minute? There's something I—I want to say. It's—it's—this is not—not just speech. It's—man—a man does not live—does not live by bread—by bread alone. That's it—that's all I can say —but that's it."

Another time Bill said, "It's as though my mind were in a series of locked boxes, and I can't get at them until you give me the key."

Probably no one ever expressed this aspect of aphasia more compellingly. The boxes are there, filled with whatever has been organized in them through the years, but the keys are lost.

Another time, Bill said: "Did you know that aphasics can't lie? If you ask me something, I have to tell you the truth. I have no—no—no—. (No alternatives?) Yes, that's it. Aphasics have no alternatives."

Long before reading was rewarding, Bill found a congenial atmosphere in the hospital library. He played records in the music room for hours at a time. He said at first he did not know one composition from another, but music made him feel peaceful. One day, however, listening to a record he had played over and over for no conscious reason, Bill suddenly realized it was something his mother played on the organ. Gradually more and more discrimination and recognition returned. Eventually he was able to hear music, know it was the Beethoven Fifth, or the Grieg concerto, and to recall familiar themes. One day he invited the clinician to a program of rare old records he culled from a collection donated to the library, and his program notes were informed and interesting.

An occupational therapist introduced Bill to oil painting. He had never painted before, but it intrigued him. He showed a subtle sense of color, but he copied pictures indiscriminately. One day, the clinician said, "Bill, why don't you paint what you see?" They walked around the hospital finding windows that offered good views of the Mississippi River valley. Bill painted the river and the hills with increasing sensitivity, then began to paint places he remembered. This became another key to the locked boxes in his mind.

As his speech became more fluent, Bill began to talk to other patients. When he found he could carry on a conversation, he talked from morning to night. He talked to anyone who would listen to him. When one person left, he buttonholed another. He had no time to read, to paint, or work on assignments. The clinician allowed him to enjoy this busman's holiday, then countered by giving him a simple task he could not perform. Bill got the point. He grinned and said, "Twisting the knife, h'm?" but he went back to work.

Bill began to find books he remembered and to enjoy rereading them. From this he went on to reading new books by writers he remembered and liked.

He had periods of marked anxiety. These always seemed to follow periods of conspicuous gain. It was as though he looked back and realized how impaired he had been, and then looked forward, and knew how far he had yet to go. He became obsessed with trying to assign percentages to recovery in various areas. The clinician reviewed the tangible evidence of progress whenever this happened, then suggested he stop taking his temperature every hour, and use his time and energy doing things that were productive.

Bill was good at evaluating treatment procedures. The clinician told him the reason for each suggestion she made and encouraged Bill to judge its usefulness for himself. He could never be induced to work seriously at arithmetic. He figured he could brush up on it if he needed to, and that he'd probably always use a calculator anyway. The clinician acceded, considering that language should come first. Later, on a job, Bill had trouble making change rapidly, but he evolved a technique for dealing with it and improved because it was important to him.

When Bill left the hospital eight months after admission, he scored at the 99th percentile for adults on the Ammons test. His Binet vocabulary level was Superior Adult III. Reading vocabulary tested at the ceiling for college graduates, and spelling was a little beyond 11th-grade level. Bill's reading rate was 350 words a minute, and he could talk about what he read. His speech sounded normal in most situations, and he could discuss almost anything that interested him. He had, in fact, a good fund of information and anecdote. Writing was of literary quality, although still slower than normal.

There were other aphasic residuals. Bill sometimes failed to communicate in situations that were important to him. He spent hours rehearsing what he wanted to tell someone and then became so involved in the effort to execute his plan that he could not listen. He could tolerate no interruptions, because he was afraid he'd forget what he wanted to say. He lectured at people without regard for appropriateness of time or place, the reactions of the listener, or practical considerations he had overlooked. Bill was in fact prone to overlook practical considerations because he had been insulated from them too long. Afterwards he was aghast at his obtuseness, for he was naturally a sensible and considerate person. When his wife understood it was anxiety that made Bill so obdurate, they were able to work the problem out together.

Long before Bill left the hospital, the social worker and vocational psychologist began to plan with Bill and his wife for the next step in his rehabilitation. The plan they evolved provided adequate housing, family maintenance, and a program of combined language and vocational training for Bill. Bill selected a program that would prepare him for a job he liked and could perform in spite of physical limitations. The counselors explained that such programs were designed to keep families together through periods of emergency and were tax-supported, but statistics showed that their cost was more than returned to the state in taxes paid by beneficiaries. This seemed reasonable to Bill and his wife, but relatives were irrevocably opposed to any plan that involved an organized charity, and in the end it was abandoned.

Bill made the final decision. He thought that if he went to his parents' home in California he could enroll in a similar vocational program and send for his family when he could make a home for them. This was not an easy sacrifice for Bill or his wife, but the situation had become one of intolerable conflict, and neither of them thought the separation would be for very long.

TEN YEARS LATER

Bill's high hopes did not materialize. The program he hoped to find did not exist in the California area where his parents lived. He received some help in a nearby Rehabilitation Center, but no vocational training. He fell getting out of a car and injured his good leg. His parents were not well. The separation from his wife and children lengthened. Bill's courage gave way to depression as he investigated one job after another and found he could not perform them because of some physiological incapacity. A gradual estrangement grew between Bill and his wife. In his hopelessness, Bill rejected her efforts to reach him, although she made a trip to California and tried to find a job there. The slow ravages of time, distance, and despair did their work, and the marriage ended in divorce.

Slowly, Bill found his way out of the depression that had engulfed him. He found a job in a specialized shop whose customers were suburban commuters. Thus it offered lulls during the day when Bill could sit down and rest between rush periods. These were literally rocking chair intervals, and they spelled survival for him.

Bill still enjoys reading and music and painting. He grew up with a passion for boats, and a few years ago he acquired one. He enjoys people, and from time to time he finds a new friend with congenial interests. Once when Dr. Schuell was in California, they spent a Sunday morning browsing in places Bill knew, and the afternoon in a Chinese restaurant talking over endless cups of tea. Bill is not a very good correspondent, but his letters, when they come, are literate and communicative. They are informed with humor, with appreciation of the life that flows about him, and the kind of acceptance he has won.

TO ROUND OUT THE PICTURE

Although Simple Aphasic patients present milder aphasia than patients in Sensorimotor, Auditory, and Irreversible groups, there is a range of severity within the category. Bill had moderately severe aphasia, as Simple Aphasic subjects go. The outcome was complicated by persisting hemiplegia, reduced physical capacity, and relentless economic pressures. Recovery of language nevertheless followed a characteristic Simple Aphasic course, and Bill made consistent and excellent progress in spite of receiving no treatment the first 22 months.

Although Bill needed continued treatment, he had made significant gains and was functioning as an intelligent and literate person when he left the hospital. Continued hospitalization was not the answer for him. He was not ready for complete independence, but he needed the stimulation and challenge of a more normal environment and contact with reality beyond hospital walls. He made the choice he thought best for his family.

Some Simple Aphasic patients have presented milder aphasia. John Tolley came into the hospital for seizure control two years after he had received a head injury in Korea. He showed no obvious aphasia. An alert resident referred him to the Aphasia Section because there was a history of transient aphasia in his army record. The examiner found only minimal reduction of vocabulary and of verbal retention span. She explained this, saying it was undoubtedly a result of the head injury, but the effects were so mild she would not have detected them without examination. She added that there was nothing to worry about if he was getting along all right, but there were things he could do if he wanted to. Then John began to talk.

He said he could not remember much that happened after he was hurt. He had never heard of aphasia, and did not know he'd ever had any trouble with his speech. He said when he left the hospital he went back to his home town. He met people he'd known all his life, and could not remember their names. He could not remember addresses or telephone numbers. One night he got into a card game, and discovered he could not keep score. A few days later he tried to balance his check book, and found he did not know how. He listened to the news on the radio but could not remember what he had heard. He read the paper, and did not know what he had read. He thought he was losing his mind, and lived in terror that this would be discovered and he would be committed to an institution. He avoided his friends and crossed the street if he saw anyone coming he knew. He did not dare look for a job. He said he had stayed home and watched television for two years. He added, "If anyone had told me what you did two years ago, it would have made all the difference in the world." The moral, of course, is that aphasia should not be ignored, even when it is mild, or when spontaneous recovery appears complete.

Spontaneous recovery does occur and is often dramatic when it happens. Patients are able to do tasks each day they could not do the day before. It is a far different clinical course from that of patients with persisting aphasia, where gains occur slowly, as a result of persistent effort over long periods of time.

APHASIC IMPAIRMENT IN SIMPLE APHASIA

These subjects show impoverishment of language in all modalities, without specific perceptual, motor, or sensorimotor involvement. Impairment ranges from mild to severe on initial examination.

This impoverishment is characterized by reduction of vocabulary in all modalities, varying in severity from patient to patient. With moderate or moderately severe impairment, mispronunciations occur in speech. These mispronunciations are inconsistent, in that sounds and words are pronounced correctly at one time and incorrectly at another. Sounds and combinations of sounds with complex movement patterns are often substituted for relatively simple ones. In some subjects this impairment is so severe that speech is unintellible, or deteriorates into jargon after a few words. These errors, however, can be corrected readily by ear, and some speech is usually present, or emerges early, that sounds normal. This kind of impairment appears to be related to a disturbance of auditory feedback mechanisms and impaired recall of learned auditory patterns.

Simple Aphasic subjects usually have difficulty finding words. Sometimes the patient cannot find the word he wants, and unless the listener can guess what he wants to say he is lost. If the listener guesses right, the patient invariably recognizes the word at once. As language increases, the patient is often able to substitute one word for another, and communication does not break down.

The most common error in word finding is the substitution of words associated in meaning with the intended word. In the beginning the patient often does not recognize such errors. As improvement occurs, however, he tends more and more to reject the wrong word, and to continue searching until he finds the word he wants to use. He might say, for example, "I used to go fishing out at Round Lake, no, Long Lake, no, that's not right—Square Lake, that's it, Square Lake."

Sometimes a Simple Aphasic patient is considered disoriented because he says *Tuesday* for *Wednesday, Mississippi* for *Minnesota,* or calls his *wife* his *mother.* Other patients have been diagnosed as mentally confused because they forget what they have been asked, what they start to say, or what they are told to do. Simple Aphasic patients sometimes sound confused, also, because it is easy for them to follow a chance association and go off on a tangent. An aphasic patient might say on being questioned that his doctor is a lawyer, and that he goes to court, but asked if the doctor goes to court, he will reject it, and probably correct his statement and say he goes to the hospital. He will not, however, persist in the belief that he spent the morning out in the 10-acre field instead of on the ward, or that his doctor is the man who runs the sawmill down the road. The aphasic patient, moreover, soon learns to stop and ask a question to reorient himself, such as, "What did you ask me, again?" or, "What was I talking about?" or even, simply and descriptively, "I lost it."

In these patients, auditory comprehension is usually good for short language units, but errors increase as materials increase in length. Retention span increases gradually with controlled auditory stimulation, and this improvement is reflected in all language modalities.

Simple Aphasic patients tend to write in much the same way as they talk. As more language becomes available, writing improves, both in vocabulary usage and in structure of sentences. Reading improves similarly, and most literate patients are able to read stories, magazine articles, professional journals, and books before they leave the hospital.

TEST FINDINGS

TESTS FOR AUDITORY COMPREHENSION

On tests for auditory comprehension, Simple Aphasics showed the lowest percentage of errors, averaged over the nine tests, of all diagnostic groups except persisting Dysfluency patients, on both initial and final testing. They also showed the highest percentage of improvement on auditory tests except for the Dysfluency patients.

On the Ammons *Full-Range Picture Vocabulary Test,* their mean was at the 25th percentile for adults on initial testing, and at the 45th percentile on testing after treatment. This exceeded the performance of the other diagnostic groups except for the persisting Dysfluency group. In individual subjects, reduction of auditory comprehension ranged from mild to moderately severe but did not usually affect common words.

Reduction of auditory retention span was indicated by increase of errors as materials increased in length. For example, the percentage of error was 13% on auditory comprehension of a short paragraph, and 30% on a longer paragraph, on initial testing. On final testing, these percentages were reduced to 3% on the short paragraph, and 13% on the long one.

VISUAL AND READING TESTS

On visual and reading tests, Simple Aphasic subjects obtained the lowest mean error of all diagnostic groups except for persisting Dysfluents on all tests, on both initial and final examination, and exceeded all groups except the Dysfluents in percentage of improvement.

Simple Aphasic subjects made no errors matching colors, pictures, or forms, and only minimal errors matching letters, matching words to pictures, and matching printed to spoken words. Superiority of this group on reading tests was clear and unmistakable.

Errors reflected reduction of reading vocabulary to some extent, but primarily they reflected reduction of verbal retention span. On initial testing, the percentage of errors was 33% on comprehension of a short printed paragraph, and 60% on a long one. On final testing, these percentages were reduced to 20% and to 38%.

SPEECH AND LANGUAGE TESTS

There were no significant differences between Simple Aphasic and Visual subjects on speech and language tests. They exceeded the performance of the other diagnostic groups by wide margins.

Simple Aphasic subjects made only minimal errors repeating single words, and no errors counting to 20 or naming the days of the week. More difficult tests reflected the tendency of language to break down as longer or more precise responses were required. This is demonstrated in percentages of error, on initial and final testing, on the following characteristic tests:

	Percent of initial errors	Percent of final errors
1. Naming common objects	22	1
2. Expressing ideas (three things done during day, and three things a good citizen should do).	38	12
3. Explaining similarities*	53	33
4. Explaining common proverbs*	78	55

*No longer in the test battery.

On expressing ideas, most Simple Aphasic subjects, like Bill, had partial success but could not complete the task.

On explaining similarities, the nature of the response changed as patients acquired more language. Test procedure was to give examples, then use the form, "Knife and fork. How are they alike?" for each item. Patients with the most severe reduction of languages tended to state differences. This appeared to be because they could not retain both the terms and the instructions simultaneously, and deal with them all at once. They tended to deal with each item separately, and say something like, "Knife—cut —fork—eat," then stop. A little later, the same patient might reply, "Airplane, fly— car, go—" or, "Go east—go west," with similarity implied. On final testing, most patients had enough vocabulary to produce words such as *utensils, transportation,* or *directions,* at least sometimes.

We observe such changes too often, coming about in too short a time, for us to consider the early responses defective because of impairment of abstraction, except insofar as abstraction requires more language than producing simple associations. On factor analysis, similarities had a high loading on language (91), and relatively low loading on recognition of stimulus equivalence (16).

Explaining proverbs had its highest loading on language (79), but it also had a relatively high loading on recognition of stimulus equivalence (45). Performance on this test also improved as language increased. Patients who initially explained, "Don't put all your eggs in one basket," by saying, "Eggs might break," frequently said something like, "Don't put all your money in one place," on final examination. It would appear as though part of the difficulty was that for the patient with limited language, the stimulus *eggs* produced the common association *break*, and nothing more. With more available language, the patient could draw upon a larger field of analogy, and elaborate the response.

VISUOMOTOR AND WRITING TESTS

Simple Aphasic subjects obtained the lowest mean number of errors on all visuomotor and writing tests on initial and final testing and showed the highest percentage of improvement. They made only minimal errors on drawing and copying tests, performing much like normals.

On typical writing tests, percentages of errors on initial and final testing were as follows:

	Percent of initial errors	Percent of final errors
1. Written spelling (to sixth-grade level)	26	16
2. Spontaneous sentences	43	16
3. Spontaneous paragraph	59	33

Here, again, we see the tendency for errors to increase as responses increased in length.

NUMERICAL RELATIONS AND ARITHMETIC PROCESSES

Simple Aphasic patients made only minimal errors on tests such as making change, setting a clock, and selecting the correct answers to simple numerical combinations.

Simple Aphasics performed better than all other groups except Persisting Dysfluents, both initially and finally, on solving arithmetic problems and made the most improvement. On this section of the test, the initial error was 43% for Simple Aphasic patients, and the final error was 24%. In most cases no work had been done on arithmetic, but it improved spontaneously as language increased. This is not meant to imply that work in arithmetic is undesirable or unnecessary for aphasic patients. In the relatively short period of hospitalization, patients usually had all they could do to work on language. Patients with the mildest aphasia were tutored in arithmetic. Tutoring was available in educational therapy for any patient for whom it seemed advisable. However, except for simple naming and counting activities, arithmetic is usually less threatening after functional language has become reasonably adequate, and probably should be deferred until this goal is reached.

NEUROLOGICAL BACKGROUND

The average age of Simple Aphasic subjects was 38 years. This was significantly younger than in other diagnostic groups. However, 21% of these subjects were over 50, and 19% were also over 60. This indicates that age itself is not an essential consideration in diagnosis or prognosis in aphasia.

Simple Aphasics had the highest educational level of all diagnostic groups. The average patient had some training beyond high school but did not have a college degree. These patients did not differ from other groups in occupational level, however. The difference in educational level was probably due to the relatively high proportion of younger patients in this group.

We see no evidence of any relation between education and severity of aphasia. The relationship between education and recovery from aphasia appears indirect and equivocal, although there is undoubtedly a relation between educational achievement and the value placed on communication skills.

If language imposes its patterns on the brain and is one of the principal means by which the brain is organized, then language has a biological function. It determines the very structure of the brain itself. The unavailability of these complex patterns is more crippling, in the basic biological sense of what man is, than dysfunction of an arm or leg. The literate aphasic is aware of this, as Bill was, when he said, "It's as though my mind were in a series of locked boxes, and I can't get at them until you give me the key."

Bill reacted to hemiplegia. He was sensitive about wearing a brace and tended to hide it when he could. When the clinician became aware of this, she made a point of examining the brace matter-of-factly one day, and asking how much it helped, and what he could do with his game leg. The next day, Bill hauled it comfortably up on a chair, grinned, and said, "I've decided it's a pretty good old carcass, after all, to have taken all it's been through." He always had to be pushed, however, to work in physical therapy, because he wanted to spend all his time on the intellectual pursuits that were essential to him.

Probably vocational dependency on language increases, also, as a function of education. As a result of all these factors, aphasia is more threatening to highly literate people than to those whose interests and needs place lesser demands on communication. There is more anxiety and less ability to tolerate even mild residual deficits. Sometimes this results in a higher level of final achievement, but it also results in greater frustration and discouragement, which can be a hindrance to recovery.

Unless an aphasic patient is willing to make some mistakes initially, his verbal output will probably not be large enough to produce improvement. It is necessary to get language processes functioning before errors can be reduced, and making errors is part of this process. This is often difficult for the educated aphasic to accept emotionally, although the theory makes sense to him. One of the advantages of practice with machines such as the Language Master* is that it permits the patient to make mistakes unobserved.

The patient who is satisfied if he can talk a little to his family and friends, read the headlines, and sign his name has an easier time reaching his goals than the boy who wants to go back to college, or the man who wants to return to his profession. These goals, too, have been achieved, but at a higher cost.

The patient with a lower level of aspiration views his progress differently from the beginning. He is more willing to think he's doing pretty well when he is. Instead of trying, like Bill, to compute percentages of recovery, he is more inclined to say, in the words of one patient, "Go home—look after farm." He added, "Talk good enough now. Most people—talk too much."

The etiology of aphasia was head injury for 15% of Simple Aphasic patients in the present series, neoplasm in 5%, toxic processes in 5%, and cerebrovascular accident in 76%. Although the incidence of cerebrovascular accidents was significantly lower in this group than in the Sensorimotor and Irreversible groups, it was still a very high percentage. The fact that all etiologies were found in all diagnostic groups supports the hypothesis that aphasic findings are determined more by the locus and extent of the lesion than by its nature.

Nineteen percent of the cerebrovascular accidents for Simple Aphasics were complete thromboses of the internal carotid artery. As one would predict, there were no complete thromboses of the middle cerebral artery in this group.

There were only six cases of complete thrombosis of the middle cerebral artery confirmed by angiography or autopsy, in all seven diagnostic groups. All of these patients showed severe aphasia. There were 14 cases of confirmed thrombosis of the internal carotid, and these patients showed all degrees of aphasic deficit from mild to extremely severe. This is admittedly a small series, but the findings are understandable anatomically. When the middle cerebral artery is occluded, little or no collateral circulation can be established. If the occlusion is proximal to the circle of Willis, on the other hand, there may be adequate collateral circulation beyond the lesion. There are known to be wide individual differences in collateral circulation, probably depending on both the configuration and the condition of cerebral vessels.

A detailed report of neurological and medical data for each of the diagnostic groups can be found in Table 6 in Appendix 2. The findings can be briefly summarized for these patients as follows:

Simple Aphasic patients in general showed the mildest neurological involvement of all diagnostic groups, although some, like Bill, presented a relatively severe hemiplegia. They showed no incidence of visual field defects, and a low incidence of reduction of sensation and hypertension. In incidence of complicating conditions, as in severity of neurological involvement, the situation was generally favorable for these patients.

*The Language Master is a playback instrument designed to utilize short tapes mounted on nine-inch cards, which contain the same materials in printed form. The patient places the card in a convenient track to listen, and by this simple operation can hear any unit as many times as he wishes. At present it is manufactured by Bell and Howell.

Self-care and ambulation scores were based on functional skills, such as dressing, eating, getting from bed to chair, and from chair to standing position, going up and down stairs, and speed and distance in walking. A maximal score could be obtained whether the patient used one or two hands, or used a brace or cane or both.

All Simple Aphasics received maximal scores on final evaluation of self-care activities. Seventy-three percent walked without assistance initially, and all received maximal scores finally.

Thirty-three percent of these patients either went back to school, took special vocational training, or resumed gainful employment. This percentage seems low compared with the 60% found in the Sensorimotor group. There is a reasonable explanation for this difference. The average period of hospitalization was about six months shorter for Simple Aphasic patients than for Sensorimotor patients. A further consideration was that many Simple Aphasic patients hoped to return to their own occupations, although perhaps with modifications that permitted them to work under less pressure. This was clearly impossible for most Sensorimotor subjects, who had to settle for jobs with low language requirements.

The majority of Simple Aphasic patients, like Bill, went home to work on their own, until more recovery had taken place. They were able to talk and listen and to read and write, and they knew how to work independently to obtain continued improvement.

This planning was realistic, since a good deal of reinforcement of recovered functions is necessary before they are dependable in situations of stress or anxiety. One patient enrolled in a college speech course in his home town. Another spent a winter in California and then went back to his job as a contract engineer.

Another patient was a retired judge of the state supreme court. Before he received treatment for aphasia he would not talk to his children over long-distance telephone and refused to see friends who came to his home. In the hospital he became the valued friend and adviser of all the younger patients, who respected and loved him and sought his counsel. On discharge, he attended his daughter's college commencement and asked to be introduced to the college president. When he returned home he went to see his old friends and enjoyed talking shop with them. He subsequently suffered another stroke and died without regaining consciousness, but the last months of his life were happy ones, and this was important. Actually the treatment he received in the hospital was more than justified by the good he did for other patients. The essential consideration, however, is that life and death are unpredictable, and our course is the simple one of treating all patients we know how to help.

A FUNCTIONAL SCHEMA FOR SIMPLE APHASIA

Simple Aphasia is characterized by a reduction in available vocabulary and verbal retention span, the root symptomatology for all types of aphasia. This is clearly due to an impairment of those processes needed to formulate propositions in the *symbolic mode,* as illustrated in Figure 10–1. Because this group of aphasics exhibits no other complicating conditions, only the symbolic component of the functional schema is designated. For the Simple Aphasia patient, the ability to assimilate or express knowl-

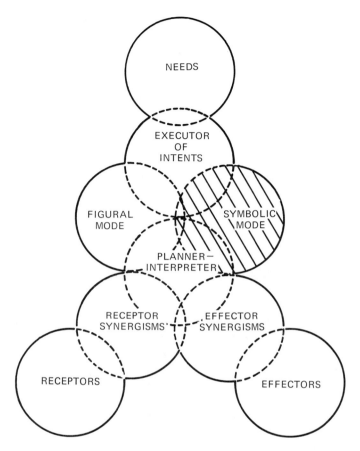

Fig. 10–1. Functional schema for simple aphasia.

edge by description is impaired. Hence he has difficulty both in producing and comprehending symbolic communiques.

This means that such patients have difficulty across all language modalities, including
formulating thought processes in the symbolic mode, although they exhibit no impairment of hearing, seeing, or articulation. For instance, the Simple Aphasic has no
difficulty effecting the synergisms involved in saying or hearing words; both the articulatory as well as auditory plans for speech are intact. His major difficulty is attempting
to retrieve, remember, or recognize language since all these functions depend upon the
ability to formulate propositions in the symbolic mode, which is impaired.

chapter **11**

APHASIA WITH CEREBRAL
INVOLVEMENT OF VISUAL
PROCESSES

Martin Greshwin was graduated from college with honors in history before the beginning of the Korean War. Martin had a serious and practical mind. He was a quiet responsible boy who sometimes surprised one by his decisiveness and tenacity, and by his subtle sense of the absurd.

During the winter of 1952 when Martin was on naval duty in the Pacific he developed an upper respiratory infection that hung on for several weeks. In mid-March he began to have severe frontal headaches, and on March 23rd, he developed double vision.

Funduscopic examination showed papilledema and a small perivascular hemorrhage. The only clinical findings reported were bilateral weakness of the sixth cranial nerve, and supranuclear paresis of the right eighth. Air studies showed the ventricular system shifted to the right and displacement of the left temporal horn. A left fronto-temporal craniotomy was performed on April 2, 1952, but no pathology was found. The final diagnosis was acute infectious encephalitis.

There was no mention of aphasia in the medical record before surgery, and there is good evidence that no aphasia was present. Martin wrote a long letter home the night before the operation, and he could not have written such a letter at any time during the following year.

From Japan, Martin was evacuated to a navy hospital on the west coast, and in August transferred to the Minneapolis VA Hospital for treatment of aphasia. Neurological findings on admission were mild weakness on the right side of his body, a bilateral visual field cut consisting of an upper right quadrantanopsia, and aphasia. At this time he was 24 years old.

INITIAL FINDINGS

Martin had a hospital pallor, and he looked ill. He still bore the marks of brain surgery, an area of swelling, and a cranial depression. Later he said if they'd cut off the bump and put it in the hole, he'd be all right. When he first came to the clinic, however, he was unable to talk this much, had no inclination toward humor, was tense with anxiety, wary of everyone, and a little cross.

Since Martin had been bored as well as anxious, he began to enjoy the challenge of the examination. He was a young man who liked to use his mind even when it did not work very well. He did not know how to give up, and he never wanted to leave any part of a task, even on testing, until he had mastered it. The clinician, seeing that he became relaxed and peaceful while he worked, did not hurry him, and gave him all the answers he wanted.

On auditory tests, Martin showed reduction of vocabulary and of auditory retention span. He could point to pictures of common objects when they were named by the examiner, but on the Ammons *Full-Range Picture Vocabulary Test*, he scored below the first percentile for normal adults. This indicated that in general Martin understood only the most common words he heard. He could repeat sentences of four or five words, but no longer sentences. He followed directions five or six words long, but not longer directions. He responded correctly to some questions on the content of a short paragraph read aloud to him, but could not follow a longer paragraph.

Although his performance was suspiciously slow, Martin made no errors matching letters, or matching words to pictures. He worked in a perfectionistic manner and was unwilling to make a choice until he had satisfied himself that it was correct. He made errors pointing to letters named by the examiner and reading letters aloud. On tests for reading comprehension, he had no better than chance success on simple sentences. He grasped the main ideas of a short narrative paragraph, but not of a longer one.

Martin had no difficulty repeating words, counting to 20, or naming the days of the week, but he could not name the months of the year and was able to name only 7 out of 18 common objects. Usually he said, "I don't know," but he called a *cup* a *pitcher*, a *pencil* a *stamp*, and a little *boy* a *man*.

Responses to simple questions indicated further difficulty in finding words. Answers were vague, and showed perseveration, although associations sometimes occurred. For example:

What do you shave with? *Anything you. . . .*
What do you write with? *Anything you can get . . . with your money.*
What do you dig with? *Anything you can get.*
What do you drive nails with? *Pound.*

What do you shoot with? *Go bang.*
What do you cut with? *Anything that will allow itself to be cut.*

He could not rhyme, but offered, "Oh, well, he gets by well." The following are examples of definitions he gave.

robin: A story about a bird.
island: An island was a—that's a—can see from their back yard— (Where is the island?) In the lake.
bargain: A bargain was a device that helped their routing or their writing.
courage: The start of courage gave help to their—I know what it means. Getting him to get used to out of his ability—and make the thing work.

He could tell three things he had done during the day, but not three things a good citizen should do. He could not give sentences using common words, or explain similarities or proverbs. Although his spontaneous speech was often vague and incoherent, it was usually possible to trace the skeleton of thought behind it, as in the definition of *courage.* Speech broke down because he could not find the words he wanted, or arrange them readily to achieve continuity.

Copying and drawing were only mildly impaired. No gross distortions were evident. However, on writing letters to dictation, there were confusions of letters with similar visual configurations, and occasional mild distortions of letter forms. Responses were often hesitant and uncertain. He could not think what *u* looked like, and finally printed a distorted ⊔ below the line, although he had previously been writing in script. He could not recall *z*, in print or script.

Spelling tested at second-grade level. Martin was surprised when he could not write a word, and persisted, trying to help himself by sounding it to himself. He wrote *trame* for *train*, and *choot* for *shout.* He could not write sentences spontaneously or to dictation.

Arithmetic was surprisingly good, although he could not work problems that involved fractions or decimals.

To summarize the findings: Martin showed moderately severe aphasia characterized by reduction of vocabulary and reduction of verbal retention span reflected in all language modalities. He could not deal with long language units in any modality. In addition, he showed involvement of visual processes, reflected in mild impairment of discrimination and recognition, and somewhat more severe impairment of recall of learned visual symbols.

THE COURSE OF RECOVERY

It was obvious to Martin that there were things he needed to improve, and like the sensible person he was, he wanted to begin. Like most aphasic patients, he was far less anxious when he knew what was wrong and could focus on definite problems. He made excellent progress from the beginning. He lived near enough to go home weekends, and his mother reported happily that he was more like the old Martin every time he came home.

We used repetition and oral spelling of words, and repetition of sentences. We also used short paragraphs, reading them in unison, until Martin was able to read them alone. At first the clinician asked questions on content; then Martin began to tell as much as he could about what he read, and the clinician asked questions about the rest.

He practiced writing letters of the alphabet, spending most of his time on the ones he had trouble with, and writing letters and words to dictation.

By the end of the first month, Martin had made significant functional gains. He was repeating sentences seven and eight words long. He named 14 out of 18 pictures correctly instead of 7, and responded to questions by saying you shaved with a razor, wrote with a pencil, dug with a hoe, etc. He could formulate sentences using given words, and tell three things a good citizen should do. Spontaneous speech was usually appropriate and coherent. Reading vocabulary tested at seventh-grade level. Martin could read a short paragraph and answer questions about its content. Spelling tested at fourth-grade level, and Martin could write simple sentences both spontaneously and to dictation.

Martin had now spent a little over six months in various hospitals. He accepted the situation without complaint, but he did not make friends. He was reserved and a little shy, as well as aphasic. He came to the clinic and went to the dining room, and studied, and slept. It occurred to the clinician that with a little guidance Martin's mother, who was a sensible and intelligent woman, could do everything the clinician was doing, and that Martin would be happier at home, and probably receive more general stimulation. This seemed a good idea to everyone, and Martin was given a 30-day leave.

Martin's mother received specific instructions, materials to use at home, and demonstrations of procedures. The clinician urged her to send weekly reports, and to write about any problems she encountered. The following are excerpts from her letters of this period.

> I think the fact that Martin and I have enjoyed our work this week is probably the most significant part of this first report. He seems very relaxed, full of humor, and shows much interest in outside activities.
>
> It is difficult for me to judge what progress has been made, but I feel he reads more easily. I am sure he is doing better in forming sentences, because I have the written record to look at. We talk about the words before he writes the sentences. It seems that a detached word has very little meaning for him, but after discussing its various uses, he can write a good sentence. He seems to enjoy this approach, but if it is giving him too much help, just tell me.
>
> In his outside activities he has gone to two football games, goes daily to the YMCA to use their apparatus in the gym, and visits with people downtown.
>
> He has not yet taken the car alone, but drives very well now—even backs into parking space at the curb.

A week later, she wrote.

> Our work has gone along very satisfactorily. The reading has not shown marked improvement, and Martin is still confused by some letters of the alphabet. . . . I think he gets more out of the newspapers lately. At first, he didn't care to discuss what he had read, but now talks about the sports news quite freely.
>
> I have had a few friends in for a cup of coffee several times, and Martin comes in, greets them, and visits very naturally.

He still works out at the YMCA almost daily. He also walks at least 20 blocks a day. At first, four or five was all he cared to do, but he is much stronger physically than he was.

I used to be fearful that he would fall going downstairs, because he stepped so heavily on his right foot that it affected his balance. He has complained for months that his foot is always 'asleep' and has no feeling in it. Since he walks more, he seems to coordinate better, and I notice less stumbling.

At the end of the month, Martin returned to the hospital. His general psysiological condition had improved, and he was relaxed and responsive and full of little quips. He had made measurable gains in all language modalities. On the Ammons test, he tested at the 30th percentile for adults. Reading vocabulary tested at grade level 7.6, and paragraph comprehension at grade level 5.4. Spelling had advanced to sixth-grade level. Both oral and written formulation had improved. Since the plan had worked so well, everyone agreed it should be continued. Martin was given new materials that were a little more difficult, and he went home for another 30-day period.

He continued to make steady progress. His mother wrote:

> Martin is now busy writing a letter to his sister. It is taking him longer than it used to take him, but the sentences are his. They sound like a letter he might have written a year ago. He uses the dictionary to check spelling, and asks for no help. I am elated over his success.
>
> The reading showed improvement this week. We are using "A Child's History of Art" by the former headmaster of the Calvert School in Baltimore. It is written for fourth, fifth, and sixth grades, and is interestingly presented. We were reading about Italian painting. It seems less juvenile, and I think he is more enthusiastic about it. . . . He now has his driver's license, and drove me to Rochester and back one day last week. He did very well.

Toward the end of the month, she wrote, "I think his vocabulary has grown. He still talks slowly and hunts for words, but he no longer substitutes 'whoopla,' or 'thing-amajig.' Also, he is aware of tenses of verbs, singular and plural, and gender, all of which meant nothing at first."

She reported that he asked for Churchill's latest book for Christmas, and added, "I'm sure he doesn't expect to read it right away, but at least he is not down-hearted."

In the same letter, she wrote, "He is beginning to go out with young people more and more. At first he was ill at ease with them and refused all invitations."

Martin returned to the hospital on schedule the middle of November. Again, all the findings were favorable. He scored at the 59th percentile on the Ammons test. On reading tests, he scored at the 10th-grade level on sentence comprehension, and at grade level 9.7 on paragraph comprehension. Spelling tested close to seventh-grade level. Functional speech sounded normal. Both oral and written formulation were more accurate.

But this time Martin did not receive another pass. His X-rays had arrived from Japan and been studied by the doctors, who decided to do more studies. An angiogram showed displacement of the left middle cerebral artery anteriorly, laterally, and upward. An electroencephalogram showed a slow wave focus over the left tempero-parietal area. A sleep study showed spikes in the left parietal lead. The eventual decision was to operate again.

Martin, of course, was game. His mother had come up at the end of the week expecting to get further recommendations and materials for working at home. She had made no arrangement to stay over the weekend, and since her younger son had remained at home, she could not decide what to do. Martin said, "Mother, go home. Go home and take care of John. There is nothing you can do here if you stay." She followed his advice, saying he sounded just like his father, who had been dead for several years. However, she returned the day of surgery.

The surgeon found a series of multilocular cysts in the left temporal lobe, with thin intervening walls. The walls were broken down, revealing one common cavity. The floor was lined with tumorous tissue, which was interpreted as astrocytoma, on frozen section. This was removed until the surgeon felt that excision was going so deep into the middle fossa that it should be discontinued. There was nothing hopeful about it.

When it was finished, the clinician said, "I am going to tell his mother the operation is over. Tell me exactly what you want me to say."

The surgeon replied, "She knows you better than anyone else. Tell her all you can."

Not much had to be said. There were physicians in the family, and Mrs. Greshwin asked only three questions. She asked if they had found the tumor, if they had removed it all, and if it was malignant. The clinician said, "They think so."

Later she asked the surgeon how long Martin could be expected to live, and was told that the average expectancy was about two years. She decided that Martin should not be told, and that we should continue to work for recovery of speech, because she thought he would be happier doing something constructive. She said, "We have to rehabilitate him as much as possible. Anything else would be unthinkable."

Her final decision was to tell no one that surgery had not been effective. She thought people would not be able to help watching him, and that Martin would sense that something was wrong. A long time afterward, when the strain had become too great, she relaxed this rule. The clinician had been urging her for some time to find someone close at hand she could talk to, and she did. She went to a relative who was a physician. He respected her confidence and was extremely supportive. Realizing that this was too great a burden for anyone to carry alone, he made appointments for her to come to his office regularly to talk to him.

THE POSTSURGICAL COURSE

Two weeks after the operation in November, Martin was almost as aphasic as he had been on admission to the hospital in August, but there were no new findings. The clinical picture was the same as it had been initially. By January 20th, he had reached approximately the same performance levels he had reached during the first two months of treatment, in all language modalities. This meant he had progressed almost twice as fast as he had the first time, but was still about a month behind the presurgical level. He was discharged from the hospital again, to continue to work with his mother at home. He was called back at two-month, then three-month, and finally six-month intervals for the next three years.

Martin worked faithfully and demonstrated measurable gains on each admission. By June 1953, he tested at the average adult level on the Binet Vocabulary Test. Reading vocabulary was on high-school level, and paragraph comprehension and spelling reached the ninth-grade level. Martin was writing monthly letters to the clinician to report his own progress:

May 2, 1953

Dear_____:

Yes, it is still raining out, cold and dreary. This first month went by in a hurry. In fact, it really doesn't seem that it has been a month, but I guess that it has. Since you spent two weeks in Chicago, I dare say you found that time does fly by.

John has had his boat on the river for about two weeks. We have had poor weather for riding in the boat, though, so I haven't gone out with him yet. I still enjoy playing golf more than I do boating so you will know which side of the city to look for me.

Dr. Hull has been giving me help in speech for the last two weeks. He is very interesting to work with. He taught at Wren College until two years ago, at which time he was retired, for he was 65 years old. I enjoy knowing him a great deal.

In half an hour the Kentucky Derby will be run. I choose the horse second from the left.

Sincerely,
Martin

Dr. Hull, a retired psychologist, was a family friend. He had kindly offered to work with Martin, and carry on the same program, if this was acceptable. Mrs. Greshwin thought this would be both a rewarding association and a stimulating change for Martin, and the clinician agreed. This turned out to be the case. Later Dr. Hull added tutoring in mathematics to the program, which was a subject Martin had always enjoyed.

The following fall Martin began to work part-time in the office of one of his uncles. He checked various kinds of records, and his work was accurate, but slow. He could not have worked competitively for this reason and the fact that he continued to fatigue easily. He always required a rest period during the middle part of the day.

In March of 1954, Martin wrote:

March 7, 1954

Dear _____:

Swish!!!! Don't worry, that's just me in my new car. I bought it just last week. It's a Nash Rambler—a hard top; very snazze.

My volley ball team made the paper Saturday night, because we are leading the league. We won two out of three games, twice last week, that put us ahead of the league. I am getting to be much better at playing volley ball, than I was when we started the season.

Dr. Hull is still tutoring me in speech. I think it is going all right. You can decide at the end of next month, which is when I will show up to be checked.

Love,
Martin

Martin had some money of his own, and during this period he managed his own investments. He used such acumen that everything he bought doubled or tripled in value within a two- to three-year period, and some purchases increased at an even higher rate.

In April 1955, Martin scored at the 75th percentile for adults on vocabulary recognition, on the Ammons test. His Binet vocabulary level was Superior Adult II. Reading vocabulary tested at grade level 18, and paragraph comprehension on the Iowa Advanced Reading Test was at the 94th percentile for college freshmen, on an untimed test. Spelling tested at 11th-grade level, and arithmetic at 12th. Spontaneous writing was excellent, but slow. Martin wrote a paragraph with no errors, but achieved only 35 words in five minutes. On testing, he showed many signs of superior intelligence. The examiner reported, "Although he could understand materials presented in college classes, he could not keep up with lectures or reading assignments, or pass ordinary written examinations."

Formal tutoring was discontinued shortly after this. Martin had enough to do to keep busy, and was engrossed with events taking place in the family. Besides, he needed a respite. There had, of course, been breaks in the routine before, for holidays and vacations, but aside from these the program had been intensive and continuous. If it could be avoided, we did not want him to become discouraged and depressed from being kept at school too long. Dr. Hull was going away for the summer, and it was easy to compliment Martin sincerely on his work, and to tell him that all he needed now was to continue reading books that interested him to increase his reading rate, and to continue writing. He had been keeping a diary, and he wrote letters frequently. Everything continued to go well for almost a year, and his letters indicated that this was a happy time for him. He became interested in photography the next winter, and wrote about colored pictures he had taken, of his own activities, and those of other members of the family.

THE COURSE OF REGRESSION

The first signs of regression were observed in April 1956, when Martin returned to the hospital for reevaluation. This was about four years after the initial symptoms, and three and a half years after surgery in Minneapolis.

On tests for auditory comprehension, Martin pointed to common objects when they were named by the examiner, but made errors pointing to objects named in series of two, and could point to no objects named in series of three. He repeated four digits correctly but not five, and had trouble following long directions.

He complained of headache and dizziness when asked to perform visual tests. He had no difficulty on reading tests, however, until he came to comprehension of a long paragraph. On oral reading, he misread words occasionally, such as *he* for *we*, and *there* for *they*. He had not done this for a long time.

On naming objects he said *table* for *chair*, and could not think of the word for *car* or *tree*. He could not define *repair*, and he defined *leather* as *cloth*, then added it had leather in it. Asked to tell three things a good citizen should do, he replied, "A citizen would work hard, play hard, and keeps well account of things that has been accomplished." Martin had given no responses as disorganized as this for three years.

He made errors copying letters and writing letters to dictation. He wrote simple sentences correctly, however, both spontaneously and to dictation. He spelled *climbing* phonetically, omitting the *b*.

On standardized tests, comparison of scores with those obtained a year earlier showed the following changes:

	April 1955	April 1956
1. Ammons Full-Range Picture Vocabulary Test	75th percentile for for adults	45th percentile for adults
2. Binet Vocabulary	Superior Adult II	13-year-old level
3. Iowa, Reading Vocabulary	Grade level 18	Grade level 13
4. Iowa, Paragraph Comprehension (untimed)	94th percentile for college freshmen	45th percentile for high-school
5. Wide Range Spelling	Grade level 11	Grade level 6.5
6. Wide Range Arithmetic	Grade level 12	Grade level 5 +

The examiner noted: "On easy tasks the patient performed well, and showed the critical ability and the perseverance that has previously characterized his work. As tasks become more difficult, he grew anxious, developed headaches, and wanted to give up and leave the situation. He had not exhibited behavior of this kind previously, even when he was severely aphasic. If an easier task was presented, he again became alert, responsive, and attentive. The discrepancies between performances now and performances a year ago are too consistent and too great to be accounted for by discontinuation of formal treatment. It seems more probable that the obtained performance represents his present capacities."

The examiner took the findings to the neurologist who had Martin's case, saying, "I wish you'd look at these and tell me what you think." He said he would examine Martin again. The only change found on careful neurological examination was that the visual field defect had progressed from the right upper quadrant to the entire right half of the visual fields.

When Mrs. Greshwin was told that there were indications of extension of the lesion, she reported observations that confirmed this impression. She thought Martin had a more difficult time following conversations, missed more of what he was told, took longer to respond, enjoyed radio, television, and reading less, and could not do many of the things he had been doing. Fortunately, Martin seemed to want to do less, and to be relatively contented.

In October, Mrs. Greshwin wrote that there were further changes, and added, "I wish you could come down. It would please Martin, and I'd like to have you see what is happening for yourself."

This was arranged. Martin was pleased, and it was a happy time. There were differences. For one thing, there was loss of recent memory. This is something quite different from aphasia, and Martin had never shown this kind of behavior before. Over and over again he did something, then said, "I can't remember if I took my medicine," or whatever it was.

His mother had become concerned about his driving, although he had shown no signs of not being the excellent driver he had always been. She had discussed this with Martin, putting it on the basis that she thought he did not see as well as he used to, and that he should not drive until his eyes had been examined again. Martin agreed, though reluctantly, and they had made an appointment with the ophthalmologist, and taken the car to the garage for overhauling to reduce temptation. Martin asked over and over all day if he shouldn't go and get his car.

Each time, his mother said patiently, "No, Martin. I don't want you to drive until you have had your eyes examined."

Each time Martin protested, "There's nothing wrong with my eyes. I see all right."

His mother answered, "I don't think you do, and no one would feel worse than you, Martin, if a child ran out from the curb, and you didn't see him. You can't take that chance."

Martin would answer reasonably, "Of course not. We'd better get my eyes examined," and she would tell him again he had an appointment for the following Tuesday.

Martin was satisfied, but five minutes later he asked, "Shall I go down and get my car?"

Occasionally, too, he found himself at a loss when he tried to perform some accustomed activity. He took a coke out of the refrigerator, and stood bewildered, with the coke in one hand and a bottle opener in the other, saying, "I seem to have forgotten how we do this," then added to himself, "I must try harder."

All of these things pointed to generalized and widespread brain damage, and Martin returned to the hospital at the end of the month. The last test was administered in November 1956. Testing had to be done a little at a time, because Martin fatigued easily. When he was asked what bothered him, he replied, "Right now I get very tired in the afternoon. I have trouble getting everything done. Keeping my mind on what you're doing."

On auditory tests, Martin made errors pointing to common objects named by the examiner, pointing to letters named by the examiner, and following simple directions. He scored at the 25th percentile on the Ammons test. He could repeat three digits, but not four, and no sentences longer than four or five words. He could not follow with comprehension either the long or short paragraph read aloud to him.

On visual and reading tests he made errors matching letters, matching words to pictures, and matching printed to spoken words. Reading comprehension broke down on the level of simple sentences and a short narrative paragraph. He was unable to follow a long paragraph at all. On oral reading, many words were misread.

On speech and language tests, Martin was able to name only 6 out of 18 objects. He called a *cup* a *saucer*, a *boy* a *group*, a *flower, leaves,* and for *girl* he said, *they talk.*

He made errors answering six out of eight simple questions, such as "What do you do with a hammer?" and "What do you shave with?" He said you ate with your fingers, and added, "That was so hard."

Examples of attempted definitions are the following:

robin: A bird.
island: A body of water.
motor: Don't know.
bargain: You get food in the store. He will give you a little saving in price.
courage: Excellent courage is—courage is excellent—looking out to one another.
repair: Looking out to one another—no, that's not right. That's what he gets.

Looking out to one another.
leather: Leather. Leather. I don't know.

He described a picture of children flying kites as follows: "One of the—it's a girl, looks out, and the boy is over the—uff, I have such troubles describing this—I'm not making anything that's worth anything—the boys are—the first two boys went out and flied the kites but the second boy got in the wrong wires. There's a—right there." (The boy in the wrong wires referred to a boy trying to get his kite out of a tree. There were no wires in the picture.)

Drawing and copying were very defective, and Martin could not write letters of the alphabet or simple words to dictation. He wrote *nam* for *man*, and *day* for *dog*.

He could make change and select the correct answers to simple arithmetic combinations, but he could not do simple problems involving tens and hundreds.

He could not draw a man, and he reversed the arms on assembling the Wechsler mannikin. He could not assemble the head.

To summarize the findings, Martin again showed a moderately severe reduction of vocabulary and verbal retention span on tests for auditory comprehension, tests for speech and language, and reading tests. On both reading and writing tests he confused letters and words with similar visual configurations. Recall of learned visual patterns, both letters and words, was more severely impaired than on original testing. In addition, spatial disorientation was present, which had not been observed on previous testing. Martin was now having difficulty finding his way about in the hospital, which he had not had before.

Some readers may feel that it was unnecessarily cruel to submit Martin to a battery of tests when it was no longer possible to stay ahead of the destructive processes now operating.

However, in the first place, it is necessary to study processes of regression as well as processes of recovery. Detailed observations of both processes help the clinician to have confidence in the first signs of regression that occur, and in some cases this could lead to successful intervention before greater damage is done.

Moreover, it was not a traumatic procedure. Martin was used to coming back to the hospital for testing. He would probably have been more perturbed if testing had not been done as usual. He expected the clinician to want to know everything about him, and found this supportive. He knew he was not well, and he wanted the clinician to tell him this was why he was having trouble, and he needn't worry about reading and writing when he was feeling so badly. Martin was like a sick child now, wanting reassurance, and he trusted the clinician. He did what she asked as a matter of course. He was pleased when she said something was good. He accepted encouragement when he was trying to perform a task, and he accepted it when the clinician said he'd done enough for now. He usually said he thought he'd go rest, but would come back again tomorrow.

Martin went home. He entered the local hospital just before Christmas. Sometimes he was well enough to go home for a while, but gradually being home mattered less and less to him. Sometimes he knew the people who came to see him and was happy that they had come. Sometimes he thought he was away at school, or back in the navy, surrounded by friends of those days. Finally he lapsed into coma and died in April 1957.

FURTHER OBSERVATIONS

Visual patients show language impairment characterized by reduction of vocabulary and reduction of verbal retention reflected in all language modalities. They differ from simple Aphasic patients only in showing impaired visual discrimination. Resulting disturbances are reflected in both recognition and recall of learned visual patterns, and thus they affect both reading and writing. Impairment may be mild, resulting in only occasional confusions between letters and words with similar visual configurations, or it may be severe, resulting in complete initial loss of recognition and recall of learned symbols.

Factor analysis showed that recognition of pictures and objects was affected, as well as recognition of letters. The Ammons test, for example, loaded a little higher on the factor we identified as visual discrimination (on matching, recognition, and recall) than on language, although the difference was small. To the investigators, this seemed to indicate that processes involved in matching, recognition, and recall of letters and words were not essentially different from those involved in other perceptual learning, although learning of symbols is probably of a higher order of complexity.

In the final stages of the disease, Martin became almost blind, although the entire sensorium was so clouded that it was hard to know how much he actually saw. The additional spatial disorientation he incurred is rarely found in Visual patients. It is more compatible with generalized brain damage than the usual Visual syndrome. Penfield and Roberts (1959) localized awareness of spatial relations and body scheme in the nondominant hemisphere, in an area that roughly corresponds to the posterior language area in the dominant hemisphere.

Drawing as well as writing, is usually affected in most Visual patients. The impairment may be of any degree, from negligible to severe.

One severe Visual patient was an art student. His drawing was at first extremely distorted. He could not draw a man or a house, or reproduce a wheel, when first examined. Drawing ability was recovered, however, long before he had relearned all the alphabetical forms or was reading or writing with any fluency. Probably he was not drawing as well as before. Six months later, when his writing was very good, he was offered a commission to paint a picture of an old house. He tried several times and gave it up, saying he did not know why, but he could not do it. Subsequently, however, he returned to art classes, where competent instructors still judged him a gifted painter.

In the area of visual as well as of auditory perception, the process of repeated stimulation appears to effect improvement, even after fairly serious interferences produced by brain injury. This is probably true only when impairment is confined to the intrinsic visual system.

APHASIC IMPAIRMENT IN THE VISUAL GROUP

It is important to remember that classification in the Visual group does not depend upon even severe limitations in reading and writing, which may result from a language deficit alone. There must be evidence of specific visual components in observed reading and writing deficits, compatible with perceptual involvement on a central and not a peripheral basis. If auditory comprehension and speech and language skills exceed reading and writing skills by a large margin, however, evidence of visual involvement will usually be found.

Specifically, Visual subjects confuse visual symbols with similar configurations. This confusion is based on impaired ability to make fine visual discriminations. Like other deficits in aphasia, it may be mild or severe.

With severe impairment, letter forms must be relearned one by one, in upper case, lower case, print and script. This is probably achieved, initially at least, by reinforcement of visual patterns through kinesthetic cues. Visually impaired subjects are frequently observed tracing letters in the air or on the page, to aid defective recognition or recall. Word recognition is first achieved by identifying individual letters and spelling the word. Since this is slow, there is a tendency to guess at the end of the word. *Medical* may be read *medieval*, *eternally* as *eternity*, or *paradox* as *paradise*, and so on.

Letters that look alike are often confused in reading and writing. In upper-case print, the most common confusions are *E–F, C–G, J–L, H–N–A–K,M–W,* and sometimes *P–B–R* or *O–Q*. In lower case, they are *b–d–p–q–, h–n–u–r, m–w, f–t,* and *j–y*. In script, *y* and *j* are often confused, *y* and *g*, *q* and *g*, *u* and *w*, *o* and *a*, *h* and *b*, *h* and *k*, and sometimes even *h* and *y*.

Reversals and distortions of letter forms appear. There is a tendency toward phonetic spelling, as patients try to use auditory patterns to aid defective visual recall. For this reason, words with silent letters, and particularly words with double letters, are often misspelled. When patients have enough language to be able to spell words, oral spelling is usually better than written spelling. Patients often spell words aloud correctly then write them incorrectly.

Visual subjects resemble Simple Aphasic subjects closely, except for the added perceptual deficit that Simple Aphasic subjects do not have.

TEST FINDINGS

There were no significant differences between means obtained by Simple Aphasic and Visual subjects on tests for auditory comprehension or tests for speech and language, on either test or retest. Ammons test scores were almost identical for the two groups on both test administrations.

Visual patient profiles were characterized by error peaks on reading and writing. They averaged more errors than Simple Aphasics on all reading tests, from matching words to pictures to comprehension of a long paragraph.

Visual subjects also averaged more errors than Simple Aphasics on all drawing, copying, and writing tests on initial and final testing, and showed a smaller reduction of error on all tests.

Visual subjects, for whom writing itself was uncertain, made more errors on written than on oral spelling before and after treatment. In the Simple Aphasic group, the differences between written and oral spelling were smaller, and in the opposite direction.

Visual subjects also averaged significantly more errors than Simple Aphasics on tests for numerical relations and arithmetic processes.The percentage of error reduction was significantly lower on all tests in this section for Visual subjects.

No evidence of disturbance of body scheme was found in this group.

Visual subjects made excellent recovery of language functions not dependent on visual processes. They improved in reading, writing, and arithmetic also, and sometimes dramatically. Reading and writing approached former qualitative levels. Patients read the same kind of books they enjoyed before, and wrote with as much or as little flair as they had previously possessed. Even handwriting looked much the same, in the judgment of patients and their families, when it was recovered. However, recovery was slower in reading and writing than in other language modalities, performance remained slow, and occasional inconsistent errors persisted.

Because of these residuals, it is usually inadvisable for these patients to try to return to occupations that require fine visual discriminations, such as accounting, printing, proofreading, or clerical work. Occupations requiring voluminous reading or writing are also contraindicated, probably, by the retardation of reading rate and similar slowness in writing.

NEUROLOGICAL BACKGROUND

The average age of Visual patients was 45, seven years older than the Simple Aphasics, but some 14 years younger than the average in the Scattered and Irreversible groups. Forty-one percent of these patients were over 50 years old, and 30% were also over 60.

Visual subjects averaged between 10 and 12 years schooling. They had the lowest average occupational level of all diagnostic groups, but this difference was not statistically significant. It was probably accounted for by the chance factor that no Visual patients in this series had occupations classified as professional.

Etiology was trauma for 20% of these subjects, neoplasm for 8%, and infectious process for 4% and cerebrovascular accident for the remaining 68%. Six percent of the cerebrovascular accidents were confirmed complete thromboses of the internal carotid artery. There were no complete thromboses of the middle cerebral artery in the Visual group.

Visual subjects did not differ significantly from Simple Aphasics in incidence of cerebrovascular accidents, or in incidence of complete thrombosis. Both occurred less often in Simple Aphasic and Visual patients than in any other group.

Visual patients were like Simple Aphasic patients in presenting a relatively low incidence of findings indicating extensive or severe neurological involvement. In reduction of sensation, the Visual group exceeded the incidence of most other groups, contrary to the general prediction.

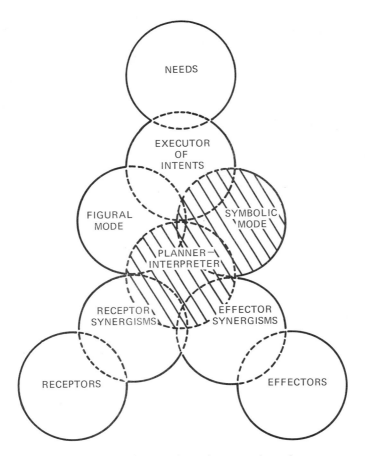

Fig. 11–1. Functional schema for aphasia with involvement of visual processes.

In general, the incidence of complicating neurophysiological conditions was significantly lower in Simple Aphasic, Visual, and Sensorimotor patients than in the other groups. The exception was in visual field defects, in which Visual patients exceeded all other diagnostic groups.

Patients in the Visual group generally did exceedingly well in self-care and ambulation. Thirty-five percent entered a program of vocational training or returned to gainful employment after leaving the hospital. This finding is important, considering the fact that 30% were over 60 and had passed or were approaching retirement age.

A FUNCTIONAL SCHEMA FOR APHASIA WITH CEREBRAL INVOLVEMENT OF VISUAL PROCESSES

Aphasics with impaired visual processes cannot be distinguished from Simple Aphasics with respect to either production or comprehension of speech. However, these patients do show disproportionally greater difficulty in processing visually presented linguistic materials. Although they make many errors in reading and writing, their ability to discriminate nonsymbolic visual patterns or to succeed at tasks involving visual–motor coordination is unimpaired. Since there is no evidence of bilateral damage that would implicate the figural component, the functional locus of their visual impairment is placed in the *planner–interpreter* component.

Of course, as stated in Chapter 6, it should be emphasized that the functional components in the schema actually represent distinct parallel functional levels which characterize analogous processes for all sensory modalities. Therefore, the locus for visual involvement of the type specified for this group of patients should be thought of as existing in the planner–interpreter component specific to the processing of symbols as figural objects in the visual modality.

chapter **12**

MILD APHASIA WITH PERSISTING DYSFLUENCY

Bob Jackson served in the Field Artillery during World War II, and was in Japan for two years during the Korean War. He worked for the telephone company as a lineman and installer from 1947 until his illness in 1965. Bob spent the Christmas holidays of 1965 in a large city hospital away from home. He was having a series of tests to determine the cause of his "black outs." His wife and five-year-old daughter were excited and happy when he was allowed to return home for the New Year holiday. He started to have seizures on New Year's Eve, and the new year found him back in the hospital with right hemiplegia and aphasia. The diagnosis was cerebral thrombosis. Bob's wife was terrified that she would lose her husband, since the stroke seemed to affect him so much more than the coronary thrombosis he had had ten years before. As Bob recovered, Mrs. Jackson felt that Bob was ready for therapy, but none was available at the private hospital. They decided Bob should go to the nearest Veterans Administration Hospital, but had some trying days searching for his Army discharge papers. Bob knew where they were, but he couldn't tell his wife.

Once in the hospital, Bob was started on a physical therapy program and was soon able to walk without help, but Mrs. Jackson was concerned about his lack of speech. She knew she was getting into the habit of talking for her husband. When it was suggested that Bob be transferred to the Minneapolis Hospital, Bob and his wife eagerly agreed, although they knew this would mean a separation of many miles for them.

The diagnosis made at the Minneapolis Hospital was cerebral thrombosis of the small branch of the left middle cerebral artery. Bob had a right facial and tongue paralysis and flaccid paralysis of the right arm. Electroencephalograms revealed a slow wave focus in the left anterior region.

Bob was first seen in the Aphasia Clinic in February, 1966. His ruddy face and gray-blond crew cut made him appear younger than his 47 years. From the first day, his therapist was impressed by his ability to laugh at himself as he good-naturedly did his best to perform well on the battery of tests.

INITIAL FINDINGS

On tests for auditory comprehension, Bob showed mild impairment. He made minimal errors in recognizing letters and was able to perform all the directions except the longest one. He could repeat five digits, but only two short sentences. He scored in the 92 percentile for adults on the Ammons Full-Range Picture Vocabulary Test. He was able to answer questions on a paragraph read to him, but made errors when he was asked to repeat sentences.

On visual tests Bob made no errors in matching forms, letters, or words to pictures. When asked to match printed to spoken words, he made minimal errors, confusing only a few words which sounded alike. He made minimal errors in reading sentences and a paragraph, but his silent reading rate was within normal limits. Bob's performance broke down in reading aloud. He was able to read only half of the words and did not attempt the oral sentences.

Bob was able to imitate all gross movements of the speech musculature, but none of the rapid alternating movements. Protrusion and retraction of the tongue and lateral movements were slow and arhythmic. He had difficulty initiating movements of the speech musculature. He was able to repeat more than half of the monosyllables; errors appeared more in the complex blends than in simple monosyllables. On longer units and in spontaneous speech he had great difficulty enunciating clearly. He performed well when asked to count, to name the days of the week, and to complete sentences, but he could not recall the answers to two simple questions such as "What do you do with a razor?" He could give only his name and his wife's name when asked for biographical information. Bob was able to name all but six pictures and could define one word—a robin, he said, was a bird.

Bob's speech was characterized by a slow rate and by labored and imprecise articulation. The cineflurography report read: "Patient seems to have normal tongue movements. He apparently has a substituting problem occurring at a cerebral level." It is interesting to note the description "substituting problem" the radiologist gave this patient's speech. It appears that the patient made mistakes with his tongue and corrected them by ear, producing a pattern of speech much like stuttering.

Bob did well except for written and oral spelling, making 50% error in written and 90% error in oral spelling. He did manage to produce one written sentence using the word *door*. He made errors in complex written arithmetic problems, but he was able to perform all other numerical tests without error. For the first time in his life Bob wrote and drew with his left hand since his right hand was paralyzed.

In summary, findings revealed a mild reduction of available vocabulary and verbal retention span in all modalities, complicated by a persisting dysfluency. His erratic performance, such as his ability to name most pictures but to give very little biographical information, was due to his unstable neurophysiological condition. Since the biographical information section of the test was given early, we suspect that the patient was making some spontaneous recovery throughout testing.

COURSE OF RECOVERY

Bob received treatment for aphasia for about three months, beginning in February, 1966. He was started on phrases using ten Language Master cards each day. We gave him ten words daily to spell aloud, to write, and to use in sentences. We read aloud with him, then asked him to read the sentences alone. He was given a short article in the *Reader's Digest Reading Skill Builder Series* to read, and asked to write answers to questions for part of his outside work. Bob made excellent progress in increasing his available vocabulary and verbal retention span, by intensive auditory stimulation. He made extremely rapid progress in reading and writing. The biggest problem was in learning to control his speech musculature for clear articulation. On March 10, Mrs. Jackson wrote to the therapist in part: "I can notice a very great improvement in Bob each time we hear from him. The first letter I received from him was nothing but pure garble, cherished only for his thoughtfulness and effort. This last week I received another that was very coherent; he told of his daily routine and didn't wander off at all. The improvement was quite wonderful. Also, each time he calls there is a marked difference and all for the better."

Bob was learning to control his speech musculature. He had to take his time and could not be hurried. What helped him most with articulation was strong rhythmic drill on consonants and blends, first in nonsense syllables, then in words, phrases, and sentences.

Mrs. Jackson sent the clinician the various forms with which Bud worked, and also lists of telephone parts used in his work. As he practiced ordering parts as if he were on the phone, Bob felt that he would be able to inventory, order, and issue supplies to line crews.

On retest in April, Bob made minimal errors in repeating sentences, and he was able to repeat five digits. He made no other errors on auditory tests. He made only one error in reading comprehension at the paragraph level, and only two errors of a possible 30 in reading sentences aloud. These errors were omission errors. Bob made minimal errors in spelling, increasing his score from the 3.6 grade level to the 6.6 grade level. He made errors in two of the sentences written to dictation and was able to write a spontaneous paragraph without error.

Speech and language tests showed that Bob no longer had much word-finding difficulty. He defined all the words without error. He did show a mild reduction of retention span in retelling a paragraph. Bob still had some difficulty with rapid alternating movements of the speech musculature; his three speech errors were caused by slowness of his tongue. He made no other errors on the speech and language section. Bob still needed to strive for control of speech movements, but speech was clear and the few articulatory errors were corrected as he made them. This made his speech somewhat slow and hesitant, with occasional but unobtrusive repetitions. He expressed his chief complaint about his condition as, "getting words mixed up in my tongue."

After an appointment with a vocational counselor, Bob was discharged in April. Unfortunately, another coronary attack has kept him from going back to work. Bob has fully accepted his role as housekeeper. His wife recently wrote from the small western town where they are now living, "He works all the time and if he didn't do such a great job keeping things going at home I wouldn't be able to work and Molly wouldn't be such a happy well-adjusted little girl. I do think God has given me two very remarkable humans to share this life with. When things are the blackest they can both find something funny in it. Bob keeps the house, yard and both of us going. It is a good life and few families are as close."

FURTHER OBSERVATIONS

Dysarthria, defined as consistent impairment of articulation or fluency, is not necessarily correlated with reduction of language. Dysarthria may reflect paralysis or paresis of the musculature—such as is found in bulbar polio, in cerebral palsy, in pseudo-bulbar disorders, or in impaired coordination and control of motor processes, as in some cerebellar diseases. When dysarthria alone is present, reading, writing, and auditory comprehension are normal. Because the patients we are discussing do not have paralysis of speech musculature but do have both aphasia and persisting articulatory problems, we have chosen to call them *dysfluent*.

What we call *sensorimotor* impairment, without paralysis or paresis of the musculature, is characterized by phonemic disintegration in conjunction with reduced auditory and proprioceptive discrimination, and is correlated with overall reduction of language. We use the term *sensorimotor disorder* rather than *apraxia*, because *apraxia* has been used in the literature to describe a wide variety of conditions and has many connotations —including ones of localization—that are no longer tenable.

We define *sensorimotor impairment* as reduction of auditory *and* proprioceptive feedback of the speech musculature.

PERSISTING DYSFLUENCY

The Dysfluent patient shows language impairment characterized by mild or transient reduction of available vocabulary and verbal retention span, reflected in all modalities, together with persisting difficulty in movements of the speech musculature. In one case which has been followed, the difficulty persisted for 18 years. Patients with persisting dysfluency must continue to exert conscious control over the speech musculature. The impairment is characterized by slow speech, distorted vowels, and often by placement errors. The patient seems, clinically, to lack proprioceptive feedback, but he continually corrects his errors in placement as he hears them. This continuing correction sometimes makes the speaker sound a little like a primary stutterer.

We believe that the types of articulatory changes Scott and Ringel (1971) observed with normal subjects deprived of oral sensory feedback, are surprisingly similar to changes found in the Dysfluent aphasic group. Further, Scott and Ringel (1971) clearly demonstrated the articulatory differences between dysarthria caused by motor weakness of the speech musculature and the type of articulation demonstrated by patients who suffer from inadequate proprioceptive feedback. Although we cannot be certain, because of differences in classification and terminology, we think Rosenbek's study (1971) of "apraxia of speech" is probably applicable here too. Such patients made errors in oral form identification and had significantly greater two-point difference limens for midline of underlip, tongue tip, and tongue blade than did normals or "aphasics."

The fact that Persisting Dysfluent patients have unilateral lesions supports the contention that this speech pattern is not a motor weakness. Luria describes this pattern as "kinetic or efferent apraxia in which difficulties arise involving inhibition of a preceding speech movement with transition to the next movement." These patients, together with the Sensorimotor patients, are often labeled "apractic." Factor analysis showed three tests with critical loadings on both the language factor and the factor involving movements of the speech musculature. Inspection showed that the motor loadings decrease in magnitude as language loadings increase. Imitation of tongue movements had the highest motor and the smallest language component, while alternating movements, requiring finer motor coordinations and control, showed slightly higher language loading and a lower motor component. In repetition of monosyllabic words, the motor loading becomes almost negligible, while the language loading shows continued increase in magnitude. These interrelations suggest that the speech mechanism is a functionally educated structure whose output is related to the organization of language, as well as to the integration of motor processes with the language system that programs and controls verbal output. Because Persisting Dysfluent patients have such a mild aphasia, they are able to learn control of the speech musculature.

In our earlier diagnostic categories, these patients were called "mild sensorimotor" patients. This group seemed to have reduction of proprioceptive feedback, without the severe reduction of auditory feedback and without the severe aphasia demonstrated by the Sensorimotor patients. One doctor wrote about a Persisting Dysfluent patient: "The patient ambulates well, reads newspapers and books. He has a partial speech aphasia particularly when talking rapidly but is generally able to express ideas quite well, although his stammering and inability to use proper words are noted." In some cases the nonfluencies have been reduced when the patient has daily practice of reading sentences aloud, then repeating them from memory, and reading a short paragraph aloud two or three times,then telling what he remembers about it. This tends to increase facility and stimulate more language.

TEST FINDINGS IN PERSISTING DYSFLUENCY

Patients with Persisting Dysfluency are less impaired in language than the other two mild groups, the Simple Aphasic and the Visual. These patients made only half the mean number of errors that Simple Aphasics made in the auditory section of the

Minnesota Test (Schuell, 1955). They had the lowest mean number of errors in the Auditory, Reading, and Writing sections of the test. On Speech and Language tests, they made significantly more errors than Simple Aphasics or Visuals, but had fewer errors than any other group. Persisting Dysfluents made a higher mean error scores on gross motor movements of the speech musculature than any other group except Irreversibles (although the Scattered Findings patients made nearly as many). On rapid alternating movements both the Persisting Dysfluents and the Sensorimotor patients made a mean number of 3.00 errors, significantly higher than the errors of any group except the Irreversibles. On repetition of monosyllabic words, Persisting Dysfluent patients made a mean error 6.57, while the mean error for Sensorimotor patients was 15.5 On retest, however, the Persisting Dysfluents were all able to repeat monosyllables without error.

NEUROLOGICAL BACKGROUND

The mean age of Persisting Dysfluent patients was 41. None were over 60 years, and 29% were under 30. This was the youngest group.

These patients averaged 13 years of schooling. Their occupations ranged from day laborer through professions, with the median being skilled laborers and clerical workers.

Etiology was trauma in 42.5% of the sample, 42.5% CVA, and 12% other etiologies. The three CVA patients had thrombosis of the left middle cerebral artery. Persisting Dysfluents had the lowest incidence of CVA's and the highest incidence of trauma.

Eighty-six percent of the Persisting Dysfluents had paresis of extremities. However, the Simple Aphasics, together with Persisting Dysfluents, had the lowest incidence of paralysis in the extremities. Seventy-two percent of the Persisting Dysfluent patients had facial paralysis, with only the Sensorimotor and Irreversible patients exceeding them. In sensory reduction, Persisting Dysfluents exceeded only Auditory and Simple Aphasics.

EEG information was available on only three of the seven Persisting Dysfluents. All three had focal lesions in the left frontal lobe. Although the neurological information was not very complete, one author (E. J-P) concluded from the information available that all seven showed obvious left frontal lobe damage. None of the Persisting Dysfluent patients had visual field cuts or abnormal mental status.

Persisting Dysfluent patients had the same incidence (28%) of hypertension as Visual patients. This was a higher percentage than Simple Aphasic, Auditory, and Sensorimotor patients, but less than Scattered Findings and Irreversible patients.

Incidence of abnormal electrocardiograms was 33% for this group, and 33% for the Sensorimotor group, which was higher than Auditory patients but lower than all other groups.

Persisting Dysfluents had the third highest incidence of involvement of palatal, pharyngeal, and tongue weakness, with one patient showing signs of each. This incidence was lower than those of the Irreversible and Scattered Findings patients, but higher than those of Simple Aphasic, Visual, and Sensorimotor patients. The limited and focused nature of this impairment clearly was not sufficient to account for the dysfluencies that were observed in this group. Six of the seven patient with Persisting Dysfluency performed advanced self-care activities on initial evaluation, as well as on final. They were all able to ambulate without assistance. None had adverse sequelae such as commitment or death. Six of the seven have achieved either gainful employment or vocational training.

A FUNCTIONAL SCHEMA FOR MILD APHASIA WITH PERSISTING DYSFLUENCY

This aphasia seems to involve a fairly mild impairment to the formulation of symbolic communiques, accompanied by a relatively severe impairment of the *effector synergism*

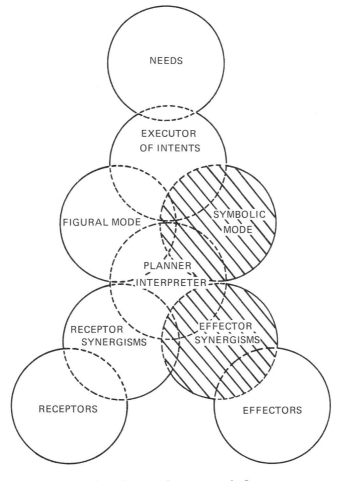

Fig. 12–1. Functional schema for aphasia with persisting dysfluency.

component, presumably due to the disruption of proprioceptive feedback from the articulation system (see Fig. 12-1). Thus, the organization of fine muscle control is faulty, even though neurological examination fails to reveal any motor weakness or any other problem with the speech musculature itself. The *receptor synergisms* are clearly intact since the patient uses this component to monitor feedback from his own speech attempts.

Consequently, the Persisting Dysfluent patient is quite able to construct plans to be used by either the *effector* or *receptor synergisms*, but is simply unable to execute them successfully. On the other hand, the patient has no trouble applying *receptor synergisms* to interpret what is received (within, of course, the limits of his simple aphasia).

chapter 13

APHASIA WITH SCATTERED FINDINGS

Dr. Thomas Bennington was a surgeon with a long and honorable record of distinguished medical service. He was a professor of surgery at a well-known midwestern university and chief of the surgical service of a large city hospital. In the past he had been president of the state medical association and a member of the state board of medical examiners. Though he was known as a brilliant exacting man, it was generally recognized that he required as much of himself as of others and that his medical standards were the same for the inmate of a state institution as for wealthy private patients.

At 69, Dr. Bennington was a tall, well-built man with a dynamic personality and active professional interests. A month before his 70th birthday, he had what was described as a mild cerebrovascular accident affecting the left cerebral hemisphere, accompanied by partial aphasia. Complete recovery followed.

Six months afterward, there was a second episode characterized by transient aphasia. A few days later, a severe cerebrovascular accident occurred. This time recovery was slow and discouraging. Six weeks after the onset, Dr. Bennington was transferred to the Neurology Service of the Minneapolis VA Hospital for its rehabilitation program.

Neurological findings on admission included severe aphasia, marked right hemiplegia, right lower facial paralysis, difficulty in swallowing, and emotional lability. Neither sensory status nor visual fields could be accurately determined. There was a history of hypertension, and indications of arteriosclerosis were found. The electrocardiogram was abnormal, with signs of an old posterior myocardial infarction. The diagnosis was cerebrovascular accident, probably thrombosis, secondary to arteriosclerosis and hypertension.

INITIAL TEST FINDINGS

Dr. Bennington was examined for aphasia eight weeks after the onset of persisting symptoms. Hospital records of this period reported resistance to treatment, hostility, and frequent catastrophic reactions. The patient appeared withdrawn and depressed.

The examiner asked if he knew where he was, and he nodded. She asked if he knew why he was in the VA Hospital, and he gave her a searching look, but did not reply. He seemed to listen intently while she explained that his doctors hoped the rehabilitation program would help him. She asked if he could talk, and he said, "Sometimes," in barely audible voice. She told him the function of the Aphasia Clinic, and he nodded again. She asked if he would try some tests, and he said, "Yes," in the same low voice.

He fatigued quickly, and frequently stopped responding in the middle of a task. The clinician persisted with the examination because she hoped to stimulate him and establish some points of contact.

There is no justification for continuing procedures when a patient is too sick to respond to tests. Sometimes, however, the aphasic patient requires stimulation before the patterns organized in his brain can begin to function. Sometimes, also, communication must be reestablished before the patient is able to integrate his resources and move toward recovery. The clinician believed that Dr. Bennington showed awareness of what had happened to him, and signs of reactive depression. She thought he needed to receive positive support and to move toward objectivity before he could begin to come to terms with what had happened. She tried to keep him working as long as possible each day, but accepted his withdrawals as signs that a limit of tolerance had been reached. He showed interest in test materials, which could be maintained about 15 minutes at a time.

On tests for auditory comprehension, Dr. Bennington pointed to common objects named by the examiner, but confused *bed* and *chair*, and *boy* and *girl*. He could not point to objects named in series of two, or of three, but when the examiner went back and named the same objects singly, responses were all correct. It is good test procedure to take a patient back from a harder to an easier task, thus underlining successful performance.

Dr. Bennington scored below the first percentile for adults on the Ammons *Full-Range Picture Vocabulary Test*. He followed short directions, but missed the four longest ones. He did not respond to any paragraph materials.

He showed no distress during this part of the examination. When he became too tired, or perhaps too threatened, he closed his eyes and went to sleep. He roused when asked if he would like to go back to his room, and usually said, "Yes," although one day he said, "I'd like to go back to my room." He was always punctiliously courteous, and the examiner was encouraged by this because it was obviously a well-integrated behavior pattern, and of a higher order than the disorganized responses that had usually been reported.

On visual and reading tests the patient consistently neglected items to the right. Occasionally he also ignored an object at the extreme left. It was clear that right homonymous hemianopsia was present. Further constriction of the visual fields was equivocal, for relevant responses were variable. The patient matched colors, pictures, and letters of the alphabet without error but made two errors matching geometric forms. He matched a few printed words to pictures, and a few printed to spoken words. There was no performance on other reading tests.

The patient could initiate phonation at will, but could not sustain it five seconds. Volume was weak, tones had a breathy quality, and he could not raise or lower pitch voluntarily.

The patient could protrude and retract his tongue and perform lateral movements, but rate was slow. He could not place the tip of the tongue on the upper or lower teeth ridge voluntarily.

The soft palate was paralyzed on the right, and the jaw deviated to the right on excursion. Nurses reported the patient choked occasionally both on liquids and solid foods, although this occurred less frequently than on admission. All diadochokinetic movements were impaired. On repetition of monosyllables, the patient made articulatory errors on 16 out of 30 words. He repeated some short phrases, but these were barely intelligible.

A few associative responses were elicited, and the patient named 11 out of 18 common objects. This was the highest response obtained on speech and language tests, although some reactive speech occurred during testing sessions. Once, when the patient was asked if he were comfortable, he nodded, and then said clearly, a few minutes later, "I'm not comfortable." Another day he shook his head no when asked if he wanted to go back to his room, but presently said, "I want to go back."

There was no voluntary function in the right upper extremity. The patient could hold a pencil in his left hand, but could not copy, draw, or trace. When asked to copy a circle, he picked up a pencil and drew a distorted half moon. He perseverated on this form on succeeding tasks. On later trials he could not produce a legible letter. Attempts were characterized by distortions, confusion of directionality, and both vertical and horizontal reversals.

On object assembly tests, the patient picked up the pieces and placed some of them correctly. He reversed the legs on the Wechsler mannikin. He placed one piece correctly on the profile, but could not decide where any of the other belonged.

He showed distress at his inability to write, but appeared relieved when the examiner told him it was too early to begin working on it, and it would be better to let it go for awhile. This was true enough. Even when patients can tolerate intensive therapy, it is preferable to start training an impaired hand with grosser movements than those involved in writing. When possible, this should be done by occupational therapists trained in administering programs of graduated activities, proceeding from gross to finer and more complex movements.

In summary, aphasic findings included reduction of vocabulary and verbal retention span in all language modalities that could be tested, some residual functional language, impairment of visual discrimination, spatial disorientation, dysarthria secondary to partial paralysis of the speech musculature, and impaired sensory control of the movements of the left hand.

Some emotional lability was observed. Only a superficial clinical relation was established. The patient had not rejected procedures, had shown no catastrophic reactions, and had gone so far as to smile on occasion. Sleep is complete withdrawal, but this occurred regularly after about 15 minutes of activity, and did not seem related to any specific preceding events. One could hope for increasing neurophysiological stability with time, since only two months had elapsed since onset.

The neurophysiological instability of the patient, his limited work tolerance, depression, and the involvement of multiple cerebral systems all pointed to a poor prognosis, but it was too soon to give up. The best procedure seemed to be a period of trial therapy with limited objectives. In such situations the pertinent question is what changes can be effected that will contribute most to the well-being of the patient. The examiner decided to try to increase auditory comprehension, stimulate more language, and improve intelligibility of speech. The rationale was that if communication could be made easier, the patient would communicate more. It was hoped that this in turn would reduce frustration and isolation, and make it possible for a deeper and more meaningful clinical relationship to develop.

The examiner told the patient she would like to try to make it easier for him to talk, and for other people to understand him. She said she thought it would be possible to get the musculature working better, and words coming more easily. He seemed to understand and was willing to go on.

THE COURSE OF TREATMENT

By the end of two weeks the patient was able to tolerate sessions of 35 minutes consistently, and on a few occasions he worked for 45 minutes.

His voice became stronger, and this carried over into functional speech. The first words of responses were usually audible, and sometimes all the words were. Articulation improved. The clinician used exercises, but also stressed a more vigorous attack on words and phrases to facilitate articulation and reduce slurring. Carryover in functional speech varied. When the patient made a strong effort, results were good. When he did not, articulation deteriorated.

At the end of three weeks, the clinician wrote in her notes: "I get glimpses of what I want. A word or phrase comes clear and strong, or for a few moments there is interest and directed effort, then it is gone. I am not sure what the inhibiting factor is. Today I said, 'Doctor, when you try for a few minutes, does it stop working for you?' He looked at me searchingly, then said, 'Yes.' This often seems to be true."

To stimulate vocabulary, the clinician used an association technique to elicit a word, then followed the response with a question to reinforce it. It worked like this. The clinician said, "The sun rises in the—," and the patient said, *"east."* The clinician then asked, "Where does the sun rise?" and he replied, "In the east." Next she said, "You carry an umbrella when it—," and he said, *"rains."* She asked, "When do you carry an umbrella?" Dr. Bennington responded firmly, "Never!" then looked up and laughed. There were moments like this, of shared amusement and enjoyment, but they were infrequent.

He began to be able to listen to short paragraphs read aloud to him, and to answer questions about content, although most responses were monosyllables. On some days, however, he just went to sleep while the clinician was reading.

He was soon able to read words, phrases, and short sentences aloud, and one day he asked to take a simply written but interesting history of locomotives back to his room.

By the end of a month he was staying a full hour, and the clinician noted that he was repeating sentences, making good conversational responses, and listening intently to excerpts from a surgeon's diary which she had begun to read to him that week without any preliminary comment. She wrote in her notes one day, "Speech was stronger and more clearly articulated than I've ever heard it, and there were more voluntary responses."

The next day the doctor asked suddenly, "Are you going to go on seeing me?"

The clinician said yes, matter-of-factly. The doctor continued to look at her, waiting, and she knew that an important question was being asked. She answered slowly that at first he was not able to do enough work to get results. She said she had realized he tired easily, and was often uncomfortable, but she thought this was better. He nodded.

She said some days were still better than other days, and she did not always know why. He was still regarding her searchingly. She asked, "Is it because you think it's no use?" He made an affirmative gesture, then began to sob painfully. He tried to apologize, but the clinician said, "It's all right. You needed to do this. You've been holding it in too long."

This was not emotional lability. It was long-restrained grief for the loss of his profession, and pent-up resentment at being a patient and helpless instead of a doctor doing his work in the hospital. This is grief that is hard for a man to express. He tries to shield his family from knowledge of it, and he does not find it easy to share with anyone. Even the clinician must wait until a question is asked in some way. Usually when the patient can ask the question he knows at least part of the answer, and has begun to make the hard adjustment.

Presently the clinician answered Dr. Bennington's question by saying, "It won't be the way it was before, but it will be better than it is now."

It was possible to go on and say that it is never easy to give up one's work, but this time inevitably comes to everyone. She said the people to be pitied were those who never found work they cared about, or received any deep satisfaction from doing. Dr. Bennington said, "Yes, that's true."

The clinician added, "But you have had it, and this is something nothing can take from you. You will always be Dr. Bennington, and your name will always be respected in medicine. You have earned an honorable retirement. You know this, don't you?"

He smiled, and said, "Yes." It was true. A few months later he was presented a medal and a citation for distinguished service by the State Medical Association.

This was a different kind of communication, and it marked a change in the clinical relationship. It was never again superficial. A good period followed. Dr. Bennington was less depressed, and an air of confidence and authority began to return. Sometimes he was so unconsciously peremptory that the clinician protested she was not his scrub nurse, which always amused him.

The nurses noted that the doctor asked for what he wanted, instead of showing anger or distress when his wishes were not anticipated. The first few times this happened it was considered noteworthy enough to be recorded. One day he said, "Please pull down the shade," very clearly, when the sun was in his eyes. The head nurse reported he responded to conversational overtures in a friendly manner, instead of ignoring them as he had done previously. On one occasion she asked if he remembered a nurse they both knew, and he asked what she was doing, and added, "She was a good scout, wasn't she?"

He enjoyed being read to for longer and longer periods. One day the clinician read Irving Cobb's (1915) description of his operation aloud, and Dr. Bennington chuckled all the way through. He was greatly amused at an account of an early operative procedure described in *The Doctor's Mayo* (Clapesattle, 1941). The clinician asked if he had ever performed this operation, and he replied, "Oh, yes, many times." She asked if he used the same method, and he laughed and said, "Oh, no. It's a fairly simply procedure, now."

Dr. Bennington's wife observed that he showed more interest in people and events outside the hospital. About this time the clinician had to be away for a few days, and Mrs. Bennington suggested she work with the doctor during this period. The clinician asked Dr. Bennington if he would like this, and he said, "Why, yes. I think it is a good idea." It worked very well.

The patient was retested after three months of treatment. There were measurable gains in auditory comprehension, in speech, and in reading. Dr. Bennington made fewer errors on the tests he had responded to before, and performed on some tests that had elicited no responses earlier. On auditory tests, he followed the short paragraph. On reading tests, he passed some items on sentence comprehension. On speech and language tests, he gave biographical information, described a picture, and defined a few words adequately. Copying was as difficult as before. Auditory comprehension was better, more language was available, and speech was more intelligible, although there were still severe limitations.

Slow improvement continued for another two or three months, although there were days that only marked time. Progress in self-care and ambulation was negligible. The patient could not maintain balance, and was never able to stand without assistance from the therapists. After long training the patient was able to eat his meals unassisted, but remained unable to perform other self-care activities.

In December, which was the seventh month of treatment, there were more and more bad days, when nothing could be obtained except a few mumbled responses. The doctor tried, but efforts to speak clearly resulted in clonic spasms of the jaw and pharynx, which sometimes spread to the arm and thorax. He still wanted to be read to, but usually fell asleep after a few sentences. Nursing notes recorded that he choked more frequently, required more help with eating, and was more lethargic.

The clinician began to think about terminating treatment. However, there were multiple medical problems, the first one of these flared, then another. There were days when the patient was ill with a cold, with a gastrointestinal disturbance, or cystitis, but hope of remission and resumed progress remained. In the meantime, the established clinical relationship seemed to mitigate discouragement and depression. This was simply maintenance therapy. The patient agreed to tell the clinician when he was uncomfortable and wanted to stop working or go back to his room. The clinician, on her part, used techniques that placed minimal demands upon the patient and enabled him to respond most easily.

During this month and the next, it was apparent to everyone that Dr. Bennington was losing ground. In February he developed pneumonia, and treatment for aphasia was interrupted. The long illness effectively severed the clinical relationship, and it was not resumed. When the clinician told the patient she did not think he was well enough to come to the clinic, he did not appear to be disturbed. On subsequent visits he knew her sometimes and was glad to see her, and at other times made little response. He never regained the ground he had lost and continued to have recurring medical problems that required total nursing care.

When he was well enough he was up in the morning and watched television, although he frequently fell asleep in his chair. He went to the gymnasium for treatments to maintain range of motion and prevent contractures, and sometimes for adapted games. His wife spent long hours at the hospital with him every day. If he felt well enough, she took him to the canteen or to the library, where they often listened to records in the music room, which he always seemed to enjoy. He talked very little, although occasionally he communicated effectively, making it clear that understanding was intact although attention was intermittent. One day he surprised his doctor by asking clearly, "Who won the ball game last night?" The doctor told him Minnesota had won, and he smiled and replied, "That's good." Continuous medical and nursing care undoubtedly prolonged his life, but the course was gradually downhill until his death from hypostatic bronchopneumonia.

AUTOPSY FINDINGS

Severe generalized arteriosclerosis was found in the coronary arteries of the heart, with focal myocardial fibrosis, and left ventricular hypertrophy.

Sclerotic changes were found in the brain, most marked in the vertebral and basilar arteries, and in the circle of Willis. Similar changes were present in the peripheral arteries.

Massive softening was found in the brain, involving the left superior and middle frontal gyrus, and extending back to the superior parietal lobule and into the superior temporal gyrus. A cystic formation extended from the subependymal lining of the ventricles to the surface of the cortex. There was total absence of much of the left lenticular nucleus and the thalamus. A second lesion, primarily cortical, involved the right superior parietal lobule.

Microscopic examination of sections showed a cyst formation, with adjacent isomorphic gliosis forming a peripheral cyst wall. The extraparenchymal vessels showed marked arteriosclerotic changes.

The final diagnosis was massive cerebral encephalomalacia and severe cerebral atherosclerosis.

FURTHER OBSERVATIONS

The outcome is fortunately better for many of these patients than it was for Dr. Bennington, but his history illustrates many of the facets and ramifications of aphasia that must be taken into account for this group.

The test findings were classical, with reduction of vocabulary and verbal retention span, preservation of some functional language, and involvement of visual and motor processes. Spatial disorientation and sensorimotor involvement of the left hand are less common, but are not incompatible with a clinical picture resulting from scattered or generalized brain damage.

It frequently happens that patients make a good recovery from a first or second cerebrovascular accident, but lose hope and give up with recurring incidents or progressive disease. The cause may be either physiological or psychological or both.

Since the course of disease is unpredictable and there may be years in which the patient's condition remains relatively stable, it is important to determine if initial apathy and withdrawal results from depression or from inability to respond. Often a trial period of therapy is the only way to find out. Depression is a realistic reaction to loss, and usually indicates more awareness and insight than euphoria, although this, too, may be a defense mechanism and cover quite different feelings.

Most aphasic patients are inaccessible to direct psychotherapy because they cannot communicate well enough. More than speech is involved, for communication is a two-way process. The aphasic patient frequently cannot talk enough to verbalize his feelings, and he frequently responds to only a small part of what other people say, which may lead to misinterpretation of what is said. On the other hand, it is almost impossible for the speech pathologist, who works with the patient's disabilities every day, not to observe what his feelings about them are, and what strengths he has to draw upon. It is possible to secure formal or informal psychiatric consultations when unusual or persisting emotional problems are present. Psychiatrists usually advise one to encourage expression of feelings, and to be as permissive and supportive as possible. Usually, with a patient who was a stable individual before his illness, this is all that is required. Confidence returns, the perceived situation changes, and adjustments to the new limitations are made.

This happened to Dr. Bennington. The depression decreased, and the aphasia improved measurably despite generally unfavorable conditions. There were too many of the latter, and they progressed too steadily for gains to be maintained. This is the reason that prognosis must always be considered guarded for Scattered Findings patients. On the other hand, this should not be construed to mean it is always poor.

Many severe hemiplegics improve enough to get about the house and yard and care for their personal needs. Only a few continue to require total nursing care. There are usually limitations that must be accepted, but many patients manage to keep busy and contented, in spite of them.

Dr. Cartier, another retired physician, once said, "I always thought when I retired I'd play golf and write a book, and now I can't do either."

This was true, but he continues to find things to enjoy. He and his wife drive to Florida every winter, and come back north in the spring. They enjoy people wherever they go. Dr. Cartier's speech is imperfect, and he cannot tell all the wonderful stories he knows, but people come to talk to him anyway, because they like to talk to him. He even refereed a golf match once, riding an electric vehicle with high enthusiasm and breakneck speed, if reports are reliable. The difference in outcome was principally due to the fact that Dr. Cartier's general neurophysiological condition was much better than Dr. Bennington's. He was not only able to maintain the gains he made, but has continued to improve during the seven years of followup. He has now passed his 74th birthday.

Many Scattered Findings patients leave the hospital, go home, and manage to keep busy and contented. A patient with visual involvement cannot drive the car or read comfortably, but his wife drives the car, and he enjoys listening to the ball games, playing with the grandchildren, and going to church on Sunday. He gets tired a little easier than he used to, rests a little more, and it takes less activity to fill a day or a week.

The most beneficial single factor is usually some kind of regular routine that structures the days, and gives the individual something to get up for and to look forward to. It should provide enough exercise to maintain circulation, and tire him enough to go to bed at night. This will be discussed more fully in another chapter.

APHASIC FINDINGS

Patients with scattered or bilateral damage, like other aphasics, show reduction of vocabulary and verbal retention span reflected in all language modalities. Impairment of language may be mild or moderately severe, but there is always some residual functional language in one modality or another.

We are using the term *functional language* to distinguish between voluntary communication and the more automatic responses that Hughlings Jackson (1879) referred to as inferior speech. In general, the latter are responses elicited by immediate external stimuli.

They include *yes* and *no* and *all right* or *I don't know*, as well as *hello* and *good-by*. They include highly overlearned serial responses, such as counting, saying the alphabet, or naming the days of the week. Hughlings Jackson (1879) included occasional, recurring, and emotionally determined utterances in this category. Weisenburg and McBride (1935) added reactive speech, to designate responses elicited by neutral external stimuli, not emotionally colored. These are usually responses that represent well-established associational connections.

This is an important kind of discrimination to make, because almost all aphasic patients recover some reactive speech. Both serial and reactive responses can be elicited readily from almost any aphasic patient, after a little preliminary practice. This is a useful thing to know, because it suggests techniques for facilitation and stimulation that work with severely impaired patients. It is important that the clinician know, also, that this does not necessarily mean that functional language will follow. The patient who has some reactive speech appears more adequate, and this is good for morale, but getting this far is merely a first step on the road to recovery, and it is by no means a decisive one.

The patient has no control over inferior speech responses; either they occur or do not occur. Functional speech, on the other hand, may be limited and imperfect, but it has at least partial utility. The patient who says *tup toffee* in the canteen usually gets a cup of coffee. The patient who says *cigarettes*, but can't think of *Parliaments*, gets cigarettes. He may or may not get Parliaments, depending upon his persistence. In fact, one patient, who smoked whatever brand of cigarettes he was offered for two months, won a package of Lucky Strikes for a prize. He was overjoyed. It seemed he had wanted Lucky Strikes all the time. He came into the clinic grinning, and saying, "Lucky Strikes! Lucky Strikes!" He never smoked anything else again, as long as he was in the hospital.

Dr. Bennington had some functional speech from the beginning. He named some pictures on initial testing, and was soon able to ask for things he wanted. Another Scattered Findings patient, who had so much paralysis of the musculature that he could not talk, carried a tablet and wrote what he wanted to say. This is functional language.

Scattered Findings visual profiles show error peaks on reading and writing comparable to those found on Visual profiles. Visual involvement may be mild or severe. Sometimes writing is fluent, but the general quality is poor. Careful exploration usually reveals that fine descriminations between letter forms are lost. Sometimes a patient admits affecting general carelessness to cover the fact that he is not sure of the difference between *u* and *w*, or *y* and *g*, or how many humps *m* has, or how you write *x* or *z*.

Scattered Findings patients sometimes complain of blurring or intermittent clouding of vision. When spatial disorientation is present, they have trouble following the line and keeping the place on a page in both reading and writing. It is not unusual to see such a patient write over a line he has previously written.

As the factor analysis suggested, spatial perception involves integration of both visual and proprioceptive information. From clinical observations it appears that sometimes one factor, and sometimes the other, is more seriously impaired. That is, sometimes the visual and sometimes the spatial component seems to play the larger role in the observed disorder, although both are involved to some extent.

Spatial disorientation appears to be reversible to only a limited degree. One young patient, however, improved remarkably. In the beginning he had trouble eating in the dining room. He picked up someone else's silver as often as his own, and knocked over his coffee or milk whenever he attempted to drink, but this behavioor soon stopped. One day in staff meeting the neurologist asked how he had managed so well. The patient replied, "I just learned that where I think it is, it isn't." Apparently the nervous system learns to correct for perceptual error, in some cases, at least.

Another young Korean veteran, James Mills, never learned to turn to the right to return to his ward on leaving the clinic, although he made this trip every day for several months. On the other hand, he saw his wife come in unexpectedly one day, at the far end of a long ward. He said, "Oh, there's Jane," and with a warm, welcoming smile, he walked directly away from her, having turned right instead of left.

Soon after Jim's discharge, the Mills built their own home. Jane wrote that as soon as they were settled, Jim improved remarkably. In a short time he was able to find anything he wanted in the house. He was soon able to dress their little girl, and take care of the lawn and the furnace.In a recent letter she said they had bought a piano, and that now, almost 12 years later, Jim is able to play again, by ear. He had tried this in the hospital and found it completely impossible.

Another patient made almost no improvement in spatial orientation, although he made a good recovery from aphasia. He had lived in the same house for many years, but he never relearned his way around it. There was a long living room with a fireplace at one end, and a grand piano and music cabinet at the other. He always turned left on entering the room and walked into the piano. His wife tried to teach him to stop in the doorway look for a portrait over the fireplace, and walk toward it, until he reached his chair. He tried patiently. Over and over, he stopped in the doorway, looked at the picture, then turned away from it and walked into the piano. He was simply not receiving reliable spatial information.

In the early days of the rehabilitation program, corrective therapists tried to teach such patients to use a cane to avoid walking into obstacles. It never worked. The patients stopped when they encountered an obstacle, as they had been taught, explored it with the cane, then walked into it. It was never where they thought it was. Thus it seems that patients who are disoriented in space may receive both visual and tactual information, but are unable to utilize either adequately to orient themselves in surrounding space, because perception of the direction or extent of their own movements is defective.

Not all Scattered Findings patients are disoriented in space. It is important to recognize these phenomena, however, because a patient who gets lost in the hospital, or in his own house or neighborhood, is sometimes judged to be generally confused or mentally incompetent. He may believe this himself, although when he knows what is wrong he may show himself to be a sensible and intelligent person, and make a reasonable adjustment to the disability. A patient cannot make a difficult adjustment when he is in a state of panic, or when people regard him as mentally defective.

The profile for this group differs from that of the Visual group in showing elevation of errors on speech and language as well as reading and writing tests. There is always some motor involvement with Scattered Findings patients. Usually some paralysis or paresis of the speech musculature is present, because they have bilateral damage. Sometimes the only involvement that can be detected is mild slurring of consonants. This may reflect paresis that is not observable on gross movements, such as protrusion, retraction, or lateral movements of the tongue. Other dysfluencies may result from impaired control of motor centers which can be due to a unilateral lesion. We do not yet have neurophysiological techniques sufficiently sensitive to explore these problems thoroughly enough for precise description, although they will probably come in the near future.

Occasionally sensorimotor involvement similar to that observed in Sensorimotor patients is found in a Scattered Findings patient, but this is infrequent. Presumably such a massive legion as this, combined with scattered or generalized brain damage, usually results in an Irreversible syndrome.

Prognosis for Scattered Findings patients is determined more by the general neuro-physiological and psychological status of the patient than by severity of aphasia. This is because the presence of complicating conditions limits the patient's ability to respond to stimulation and to exert maximal effort.

Scattered Findings patients are often chronically ill, anxious, and depressed. They have many physiological complaints. They complain of headache, blurring of vision, dizziness, chest pain, shortness of breath, and gastrointestinal or urinary tract disturbances. They don't want to talk plainer or to write better. They only want the doctor to do something to make them well. They do not worry about carrying on their usual occupations, or going back to work. They are afraid they will have another heart attack, or another stroke, or that they will die, and these things happen.

Young patients are sometimes found in this group, as a result of severe head injuries or widespread toxic or infectious processes. For these patients, too, the outlook is sometimes discouraging. The complications most common in young patients are memory defects, regressive behavior, and organic psychoses.

It is important for the clinician to realize that he is dealing with more than aphasia in all these cases. This does not mean that aphasia is not present. It does not even mean that aphasia should not be treated. It does mean that the clinician should know what is operating, and take realistic account of the limitations that are present.

This is important for the patient, as well. He should feel not rejection, but sympathetic understanding of real problems that exist, and receive the same kind of support that any other patient receives. Sometimes a patient who is aphasic and paranoid responds well to a structured program of therapy administered with firmness and authority. This gives him security, and he makes as good progress as any other aphasic patient.

When Mrs. Street was a member of the clinical staff of the Aphasia Clinic, she had a patient who used to come to her door every morning and announce crankily that he wasn't going to come today. She always said soothingly, "All right. Why don't you just come in and sit down a few minutes?" Next she said, "Since you're here, why don't we just try a few sentences?" From this point everything went smoothly until the next morning, when the patient came back and announced he wasn't going to come that day.

Many Scattered Findings patients work well with the clinician, but are unable to work without direction and encouragement. The clinician should know this, too, and set goals that can be achieved by such means. Giving assignments the patient cannot perform adequately merely fosters self-deception and destroys the integrity of the clinical relationship. This is quite different from the ruse Mrs. Street employed. She knew the grumbling patient was telling her he felt out-of-sorts and did not know why, but wanted sympathy and reassurance.

Just as there is a wide variation in severity of aphasia, there are also differences in the severity and the kind of complicating conditions that may be present, and the effect these have on performance. There are mild Scattered Findings patients who respond to treatment about the same as other aphasic patients. The important thing is careful assessment of both the aphasic problems and complicating conditions, and formulation of well-defined goals that take both into account.

TEST FINDINGS

The Scattered Findings subjects performed significantly below the level of the three mild groups and significantly better than irreversibles on all sections of the Minnesota Test. They performed significantly better than Sensorimotor patients only on tests for speech and language. The Scattered Findings group averaged the lowest percentage of improvement except for Irreversibles on all test sections.

TESTS FOR AUDITORY COMPREHENSION

On tests for auditory comprehension, Scattered Findings patients performed significantly below the three mild groups and significantly better than Irreversible patients on all tests on both initial and final examination. The Scattered Findings group averaged more errors than Sensorimotor subjects on all auditory tests except two that required repetition (series of digits and sentences of progressive length). They did not differ from Sensormotor patients on initial administration of the Ammons *Full-Range Picture Vocabulary Test*, but Sensorimotor patients made more improvement and did better than the Scattered Findings group on final testing.

VISUAL AND READING TESTS

On visual and reading tests, the Scattered Findings group performed below all except the Irreversibles on initial and final testing, and made the lowest percentage of improvement. Differences favoring Sensorimotor patients were nearly twice as large on final as on initial testing. This probably reflects specific visual deficits present in the Scattered Findings group and not in Sensorimotor patients, as well as the tendency of Sensorimotor subjects to improve in spite of severe reduction of language, and the tendency of Scattered Findings subjects to make comparatively little change.

SPEECH AND LANGUAGE TESTS

On tests for gross movements of the speech musculature, these patients again showed more impairment than Simple Aphasic, Visual, and Sensorimotor patients on both initial and final testing. Unilateral vocal cord paralysis, paralysis of the soft palate, partial paralysis of the tongue, and varying degrees of pharyngeal paralysis were reported.

On language tests, Scattered Findings patients performed significantly poorer than the three mild groups, but significantly better than the three severe groups on initial testing. Percentage of improvement was lower than for all groups except Irreversibles. On final performance Sensorimotor patients averaged fewer total errors than the Scattered Findings patients, although the difference was negligible. The Scattered Findings patients made more errors than Sensorimotor patients on tests that required short responses, but retained the advantage when long responses were demanded. In other words, Scattered Findings patients had more language than the Sensorimotor patients but tended to make more errors. Sensorimotor subjects tended to perform more accurately as far as they were able to perform at all.

VISUOMOTOR AND WRITING TESTS

On copying and drawing tests, the Scattered Findings group scored below all groups except Irreversibles on initial and final testing, and averaged less improvement than Irreversibles. Scattered Findings subjects tended to show more gross distortions, reflecting severe spatial disorientation, than were found in any other diagnostic group.

They performed better than Sensorimotor patients on all writing tests initially, because the performance of Sensorimotor subjects was depressed by severe reduction of language. However, they averaged only about half as much improvement, and on final testing ranked below Sensorimotor patients on all tests except oral spelling. Oral spelling was included with written spelling for diagnostic purposes, since discrepancies between the two performances may be revealing. Visual patients frequently spelled words aloud correctly, but wrote them defectively. Sensorimotor subjects, on the other hand, frequently utilized visual recall to write words correctly they could not spell aloud.

NUMERICAL RELATIONS AND ARITHMETIC PROCESSES

On numerical relations and arithmetic processes, Scattered Findings patients tested below all groups except Irreversible subjects on initial and final examination and showed the lowest percentage of improvement. Performances were depressed by visual and spatial disabilities, which tended to be irreversible in Scattered Findings subjects.

TESTS FOR BODY PARTS

Specific disturbance of body scheme is not readily apparent in group scores. Actually, it can be determined only by comparing the scores of an individual patient with his scores on similar tests that do not involve perception of body relations. Nevertheless, the authors are of the opinion that this specific disability is found more often in this than in other diagnostic groups, except perhaps the Irreversible group, and that some evidence of this is reflected in the group data.

Scattered Findings patients averaged more errors than the three mild groups and the Sensorimotor group in pointing to parts of the body named by the examiner, and following directions involving body parts and laterality, on initial and final testing. Sensorimotor subjects made more errors naming body parts on initial testing, but made almost twice as much improvement, and did better than the Scattered Findings group on final testing. In other words, the initial errors Sensorimotor subjects made in naming reflected reduction of vocabulary, and showed more tendency to decrease as language increased.

On drawing a man, Visual patients, who had difficulty recalling learned visual configurations, exceeded the mean percentage of errors obtained in the Scattered Findings group by a negligible difference, on initial testing. Visual patients improved significantly, however, while Scattered Findings subjects made no measurable gains, and averaged more errors on final testing.

On both object assembly tests, the easy mannikin and the more difficult profile, Scattered Findings subjects had the highest percentage of error on both initial and final testing. These tests reflect spatial disorientation as well as disturbance of body scheme. In our experience the two disabilities are closely related.

SUMMARY

Both initial and final test performances showed that Scattered Findings patients had functional language with a relatively high incidence of dysarthria. Reading and writing tests reflected impaired discrimination and recall of learned visual patterns. There was evidence of spatial disorientation and disturbance of body scheme in enough patients to differentiate the average performance of these patients from patients in other groups. In general, Scattered Findings patients averaged less improvement on retest than patients in the three mild and the Sensorimotor classifications. Measurable gains were made however, indicating that treatment was not generally contraindicated. The highest percentage of improvement was made on tests for auditory comprehension and tests for speech and language.

NEUROLOGICAL BACKGROUND

HISTORY AND ETIOLOGY

The mean age of Scattered Findings subjects was 59. This differed from the average age of Irreversible subjects by only a fraction and was significantly older than the average age in the three mild and the Sensorimotor groups.

The Scattered Findings subjects averaged between six and nine years schooling. This was the lowest average in all diagnostic groups. Some subjects were college graduates, however, and some, like Dr. Bennington, held professional degrees. The lower educational level was considered to be related to age and was attributed to the fact that 40 or 50 years ago there was less general appreciation of the need for education, less vocational emphasis on graduation from high school, and educational opportunities were more limited.

Etiology was trauma in 8% of these subjects, toxic or infectious processes in 3%, and cerebrovascular accidents in 84%. The incidence of cerebrovascular accidents was higher than in the mild and the Auditory groups but lower than in Sensorimotor and Irreversible patients. The incidence of complete thrombosis verified by angiography or autopsy was only 4%, compared to 27% in Sensorimotor and in Irreversible patients.

In general, Scattered Findings patients showed more severe neurological involvement than subjects in the three mild groups but significantly less damage as a group than the Sensorimotor and Irreversible patients. They tend to fall toward the center of the distribution. This group showed more evidence of scattered or generalized brain damage, such as bilateral neurological findings, involvement of the speech musculature, and mental changes, than any other diagnostic group. Of the other classifications, only the Auditory patients had more bilateral *neurological* findings than the Scattered group, but the Auditory patients did not show any bilateral *weakness* of the extremities.

COURSE AND OUTCOME

Fifty-seven percent of the Scattered Findings group were able to perform advanced self-care activities on initial testing and 85% on final evaluation. This was a little better than performance of Irreversible patients, but significantly below the performance of other diagnostic groups. Forty-three percent walked without the assistance of another person initially, and 70% on discharge. This was also better than Irreversible patients, but significantly below the performance of Simple Aphasic, Visual, Dysfluent, and Sensorimotor patients.

Three percent of these patients were committed to mental hospitals, 10% have incurred further episodes, and death is known to have occurred for 21% of the Scattered Findings subjects in the present series. Thus the outcome has been unfavorable for about a third of these patients in this study. This was exceeded only by the incidence of adverse sequelae in the Irreversible group. The data indicate that medical prognosis is significantly poorer in Scattered Findings and Irreversible groups than in others.

No subject in the Scattered Findings group pursued educational or vocational training on leaving the hospital, and none resumed gainful employment. Many subjects, of course, had been previously retired, but the age range was from 21 to above 65. Seventeen percent were under 50 years of age.

A further word should be said about the young patients in the Scattered Findings group. They were frequently victims of severe head injuries made all the more tragic because the patient had most of his adult life ahead of him. The outcome varied with the locus and extent of brain damage incurred. It sometimes appeared, however, that significant spontaneous recovery took place long after such changes would ordinarily be expected, sometimes a year or more after the accident.

Such a patient was David Lansing, who had been graduated from high school with honors and was planning to go away to college when he was hurt in an automobile accident.

Upon examination three months later he paid no attention to test materials, and his only response was a low moan. The examiner soothed and reassured him, and in a few day's time he seemed to recognize her, to be aware that she wanted to help him, and to show some interest in clinical materials. He soon began to talk a little, using a few common words and stereotyped phrases. At the same time his depression lifted and his personality began to emerge, and he soon made friends all over the hospital with his cheerful "Hi, there!" and "How are you doing, pretty good?"

During the next four months his language increased slowly but remained very limited. Gains were inconsistent, and progress was generally discouraging. He was then discharged to his home to test the effectiveness of a more congenial and stimulating environment for a few months.

Following this, he was referred to a university center where he could obtain intensive treatment for aphasia in a more normal environment than the hospital could provide, among other young people.

Further contacts were informal visits from time to time, with David or some member of his family. After he left the university clinic, David received further training in arithmetic, reading, and writing in a vocational high school. When last seen, his conversational speech appeared normal, and he had managed a small business enterprise successfully through the summer.

David had the strong support of an intelligent and devoted family who planned his program carefully, one step at a time, over a period of years. This was undoubtedly a tremendous factor. Undoubtedly there are still limitations. David is discouraged about them at times, but for the most part he finds his life full and rewarding. He has owned and operated his business for several summers now, and employs two high school students to help him. This is a considerable achievement, considering his condition even two years after the initial trauma. It emphasizes the

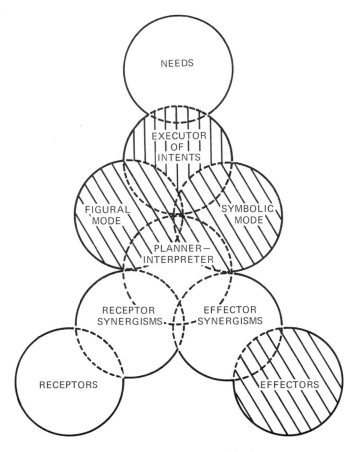

Fig. 13–1. Functional schema for aphasia with scattered findings.

need for long-term therapy, carried out in successive stages. The difference can be a boy's entire life.

A FUNCTIONAL SCHEMA FOR APHASIA WITH SCATTERED FINDINGS

Patients with scattered findings exhibit evidence of bilateral involvement insofar as they are impaired in their ability to formulate propositions in both the *symbolic* and *figural* mode. Such patients often show spatial disorientation and characteristically are afflicted with mild to severe paralysis of the articulators. Hence the *effector* component, in addition to the *symbolic* and *figural* components, are implicated in the schema depicted in Figure 13–1.

This disorder is often further complicated by some degree of either depression or confusion of intent. That the *executor of intent* component is also implicated is evidenced by the patient's unwillingness to engage in social interaction (e.g., he tends to sleep during therapy sessions, to deny the need of such, or attempts to thwart efforts to help him by other forms of resistance). The ability to execute intents is often disordered on a still finer level than indicated by the patient's attitude of resistance. For instance, he may intend to turn or reach in one direction but select the wrong set of motor commands (e.g., finer grain intents). Figure 13–1 indicates the involvement of the four components.

chapter **14**

APHASIA WITH SENSORIMOTOR
IMPAIRMENT

Charles Weston, like many young men of his generation, left college to enlist at the beginning of World War II. He had a passion for flying and wanted to be a pilot. To his sharp disappointment, he was disqualified by partial color blindness, and spent most of the war in the midwest as a physical training instructor in the Air Force. He was married while in service.

After the war, Charles worked for a commercial airline for five years. With some of his friends he bought a private plane, and qualified for a civilian pilot's license. Subsequently he learned of a position with a well-established company that offered unusual opportunities for training and advancement. Charles applied, took written tests, had a series of interviews, and a physical examination. He was selected from a field of 75 carefully screened applicants and was requested to report a week later.

On the following Friday night Charles became acutely ill and was taken to a local hospital. A lumbar puncture indicated bleeding, and an angiogram showed an aneurysm in a vessel in the left hemisphere judged inaccessible to surgery. The bleeding stopped and Charles went home, only to have a recurrence a week later. The neurosurgeon decided to ligate the left internal carotid artery to prevent further bleeding.

The surgery was done under local anaesthesia, and Charles was conscious and responsive throughout. There was no hemiplegia or aphasia before or after surgery. On the following morning, however, Charles got up, blacked out, and fell to the floor. When he regained consciousness, he was severely aphasic and hemiplegic. The doctors concluded that an embolus had lodged in a large artery, cutting off much of the blood supply to the left hemisphere.

Charles remained in a private hospital for eight weeks and then was transferred to a government hospital for further neurological evaluation. Charles' mother reported that the doctor there told Charles he would never walk or talk again. No one knows what Charles thought, but what he did was to get out of bed and try to walk. He fell after a few steps, but the doctors were impressed with his determination and gave him a cane and a brace. Charles soon was walking everywhere in the hospital and he began to say a few words.

Five months later, Charles was transferred to a third hospital for speech training. During this time Charles' wife obtained a divorce. After five months the speech pathologist left. Charles was subsequently discharged and returned to his mother's home. His mother understood that Charles needed to be occupied and independent. She exhausted the resources of the state to find treatment facilities. During one period Charles was enrolled in a class for retarded children. Since he was not a retarded child this was a disastrous experience. The teacher knew the situation was undesirable, but in the absence of other resources it seemed worth trying. Sometimes conditions that are less than ideal work out reasonably well, but this one did not.

Eventually there seemed nothing to do but accept the residual limitations and make the best of them. Charles liked music and drawing. When he could not make someone understand what he wanted to say, he drew a picture. He was an excellent driver, and he did most of the family errands. Occasionally the family took a trip, and Charles did the driving. He had a cocker spaniel and a parakeet. He taught the bird to talk. He enjoyed playing cards. He had always been popular, and he continued to see his friends.

Of their life during this period, his mother wrote: "We don't think about Charles' handicaps. We just don't see them. I try to help him by letting him help himself. I don't wait on him. Of course, I do a lot of things for him, but in a matter of fact way. Just things that have to be done—no special favors. We get along nicely, but, as we all know, Charles needs to find something to keep him occupied."

Nine years after the onset of aphasia, Mrs. Weston learned of the Aphasia Clinic in the Minneapolis Hospital, through the supervisor of speech correction in the public schools. Charles was admitted to the hospital a few weeks before his 34th birthday.

Reflecting the warm friendly qualities that had always made him a leader and the love and security that had surrounded him in his own home, Charles did not wait to be referred to the Aphasia Clinic. Characteristically, he set out to find it, and came in to introduce himself. Seeing him come into a room, smiling and limping a little, one's first thought would probably be that he had had an accident on skis, or playing football or hockey. He had an outdoor look, and it was easy to believe that he had always done a great many things well.

INITIAL FINDINGS

On tests for auditory comprehension, Charles showed moderately severe impairment of auditory discrimination, word recognition, and auditory retention span. When asked to point to letters named by the examiner, he confused letters whose names sounded alike. He scored at the 30th percentile for adults on the Ammons *Full-Range Picture Vocabulary Test*. He could repeat four digits, but not five, and sentences three or four words long. Articulation disintegrated on repetition of long words and sentences. He followed a short narrative paragraph read aloud to him without difficulty, but could not follow a longer one.

On visual tests, Charles made no errors except on matching colors,* where blue-green color blindness was apparent. He made no errors matching printed words to pictures, or printed to spoken words. He made errors reading simple sentences for comprehension, and could not follow the meaning of a paragraph on easy adult reading level. On standardized reading tests, vocabulary comprehension tested close to sixth-grade level, and sentence comprehension at fifth. Paragraph comprehension was estimated at third- or fourth-grade level. There was no performance, actually, on a standardized test, within anything approaching permissible time limits. Charles did not actually read the paragraphs. He read the questions, went back to the paragraph, and searched painstakingly for something that looked like the right answer.

Charles had no difficulty imitating gross movements of the speech musculature or repeating monosyllabic words, but diadochokinetic movements were slow. Articulation broke down on repetition of words of more than two or three syllables. Struggle behavior occurred, and there was distortion, substitution, and omission of consonants. Voiced and unvoiced consonants were frequently confused.

Charles was able to name common objects, answer questions with single-word responses, and give biographical information. Spontaneous speech consisted of single words, chains of words, short phrases, and occasional sentences. Asked to tell three things he had done during the day, Charles replied, "Got dressed—shaved—combed hair." Asked three things a good citizen should do, he answered, "Vote—25 miles per hour in car—work."

Talking about his family, he said, "Grandad watches TV," then added, "Grandad is 85 years old."

He gave the following definitions:

robin: Winter time, south—spring, robin here.
island: Warm—palm trees—small island—bananas.
motor: Car—truck—jeep—fly.
repair: Car—Army, plane—long time ago—car—tinker around—broken-down TV.
leather: Belt—cow—horse—pocketbook—shoes—hat band.

Charles made no errors on drawing or copying tests, or on writing numerals to 20. His handwriting was excellent, and his drawings were skilled. He made nine errors writing letters of the alphabet dictated in random order, tending to confuse letters whose names sounded alike. Written and oral spelling were equally impaired. He wrote *man, clock, car,* and *eggs* correctly to dictation, but no other words. He could write no sentences spontaneously or to dictation.

He could make change, tell time, and select the correct answers to most common

*Not included in the published version of the Minnesota Test.

arithmetic combinations. He could work no problems that involved more than two digits. He made no errors on tests for spatial relations or body scheme.

Analysis of test findings was a little more difficult than usual, because Charles had been trying to learn to talk for nine years, with and without formal training.

The auditory findings were clear. Charles had trouble making fine auditory discriminations. He understood the meaning of most common words and most ordinary conversational units of speech. He began to make errors when less common words and longer units of connected speech were presented.

There was no evidence of impairment of visual discrimination except for colors, and this was congenital. Reading comprehension was impaired by reduction of vocabulary and verbal retention span.

Superficial observation of Charles' conversational speech could lead to the inference that articulation was normal and word finding intact. His disability might, in fact, be classified as "syntactical aphasia." But any clinician who has followed a severe Sensorimotor patient through the course of recovery knows that short, highly-reinforced language patterns are articulated normally, once they are acquired. Charles used many words, but they were all the most common words in the language. Their patterns were well organized, and they were produced easily and automatically. When Charles was asked to repeat longer words, less common words, or unfamiliar sequences of words, his articulation broke down.

When asked to define words, or perform other tasks that required longer and more specific responses, Charles tended to produce chains of common associations. He was frequently unable to find the precise word he wanted. He could not say a robin was a bird, a motor an engine, or that repair meant to fix something. He said what he could, kept searching, and pulling out further associations. Structural forms appeared when he combined words. He "got dressed, combed hair," and said "tinker around" to express the idea of repairing a car. He had trouble generating language, certainly, but structural rules operated when he combined words at all.

There was no evidence of impairment of visual processes. Matching, copying, and drawing were all good. Spelling vocabulary was reduced far below vocabulary level in auditory comprehension, reading comprehension, or speech. The examiner believed this discrepancy could be accounted for by unequal stimulation and reinforcement. Charles talked and listened every day. He saw printed words every day, but he had long since given up trying to write. If this were the correct explanation, spelling could be expected to improve with systematic training.

Most Sensorimotor patients can learn to write a list of words easier than they can learn to say them or read them correctly. They rely on visual recall, and reproduce the words accurately, with all the silent letters intact, long before they can spell them aloud. The only trouble is that the patient tends to write *light* for *lamp*, *table* for *chair*, or *eat* for *dinner*, because he has no phonetic concepts. Since auditory and proprioceptive discrimination are both defective, phonetic concepts are extremely difficult for Sensorimotor patients to acquire. In our experience, it is better to wait until the patient has a functional speaking vocabulary and the beginning of a spelling repertoire before phonetic training is attempted, because it is such slow and difficult learning for Sensorimotor patients. These patients can respond to meaningful units of language, and with meaningful language, long before they can tell one short vowel sound from another, or recognize differences between *p, b,* and *m.* The time comes when these differences must be dealt with or progress stops, but it is better to defer this until language processes have begun to function more readily, and confidence has been restored by successful achievement. In other words, there are both physiological and psychological reasons for preceeding from easier to harder tasks.

In summary, findings included impairment of auditory discrimination and sensorimotor impairment, in addition to moderately severe reduction of vocabulary and verbal retention span reflected in all language modalities. It was important that the examiner not be mislead by comparatively high verbal output, or the comparatively low spelling level.

COURSE OF RECOVERY

We used the principle of intensive auditory stimulation for everything we did. We began with the names of the letters of the alphabet, taking one group at a time, and practicing them first in sequence, then in random order, using pointing, writing to dictation, and naming as response modes.

Beginning with a list of spelling words for each day, we spelled them aloud in unison. Next Charles repeated a number of short phrases and sentences, using each word. After this we read similar sentences, using the same words, first in unison, then Charles reading them aloud independently. We read short paragraphs aloud the same way, and Charles answered sentences about content, and then related as much as he could remember about what he had read. Outside the clinic, he practiced writing the new words until he could write each word correctly without looking at the copy, and practiced reading and writing two or three short sentences each day. He listened to sentences on the Language Master, until he could repeat them correctly, and read them unassisted.

The following session Charles read the spelling words he had practiced aloud, and used each word in a sentence. He wrote new words and review words to dictation, and the sentences he had practiced. In the beginning, we used 20 words a week with five new words each day, and reviewed the entire list on Friday.

At the end of the first month, Charles could write the letters of the alphabet dictated in random order, with an average of two or three errors. He could write about 50 words to dictation. He could formulate sentences orally, using spelling words. The records note that these sentences were short, but that about three-fourths of them were structurally correct. He wrote sentences to dictation, such as, *I ate dinner, I ate an apple, I want to go to bed,* and *I want to go to church.* He was beginning to write sentences spontaneously. He could read sentences and short paragraphs aloud independently. Retelling a paragraph about William Tell, which he had read aloud, he said, "Long ago was William Tell and son—name, Albert. People said you will—William Tell shoot arrow and bow—son, head. Then shot. Freedom again."

During the second month, Charles became able to generate longer sentences using structural words. Sometimes he made errors, but most often the sentences were correct. These examples were taken from one day's record:

my: I am going to the airport to fly my plane.
of: I'd like a cup of coffee and a doughnut.
find: I find a pocketbook.
then: I went to the bar, then I had a martini.
after: I am going to bed after dinner.
us: He is going with us.
look: Look at the storm.

These sentences were better than most of his conversational speech, but more and more sentences occurred in spontaneous utterances. Short utterances were better than longer connected responses. For example, the same week the sentences given above were elicited by presenting spelling words, Charles read a paragraph about the Mississippi River aloud and retold it as follows:

"The Mississippi—quiet country pond. Sometimes angry—spring—back up—and then thousands of dollars worth—floods. Angry Mississippi. Runs north and south."

By the end of three months, spelling tested at third-grade level, and Charles was writing sentences spontaneously every day. The clinician noted that these sentences contained words Charles had not written before. However, he still had difficulty discriminating between short vowel sounds, and on writing review words, tended to confuse *d* and *t*, *v* and *f*, and *w* and *wh*.

The next month, Charles reported that he was often surprised to find that he could write what he wished. The following are examples of sentences written spontaneously:

I will go to the football game.
I am to fly to Kansas City, Missouri.
There is much rain.
I am going to the window to look at the snow.
I wanted to see a opera.
I sent to my mother a card.
"You are right," said Father.

At Christmas, Charles went home for 17 days. He had had almost eight months of therapy. The clinician reviewed all his records to try to evaluate his progress. Speech was more fluent, utterances were longer, and structure was better. There was no question about this. Reading had outdistanced speech. Charles was reading the paper and magazine articles with good comprehension. He could write several hundred words, and short sentences spontaneously and to dictation. But the clinician wrote in her summary: "It has been and is inordinately difficult for Charles to learn names of letters, sounds of letters, and to sound words. He learns words easily visually, but he is never sure what he is writing. On review, he may write *will* for *would*, *went* for *came*, *before* for *after*, or *fly* for *bird*."

The clinician decided to concentrate on this problem when Charles returned. Errors were tabulated systematically for 50 consecutive observations during daily therapy periods for the next 10 weeks.

The daily procedure was to test first, then administer intensive phonemic stimulation, using combined auditory and visual presentations. At first stimulation consisted of spelling and sounding each phoneme, and repeating a common word beginning with the sound. The same word was always associated with each phoneme. Both long and short vowel sounds were used. If a consonant represented two sounds, both were given. *Ch, sh, the, wh,* and *ar, er, ir, ur, or,* and *ing* were given, as well as sounds represented by single letters. Since English is not a phonetic language, associations between sounds and symbols were aids to reading and writing rather than inviolable rules.

When the example was firmly associated with each phoneme, the stimulation procedure was changed. Each consonant was used with all long vowel sounds, or alternatively, with all short vowel sounds, and multiple examples of words beginning with these combinations were used. This seemed to result in accelerated spread of vocabulary in all modalities. Other techniques were used concurrently for increasing retention span, and for reading, writing, and speaking.

For the first set of controlled observations, a card was used that contained the letters of the alphabet in sequence, and the combinations previously listed. The task was to point to the symbols as they were spelled by the clinician in random order, then as they were sounded, also in random order. When the observations began, Charles had almost stopped making errors on this task, and only four were observed. There were two *t–d* confusions, one *d–t* confusion, and one *g–j* confusion. Here the first letter represents the auditory stimulus supplied by the clinician, and the second the elicited response, which in this case was pointing. This task was discontinued when a criterion of two successive trials without errors was reached.

Next, Charles was given a deck of cards, each containing one phoneme. The deck was shuffled for each administration. The task was naming the letter or letters, and producing the sound or sounds represented. For example, Charles gave the long and short sound for each vowel, the *k* and the *s* sound for *c*, etc. Ten errors were recorded before the criterion was reached. These consisted of four *p–b*, one *b–p*, one *b–m*, one *d–t*, and three *k–g* confusions.

The third task was the same except that in addition to naming the letters and producing the sounds, Charles was asked to supply a word containing each phoneme. Forty-one errors were recorded. For example, Charles looked at the card, named the letter *b* correctly, gave the correct sound, and said, on four different trials, *pay, pillow, pay, may,* for a total of three *b–p* and one *b–m* confusions. There were also three *p–b* confusions, for a total of seven confusions involving *p–b–m*, and no other errors on these sounds.

Fifteen confusions were recorded between *d–t–n–l* sounds, and no other errors. These included six *t–d*, three *d–t*, four *n–t*, one *n–d*, and one *d–l* confusion.

In addition there were six confusions of *f–v* and five of *v–f*, four of *g–k* and two of *k–g*, and one confusion of *w–h* and one of *h–wh*. Charles said *whole* for *w*, and *wheel* for *h*.

Before the criterion of two error-free trials was reached on this task, there were systematic changes. First, of course, the number of total errors decreased gradually. Second, the first responses elicited were the words associated with the phoneme during the first stimulation periods, but gradually Charles substituted words he thought of himself. Third, instead of a single word, multiple-word responses were elicited; such as *d: day, dinner, do, time; v: victory, village, vegetable, fuse; g: go, get, getting, can;* and *c(k): cake, cookies, come, can, get.* At last, Charles was beginning to be able to associate words through sound. Like most aphasic patients, Charles had not been able to produce any rhymes, on initial examination.

On the fourth task, the stimuli were the Dolch *Picture-Word Cards* (1949b) and the Dolch *Basic Sight Vocabulary Cards* (1949a). The cards were shuffled and divided into decks of 20, rotated until all the decks were used, then reshuffled. Charles was asked to sound each word, then read it aloud. Charles made no errors with vowel sounds, probably because he recognized the words. He never tried to sound a silent letter. He read *ing* as a syllable, and *ar, er, ir*, etc. in combination.

Forty-six errors were recorded. In only one instance was more than one sound wrong in a word. Charles sounded *crept, g–r–e–b–t.* Errors occurred on consonants in initial, medial, and final positions in the word. *Bake* was sounded as *pake, supper* as *summer,* and *asleep* as *asleeb.* There were nine *p–b–m* confusions, seven on *p–b,* one on *b–p,* and one on *p–m.* No significance can be attached to the fact that one kind of error occurred more than another, since distribution of phonemes was not controlled.

There were 37 *t–d–n* errors, with 13 *d–t,* nine *t–d,* five *t–n,* four *n–t,* three *d–n,* and three *n–d* confusions. In addition, *v–f* was confused four times and *f–v* once, and *g–k* once and *k–g* once. There was one *s–z* confusion, and *w* was sounded once as *u* and once as *oh.*

When criterion was reached on sounding words, the patient was asked to sound the word, then cover the card and spell the word aloud. It will be remembered that Charles could spell no words aloud on initial examination. A total of 67 errors was recorded, consisting of 28 confusions of *t–d–n,* 27 of *p–b–m,* seven of *f–v,* four of *k–g,* and one of voiced *th* and *d.*

The sixth task was to spell the word aloud when it was spoken by the examiner. Ninety-three errors were tabulated. Fifteen were confusions between *p–b–m,* 58 between *t–d–n–l,* 10 between *k–g,* and nine between *f–v.* In addition, there was one *l–r* confusion. *Stool* was spelled *s–t–o–o–r.*

The seventh task was writing the same words to dictation, without having seen or sounded them first. Seventy-one recorded errors included 42 *t–d–n–l,* 17 *p–b–m,* seven *k–g,* four *f–v* confusions, and one *l–r* confusion. Examples are listed below:

Auditory stimulus	Written response	Auditory stimulus	Written response
place	blace	whole	whote
my	buy	cut	cun
supper	summer	window	wintow
better	metter	late	lade
much	puch	ride	rite
build	puild	like	lige
both	moth	thank	thang
happy	habby	caught	gaught
afraid	afrait	come	gome
stood	stool	after	avter
dark	tark, and nark	very	fery
instead	insnead	child	chird

The eighth task was oral reading of short paragraphs. Forty-eight phonetic errors were recorded. Thirty-four of these were *t–d–n–l*, and 14 were *p–b–m* confusions. Mispronunciations recorded included *Bittsburgh* for *Pittsburgh*, *stubendous* for *stupendous*, *peacon* for *beacon*, *simple* for *symbol*, *garden* for *guarded*, *santy* for *sandy*, *suddle* for *sudden*, *wooden* for *woolen*, *minion* for *million*, and *stake* for *snake*.

Table 14–1 summarizes these data. A total of 390 phonemic errors were observed during 50 consecutive observations of performances on eight tasks of progressive difficulty. Some tasks used auditory stimuli alone, some visual stimuli alone, and one used both visual and auditory stimuli. Responses included pointing, speaking, writing, and oral reading.

Of the 390 phonemic errors, 215 were confusions of *t–d–n–l*, 98 of *p–b–m*, 36 of *f–v*, 29 of *k–g*, four of *g–j*, four of *w–h–u–o*, two of *r–l*, one of *s–z*, and one of *th–d*. Little importance can be attached to relative frequency of confusions in each phonemic group, because incidence of phonemes in words was not controlled.

The most striking observation is the difficulty discriminating between phonemes with similar loci and patterns of articulation. This difficulty is by no means limited to confusion between voiced and unvoiced sounds. *B* was confused with both *P* and *M;D* with *T, L,* and *N;* and *L* with *R,* as well as with *T, D,* and *N.* Finally, it should be noted that the same kind of confusions appeared on pointing and writing as when the patient was required to reproduce the sounds.

Similar records have been obtained from other Sensorimotor patients. This is the most complete and the purest sample secured, because it was uncontaminated by grosser auditory and proprioceptive confusions Sensorimotor patients tend to show at the beginning of treatment, and because enough language behavior could be elicited for analysis in various language modalities. The findings support the observations of Liberman (1957) and the other investigators of the Haskins Laboratory Group (Liber-

TABLE 14.1. Phonemic Errors Recorded on 50 Consecutive Observations of a Sensorimotor Subject

Stimulus	Response	*t–d–n–l*	*p–b–m*	*f–v*	*k–g*	*g–j*	*l–r*	Other	Total
Name of letter, sound, printed symbol	Point to printed letter		3		1				4
Printed letter	Name, give sound oral	1	6		3				10
Printed letter	Give word: oral	15	7	11	6			2	41
Printed word	Sound: oral	37	9	5	2			3	56
Printed word	Spell: oral	28	27	7	4			1	67
Spoken word	Spell: oral	58	15	9	10	1			93
Printed paragraph	Read: oral	34	14						48
Total errors		215	98	36	29	4	2	6	390

* *s–z, th–d, w–u, w–o, w–h*

man *et al.*, 1959) that proprioceptive as well as acoustic dimensions must be taken into account in any attempt to explain speech perception.

They also help us to understand the nature of the basic impairment in the Sensorimotor syndrome. Language is impaired because both auditory and proprioceptive discrimination are defective. The observations suggest that phonemic discrimination is based on continuous and dynamic feedback processes. Sensorimotor impairment is reflected in all language modalities because all language behavior required continuous incoming information from these systems.

During the last months of therapy, Charles was tutored in arithmetic by the educational therapist. He was discharged after 12 months of treatment.

Progress is slow for Sensorimotor patients, although it is steady and consistent. After seven or eight years without treatment, Charles made measurable and functional gains. These were more modest than gains usually made by Simple Aphasic, Visual, and Dysfluent patients, where fundamental language processes are more intact.

On final testing, Charles scored at the 40th percentile on the Ammons test. He made no errors pointing to letters named by the examiner. He could still repeat only four digits, but he repeated seven-word sentences without error, and followed the long paragraph easily, with only one error on questions regarding content.

There was marked improvement on reading. Sentence comprehension was at Grade Level 7.2, and paragraph comprehension at 6.5 on timed tests. On an untimed test, paragraph comprehension was at Grade Level 11.2. One of the best results of treatment, however, was that Charles was again able to read for pleasure. He read the newspaper, magazines, and books on adult level with enjoyment.

Gains were apparent on all tests for functional speech. Definitions were more precise, indicating more available vocabulary. A robin was *a bird*, an island, *land surrounded by sea*, an engine, *motor*, etc. At the time of admission Charles had been unable to generate sentences using given words, and only occasional sentences appeared in speech. At the time of discharge, he was formulating 30 or 40 sentences a day, using specified words. The following examples are taken from therapy records:

I read a whole book.
I am going south when I leave.
He wants change for a dollar.
The key is in my pocket.
An airplane circled the globe.
I caught a thief robbing the bank.
I went to the store to buy a glass.
I bought some cigarettes for thirty-five cents.
I thought I would go to bed.
My dog is waiting patiently at the doorstep.

Errors occurred on about 20% of attempted sentences. For example:

She is a thousand dollars. (is for *has*).
I like to go to the party with she. (she for *her*).
He is got my car. (is for *has*).
I wished I am a million dollars. (am for *had*).

Asked to tell three things he had done the previous day, Charles answered, "I went to school. I went to breakfast, lunch, and dinner. I listened to television." For three things a good citizen should do, he responded, "Work and pay–pay government taxes. Protect U.S.A."

Conversational speech sounded normal much of the time, although it continued to break down when Charles attempted long connected discourse.

On admission, Charles could not write letters of the alphabet to dictation, nor had he any phonetic concepts. Writing was limited to a residual of less than a half dozen words. On discharge, spelling tested at Grade Level 4.2. This score underestimated Charles' spelling ability. He still occasionally confused phonemes he could not discriminate readily, and thus missed common words. These errors reflected incomplete learning of phonemes, and could be expected to decrease with continued practice. On the same test, Charles wrote a great many words on sixth- or seventh-grade spelling lists correctly. He wrote sentences of five or six words correctly to dictation, and sentences of seven or eight words spontaneously. Examples of spontaneous sentences were the following:

It's cold in the car.
She have done the work.
She is inside the house.
I am sure I am going to town.
I might go to the show today.

He did not attempt to write a paragraph on the final test, although he had reported writing long letters to his mother.

There was marked improvement on arithmetic. Addition and subtraction were excellent. Charles had not progressed to problems involving serial multiplication or long division.

THE OUTCOME

There was no reason to predict that Charles would not continue to gain more language. A speech pathologist who had previously worked with aphasic patients in a VA Hospital had moved to the city in which Charles lived, and he arranged to continue to work with her. Treatment was necessarily less intensive than the hospital program, but Charles was now able to read, which provided language stimulation and enabled him to practice independently. He was also referred to the State Vocational Rehabilitation Services for vocational counseling and training. He was urged to try to get part-time work doing whatever he could do, as a first step towards independence. The clinician realized, however, that it would be difficult for Charles to accept vocational goals below his previous ones, or to be enthusiastic about a job on a lower vocational level than jobs held by his friends.

It was greatly to his credit that he submitted to a year of hospitalization, and worked as intensively and unremittingly as he did, in spite of the discouragement he felt very often. He was away from his home, family, and friends. He didn't have his dog or his car. He didn't even have a room of his own. Nothing came easily for him, but Charles never complained nor did he stop working and trying. One cannot help being impressed by the amount of frustration many Sensorimotor patients tolerate. The slow rate of progress is especially difficult for a patient like Charles, who had always learned easily and whose achievement had always been above average.

Eighteen months after Charles' discharge, the clinician wrote and asked him if he honestly thought the year in Minneapolis had been worth the effort and the sacrifices he had made. Charles' answer is reproduced below:

Dear_____

Glad to hear from you. Been a long time.

Certainly the months I spent with you were worth while. My speech is almost "perfect." Such improvement, I can read the papers, etc., without trouble.

I have been attending the Art Institute—oil painting water colors and charcoal—even drawing women in the nude. For shame. Been going about a year and a half. I love to draw and work in oils.

Jobs are almost impossible to get. At least, for me. Someday I hope to put my art to work.

I imagine Dr. Ruth Hartley was Miss Mansfield. I liked her very much—only she left and got married.

Haven't heard from Bob McDonald since his last Christmas card. When he was in the hospital here we had him over on Sundays for dinner and to spend the day. I picked him up in the morning and took him back to the hospital at night. He enjoyed coming over and we enjoyed having him.

Best of everything and love,
Charles

FURTHER OBSERVATIONS

Except for the discrepancy between speech and writing, we began to work with Charles at about the point we end with most Sensorimotor patients, after from 9 to 12 months of treatment. With aphasia as severe as this, the first year of treatment is usually spent stimulating basic vocabulary and common structural forms, and laying foundations for further recovery of language. Usually the patient gets a functional vocabulary of common words in all language modalities. Verbal retention span increases. The patient begins to use phrases, and short sentences begin to appear. He begins to acquire a phonetic basis for reading and writing. It requires intensive daily treatment, with both clinician and patient working extremely hard, to get this far in a year. All gains must be strongly reinforced from day to day, or they are lost.

Many Sensorimotor patients are unable to repeat single words correctly at the beginning of treatment. They have to hear a word or a phrase over and over before they can reproduce it accurately. Even when this is possible, repeated stimulations are required to secure voluntary recall.

In the beginning there is comparatively little spread of language. One word does not readily elicit another. The Sensorimotor patient does not, like the Simple Aphasic patient Bill Masterson, get a key that opens a box full of stored memories. He seems to need a separate key for each small compartment in the box. In other words, the stimulus seems to activate only a minimal neural network. After language processes begin to function more efficiently, there are periods of accelerated recovery and limited spread occurs.

There seems to be little question that the key required is repeated auditory stimulation with meaningful units of language. Inexperienced clinicians sometimes fail to make stimulation intensive enough to produce recall. It is permissible for the clinician to deliberately give the patient clues to enable him to respond, and mitigate failure. That this is necessary simply means that the patient has not received enough stimulations to make the response readily available. Adequate stimulation is particularly important in this early period of treatment, when the primary objectives are to retrain the ear, reestablish auditory and articulatory integrations, and build functional vocabulary. It is important that words be placed in structural contexts from the beginning. No one ever learned to speak any language by practicing strings of words in isolation.

A Sensorimotor patient should never be permitted to struggle to produce a word. During the early stages of therapy, when the patient is learning to repeat words and phrases, he should be stopped whenever this behavior appears. He should be told to listen while the clinician says the word again, to try to hear it and think it, but not to try to say it until it comes easily. He should be told repeatedly never to try to force a word out, but to let the ear do the work. Words come out easily if the clinician insists upon this.

There is no time when systematic practice does not help Sensorimotor patients. Charles made functional and measurable gains after 10 years. Other patients have made improvement after periods ranging from two to five years since onset of aphasia.

Sensorimotor patients tend to be a persistent hard-working group. Most of them persevere until they have made a generally satisfying adjustment. One patient practiced faithfully with the help of his wife for several years. On one visit, he confessed he no longer found time for it. He had a fulltime job doing light manual labor. He was a college graduate with professional training. He knew it would never be possible to return to his profession. He and his wife were liked and respected in the community, and they had many friends. He said frankly that he preferred to play golf and go hunting and fishing than to practice reading and writing. This was realistic, and the clinician considered it a sensible and mature decision. He had fought his Armageddon with courage and was sane enough to realize that victory had been won. We do not want patients to accept unnecessary limitations, but we should want them to learn to live comfortably with themselves.

TEST FINDINGS

Sensorimotor subjects showed severe reduction of language in all modalities, with the addition of specific somatosensory impairment. This was defined as difficulty producing learned movement patterns required for speech in the absence of observable paralysis or paresis of the musculature. This impairment is considered to result from reduction of sensory information and impairment of auditory and proprioceptive feedback processes. Articulation is defective and automaticity is lost, particularly in connected speech.

There is a linguistic consistency about the articulatory errors. In general, sounds that require complicated movement patterns are more defective than sounds with simpler ones. Groups of consonants and consonant blends are more defective than single consonants. Polysyllabic words are more defective than monosyllabic words. There is a tendency to confuse sounds with similar articulatory loci. Words and phrases highly organized by practice and usage tend to sound normal, but breakdowns continue to occur when new words or longer sequences are attempted.

Test profiles show error peaks on speech and writing. They show more discrepancy between initial and final curves than those of any other diagnostic group. This discrepancy is more apparent than real. It results from the extremely high percentages of errors on speech and language tests on initial examination, when verbal utterances are limited or absent.

When Sensorimotor patients were examined soon after the onset of aphasia, they frequently had no functional speech and could not repeat. As soon as the mechanism began to work and a basic vocabulary was acquired, language was functional. As a result, there was marked improvement on language tests that do not require long responses. Test profiles reflect these changes.

On initial testing, Sensorimotor subjects sometimes appeared almost as impaired as Irreversible subjects, except that comprehension of short units and performance on nonlanguage tests was better. With intensive treatment, Sensorimotor subjects characteristically made slow, steady gains in all language modalities. These gains were retained from day to day, and from week to week. With intensive treatment and systematic practice, gains have continued over a period of years, but recovery of normal language has never been observed.

In the beginning, there is literally nothing a Sensorimotor patient can do to help himself recover language. *He is absolutely dependent on intensive, controlled auditory stimulation.* Unless he can have this daily, it will not help him. This poses an economic problem. The only way it can usually be resolved is to train someone in the family to work with the patient every day, carrying out the clinician's instructions from one week to another. This often works remarkably well, if someone is available who can assume the role of therapist, and whom the patient can accept in the role. Needless to say, the untrained clinician needs continued help and encouragement.

TESTS FOR AUDITORY COMPREHENSION

Sensorimotor subjects scored considerably below the mild patients on tests for auditory comprehension on both initial and final examination. Best performance was on pointing to common objects named by the examiner. Sensorimotor patients approximated the performance of Simple Aphasic and Visual patients on this test, although mean scores on the Ammons test were lower.

Performance was low on pointing to letters named by the examiner. The most common error on initial testing was confusion of letters with names that sound alike. Mean scores on the Ammons test were identical for Sensorimotor and Scattered Findings Subjects on initial testing, but Sensorimotor patients made more improvement, and scored higher on retest. Sensorimotor subjects scored low on pointing to objects named in series of two and three, and on comprehension of a long paragraph, where materials exceeded retention span.

Some Sensorimotor subjects could not repeat, so there was no performance on repetition of digits or sentences on initial examination. When digit span could be tested, it rarely exceeded two or three digits on initial, and three or four digits on final testing. Performance of Sensorimotor subjects was severely impaired on all auditory tests that had length of stimulus as a dimension.

VISUAL AND READING TESTS

Sensorimotor subjects performed as well as Simple Aphasics on matching tests, making only minimal errors. Almost no Sensorimotor subjects could read aloud on initial testing. They performed below Irreversibles on this test, but made more improvement than either the Scattered Findings or Irreversible patients.

Performance on tests for reading comprehension was consistent with reduction of vocabulary and verbal retention span found in other modalities. Reading gains were most significant on matching words to pictures and on comprehension of a short paragraph. Sensorimotor subjects acquired considerable reading vocabulary during the course of treatment, but verbal retention span usually remained too short to deal with long materials.

It has been suggested that we talk about *visual retention span* in relation to reading impairment in aphasia, but this term is not an accurate description of what seems to happen. It is surely comparatively rare to remember what you read by revisualizing sentences and paragraphs on a page. There are individual differences in this capacity, but all aphasics have difficulty recalling what they read, and difficulty increases as materials increase in length. The skill required for revisualization of long units cannot be this common.

As an example, suppose last night you read an advertisement for an abridged edition of Samuel Johnson's dictionary. You may remember first that something amused you, and then recall that this was Samuel Johnson's own pronouncements about his work. Pursuing this further, you are apt to *tell yourself* that he said he understood very well what was required, knew very well how to do it, and had done it extremely well. The recollection may be mixed with amusement, with envy of such sublime assurance, and with a mental picture of Samuel Johnson, a coffee house in London, or a fragment of a page from the dictionary. It does not seem essentially different from the plea you heard on FM radio a little later to introduce your teenager to Chanel No. 5 and which returns to consciousness mixed with whatever private associations you have with Chanel No. 5 or with expressions on the face of your teenager that indicated he could get along without Chanel No. 5.

The point is that the pips that come from the cochlea and the retina are selected and integrated and associated and interpreted before they are stored in memory. This interpretation is compatible with results obtained on factor analysis, where comprehension of a paragraph read aloud by the examiner and comprehension of a paragraph read silently by the patient both had high loadings on Factor I, which was considered a general language factor.

In other words, it would not matter if the aphasic patient read Johnson's statements himself, or someone read them to him. If he could not retain a verbal sequence of more than five or six units, he would have forgotten who said what about what and who did what very well before the final period occurred.

There is, of course, such a process as visual recall. We would conjecture that it operates with shorter units, with letters, and to a lesser extent, with words. This process probably operates, in fact, when the Sensorimotor patient who can neither name letters nor point to letters named by the examiner writes a word he cannot spell aloud. This is always, however, a limited compensation, and relatively undependable.

SPEECH AND LANGUAGE TESTS

Sensorimotor subjects did not differ significantly from Simple Aphasic and Visual patients on tests for imitation of laryngeal, palatal, or jaw movements, or in incidence of difficulty swallowing. There was no evidence of any paralysis or paresis of the speech musculature, although there was difficulty initiating and controlling movement patterns. The patient sometimes behaved as though he did not know where the tongue was in the mouth, or how to move it in a given direction or to a given position. Sensorimotor patients averaged more errors than Simple Aphasic and Visual groups with differences of increasing magnitude on: (1) imitation of tongue movements, (2) rapid alternating movements involving repetition of syllables, and (3) repetition of monosyllables.

On factor analysis, a negative correlation was found between the loadings of these three tests on Factor 4, the only movement factor identified, and Factor I, the general language factor. The movement factor decreased in importance as the language factor increased.

In the Sensorimotor group, the mean percentages of error on these tests, on initial and final examination, were as follows:

	Initial	Final
Imitation of tongue movements	11%	9%
Rapid alternating movements	41%	9%
Repetition of monosyllables	66%	26%

This suggests that for Sensorimotor patients, certainly, the principal difficulty is in reproducing learned movement patterns, and that this difficulty increases as language loading increases on tasks, and decreases as language is recovered. This is what we have labeled sensorimotor impairment, and is defined as difficulty producing the learned sequences of movements required for speech, secondary to reduction of auditory, tactual, and proprioceptive information, and defective feedback processes.

On all 14 tests requiring voluntary language, Sensorimotor patients performed below the level of all groups except Irreversible patients, on initial testing. However, Sensorimotor patients made more gains than either Scattered Findings or Irreversible patients. On final testing Sensorimotor patients exceeded the performance of Scattered

Finding patients on eight language tests, although Scattered Findings patients maintained their superiority on six tests that required long responses.

Sensorimotor subjects made consistent and measurable progress, and gained functional speech, although language did not approach the levels of Simple Aphasic, Visual Dysfluent, and Auditory patients. After from six to nine months of intensive treatment, Sensorimotor subjects usually communicated with common words and phrases, though short sentences were beginning to occur and appeared with increasing frequency as recovery progressed.

Articulation errors were consistent, in that they increased in relation to complexity of the motor pattern and the length of the response. Words and phrases that were readily available tended to sound normal, but articulation continued to disintegrate when new words and longer units of language were presented.

Word finding errors occurred as well as errors of structural usage, and a relationship between the two was apparent during all periods of recovery.

VISUOMOTOR AND WRITING TESTS

Copying and drawing were usually intact in Sensorimotor subjects. A Sensorimotor patient might write *it* for *in*, or *to* for *do*, because he could not make the required phonemic discriminations. He might write *money* for *dollar* or *window* for *door*, because he could make neither semantic nor phonetic discriminations between the two words. In general, he tended to write much as he talked.

NUMERICAL RELATIONS AND ARITHMETIC PROCESSES

Sensorimotor patients tell below the performance of Simple Aphasic, Visual, and Dysfluent patients on tests for numerical relations, but significantly exceeded the performance of Scattered Findings, Auditory, and Irreversible patients, on both initial and final testing. The comparatively good performance of Sensorimotor subjects in arithmetic was attributed to ability to utilize visual cues. This ability served better in arithmetic than in reading because units tended to be shorter and span was not involved.

It was sometimes fascinating to watch a Sensorimotor patient work a problem such as 7 + 4 + 12. Over and over, a patient was observed to say something like, "Eight and three is thirty–three, and ninety–nine, a hundred five," and write down *23*.

TESTS FOR BODY PARTS*

There was no evidence of specific impairment of body scheme in Sensorimotor patients. They made no errors assembling the Wechsler mannikin, and exceeded the performance of all groups except Simple Aphasics on drawing a man and assembling the profile.

*No longer in the Minnesota Test Battery.

SUMMARY

The performance of Sensorimotor patients reflected severe reduction of language, on all sections of the test. In addition, impairment of sensorimotor processes was observed on speech and language tests.

NEUROLOGICAL BACKGROUND

HISTORY AND ETIOLOGY

The mean age for Sensorimotor subjects was 43.6, which ranked between the Simple Aphasic and Visual groups, and which was significantly younger than the average age in the Scattered Findings and Irreversible groups.

The etiology was cerebrovascular in 15 out of 16 subjects, and brain abscess in one. The incidence of cerebrovascular accidents was significantly higher than in any group except Irreversible patients.

Forty percent of the cerebrovascular accidents in Sensorimotor patients were described on angiography as complete thromboses of the internal carotid or middle cerebral arteries. This was the highest incidence in any clinical group. Irreversible patients were second, with 27 %. It is possible that this figure is low. Fewer angiograms were probably performed on older patients, some of whom had had previous strokes and many of whom had other complicating conditions. Ligations of the internal carotid were performed in four Sensorimotor cases. In two of these, aphasia and right hemiplegia followed surgery.

INDICES OF SEVERITY

Hemiplegia was present in 56% of the Sensorimotor subjects, and hemiparesis in 38%. The incidence of paralysis was higher than in any group except Irreversible Aphasics.

Significant positive correlations were found over the entire population between severity of motor involvement and severity of aphasia indicated by clinical ratings. Present data do not confirm the assumption sometimes made, that if motor recovery is good, language recovery will not be, and vice versa. This theory is based on the hypothesis that aphasia results from cortical lesions, while paralysis of the extremities results from subcortical damage. Since the hypothesis concerning aphasia is not tenable, there is no longer any reason to predict an inverse relationship.

Sensorimotor and Irreversible patients showed extensive and severe neurological deficits on all dimensions. While these two groups resembled each other in severity of neurological involvement, they were very unlike in incidence of complicating conditions, from which Sensorimotor patients were singularly free. The neurophysiological picture is compatible with a massive lesion in an otherwise intact brain.

Thirty–four percent performed advanced self-care initially, and all on final evaluation. The percentages were the same for ambulation. A total of 60% of these patients undertook some kind of vocational training or returned to gainful employment, which exceeds all other diagnostic groups. This is another remarkable finding, in view of the severe neurological and aphasic residuals with Sensorimotor impairment, but it is not particularly surprising to people who have worked with these patients.

Characteristically, these patients exceed whatever assignments they are given, put in long hours of daily practice, and attempt any kind of work they can do at a given time. They appear to channel all their resources and drive single-mindedly toward recovery.

The percentage of positive vocational adjustments was increased by inclusion of some patients with comparatively mild involvement, and by the fact that the period of hospitalization was usually longer for Sensorimotor patients than for other diagnostic groups, because it usually took longer for these patients to achieve maximal hospital benefits. On the other hand, the determination of Sensorimotor patients to achieve independence in spite of severe limitations cannot be discounted. Perhaps the seriousness of the disability makes it simpler for these patients to accept altered goals. They tend to settle for what is possible because the only alternative is to give up.

Sensorimotor patients usually achieved ambulation with a brace and a cane, and went on to develop speed and distance in walking. They achieved total self-care with the nonparalyzed hand, which was usually the left, and often acquired considerable manual dexterity. They achieved functional communication with limited language, talking in words and phrases and effortful sentences. They went from positions that required knowledge and trained skills to jobs on an assembly line, usually in a small factory that would hire disabled persons, or to some other kind of light manual labor. They made good employees when they could find jobs, for they had far more invested in successful job performance than the average individual. Achievement was often heroic.

There can be complicated family problems when no jobs are available, and the patient, who has always been active, does not know how to fill his time. He wants to be independent and useful, and in his frustration he may become hostile or despondent. This is a particularly difficult problem for a patient whose interests have been chiefly intellectual, and who never liked manual activities. There are no easy answers. Each case requires individual planning and counseling.

Another kind of family problem may arise when there are adolescent children in the home. The parent with limited language may feel that he has lost contact with his children and has no control over them. In his effort to fulfill his parental role, he may become excessively stern and demanding. As a result, a boy or girl may feel that whatever he does is wrong, and that the parent no longer loves him. This is a heavy weight for an adolescent to carry. Growing up is difficult enough, at best, and in these cases the problems are more acute because of the trauma inflicted by the parent's illness, his altered condition, and resulting changes in family circumstances. Usually both the patient and other members of the family require help to understand what has happened, and to learn to live with it.

One Sensorimotor patient who made a successful readjustment wisely decided to leave the management of the older children to his wife. Fortunately, she was able to accept this responsibility and serve as a successful liaison. The father felt the loss of his former close companionship with his children, but chose this course rather than risk further damage to family relationships.

Sometimes one child adjusts to the changes more easily than another, and seems to know instinctively how to communicate with the aphasic parent, and how to please him. This, of course, increases the unhappiness of the children who adjust less readily, and they may feel left out or discriminated against. If a hospitalized patient can have some periods at home before final discharge, some of the problems can be anticipated, insights can be developed, and both the patient and the family can receive some preparation for dealing with the exigencies of daily living.

It can be anticipated that a good many patients with massive lesions will develop seizures when scar tissue begins to form. The physician should prepare the patient and the family for this contingency. Usually, in fact, he does, but sometimes this is overlooked. The occurrence of a seizure is more frightening than it need be when people have no idea what is happening, and think perhaps that the patient is dying, or having another stroke.

A FUNCTIONAL SCHEMA FOR APHASIA WITH SENSORIMOTOR IMPAIRMENT

Aphasia with sensorimotor impairment, as the name implies, involves disorders in both the reception and production of speech. Due to a major lesion, feedback from the proprioceptive and auditory systems is disrupted. Consequently, the patient typically exhibits greater difficulty in articulating or comprehending complex speech. However, with extensive training the patient tends to improve with time, so that language of increasing complexity can be processed (up to the limits of the Simple Aphasic patients).

This suggests that although the *receptor* and *effector synergisms* are severely disrupted at the early stages of the disorder, they can often be reintegrated through training. Since the *planner–interpreter* component is essentially responsible for the coordination of the receptor and effector synergisms, it too must be involved in the disorder. The limits placed on the remission of symptoms associated with the sensorimotor impairment (up to that permitted by the patient's aphasia) are dependent upon the degree to which the existing lesion allows restoration of the normal functioning of the planner–interpreter component. Hence, these three components, in addition to the *symbolic mode,* are designated in the schema for this disorder in Figure 14–1.

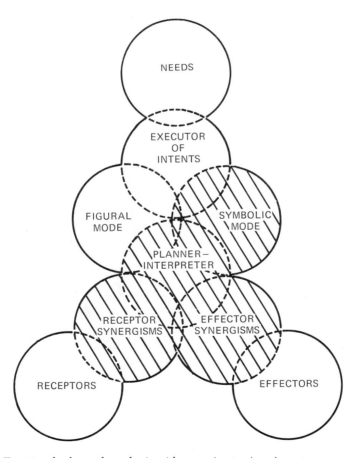

Fig. 14–1. Functional schema for aphasia with sensorimotor impairment.

chapter **15**

SEVERE APHASIA WITH
INTERMITTENT AUDITORY
IMPERCEPTION

Bill Williamson was a successful manufacturer's representative for an agricultural products company. He had an affable personality and self-confident bearing which made him popular with his friends and customers. Bill and his wife had five children, the last one born at the time of his illness. Two days before surgery for an adrenal tumor, Bill had a cerebral hemorrhage. Because the hemorrhage was secondary to the tumor, Bill was operated on schedule. Postsurgical recovery was normal except that confusion, agitated behavior, and severe aphasia made Bill difficult to handle, so he was moved to a chronic disease hospital for convalescent care. He was subsequently transferred to the Minneapolis VA Hospital for treatment of aphasia.*

Neurological examination revealed increased radial reflexes on the right side, and other reflexes sluggish bilaterally. He had minimal weakness of the right arm and leg, not detectable except on neurological examination. Cranial nerves were intact, as were all sensory modalities, except that the patient presented a right superior quadrantanopsia. The electroencephalogram showed a left temporal focus. Skull X-rays were negative, but a pneumoencephalogram showed bilateral cerebral atrophy. Brain scan indicated increased activity in the left parieto-occipital area.

*This case was first reported in the *British Journal of Disorders of Communication*, 4: 73–82, 1969, and is adapted here by permission of the editor.

INITIAL FINDINGS

Even in a somewhat small hospital uniform, Bill was an attractive gentleman, looking younger than his 48 years. When first seen he was intent on doing well, but laughed easily at the mistakes he recognized. That he had difficulty understanding what was said to him was evident. He made three errors in recognizing common words, 15 errors recognizing letters named in random order, and could not point to any items named in a series of two or three. He missed three of the 10 sentence-length questions. He was able to follow only three directions: "Open the box," "Give me the key," and "Which one do you eat with?" Although he missed longer items because retention span was reduced, he also missed the very short direction, "Ring the bell." It has been observed that patients with intermittent auditory impairment often miss short directions, and comprehend longer materials that offer more contextual cues. If verbal stimuli are too long, however, the patient will not understand because retention span is reduced. This discrepancy is illustrated in this case by the fact that Bill made no errors in answering questions about a paragraph read to him, and yet he could not point to three common pictures or ring a bell when requested.

Bill was not able to repeat digits or any sentences, but this inability reflected impaired phoneme perception rather than reduction of auditory retention span or any motor disability. Bill scored in the 40th percentile for normal adults on the Ammons *Full-Range Picture Vocabulary Test* (1948), which is below expectation for a college graduate. Unlike normal and aphasic subjects in other classifications, Bill sometimes missed monosyllabic words in common usage, such as *seed* and *skill*, and responded correctly to longer words that occur less frequently in general language usage, such as *rectangular* and *perusing*. In other words, the expected correlation between word frequency and word errors did not obtain. Instead, the patient responded correctly when a word got in, or failed to grasp the word at all, in a more or less random fashion.

Bill was able to match forms and letters without error. He made only two out of 32 possible errors matching words to pictures, confusing words related in meaning. He made seven out of 32 possible errors matching spoken to printed words. On lists for sentence and paragraph comprehension, he had only chance success. He was unable to read aloud. Reading errors reflected aphasic reduction of language rather than involvement of visual processes, since the errors Bill made did not suggest impaired visual discrimination.

Reading deficit reflected the loss of phonemic concepts and restricted reading vocabulary. Performance showed awareness of relationships between printed words and referents, although semantic confusions (such as *chair* for *table* and *arm* for *leg*) occurred. More errors occurred on matching printed to spoken words than on matching words to pictures, reflecting specific impairment of auditory processes. Thus, test evidence indicated that reading impairment could be accounted for in terms of language deficit.

Bill could perform all gross movements of the speech musculature, although early medical reports indicated difficulty imitating oral movements immediately after onset of aphasia. He was able to perform all the rapid alternating movements except repeating *la–la*, but could repeat only a few monosyllabic words correctly. Most errors were close approximations, such as *pibe* for *pie*, *bly* for *lie*, and *thray* for *pray*. It is interesting to note that the patient was nevertheless able to repeat three phonetically complex monosyllables *(screw, three,* and *try)* correctly. Errors also included jargon responses *(perb* for *spry)* and perseveration of previous responses. Bill could not repeat any phrases. He was able to count up to 10, then said *jack* and could go no further. He could not name the days of the week. Sentence completion was difficult for him. He completed, *Do you think it looks like* _____*?* with *chain* (approximation of rain), and, *There is someone at the* _____, with *desk*, but could respond to no others. Here again the auditory imperception is apparent, since patients who have no voluntary speech are often able to complete sentences. Bill was able to tell his name and age, but could give no other biographical information. He was able to tell three things he had done during the day, but speech was effortful and defective. Bill was able to name only one of the 20 common objects, but when asked to describe a picture, named three or four objects in it. He was not able to produce a sentence using a given word. He defined a *robin* as a bird, but could give no other definitions. Bill's spontaneous speech was characterized by intermittent jargon and occasional approximations of the words he was searching for. He used some short sentences. When asked where he was going, he said, "Going to the . . . the . . . the (pointing to teeth) beeth!" Bill appeared to have more language than he actually had, since he used a few social phrases such as, "How are you today?" fluently and appropriately.

Bill was able to copy Greek letters and a wheel without error. He wrote *1,2,3* but was unable to write any remaining numbers. He made three minimal errors copying letters, but could write only *b, a,* and *q* to dictation. He could perform no other writing tasks.

Bill made minimal errors making change and setting the hands of a clock. He made four errors out of 12 identifying correct answers to simple arithmetical combinations and could not perform on more complex problems. These errors reflected a language deficit.

To summarize the findings, Bill showed severe aphasia reflected in all language modalities, complicated by partial or intermittent auditory imperception. Although speech attempts often resulted in jargon and groping movements of the articulators, forcing, and articulatory errors, the presence of some connected speech that was well-articulated, natural, and fluent led us to postulate that this behavior resulted from loss of auditory, rather than somatosensory, control.

THE COURSE OF RECOVERY

We provided intensive language stimulation using combined visual and auditory presentation of materials. We used repetitive stimulation to facilitate both recognition and recall, controlling the length of the language unit. In Bill's case we began with single words, but put the words in context of phrases and short sentences as soon as easy repetition was possible. We required a response to each language unit presented. In order to prevent struggle behavior we instructed Bill to *listen*, try to *hear* the word, and *think* it. This is particularly difficult for the auditory patient, who seems to need to listen effortfully, to "turn on" his auditory system actively for the sounds to get in. One day when Bill was given the word *ears* he automatically responded, "Listen, Bill!" as he must have told himself to listen so many times.

We asked Bill to point to one of four visual stimuli as the clinician named them in random order. First we used the word and picture together, then the word alone, then the picture alone. We did this because repetition was difficult to obtain, and this helped him learn to listen and give him a measure of success at each session. The same 10 words we asked him to repeat each day were used in this way. The goals to be achieved, in this order, were: (1) repetition; (2) naming; (3) reading; (4) writing; (5) connected speech; and (6) phoneme discrimination. Desired movement was from shorter to longer and more varied language units, and from elicited to more voluntary responses.

Using Language Master cards, the therapist said the word for the patient, and waited for a response each time, until the patient could repeat the word correctly. Then Bill was asked to copy the word, saying the letters (at first with the therapist's help) as he printed the word. Bill practiced the same words, using the Language Master outside the therapy session. He was shown how to put the card through, listen, repeat, and then write the word. The following session Bill was given an opportunity to name the picture without auditory stimulation when he could. At first he could name none of them, or perhaps only one, but gradually they came.

Articulation errors decreased on successive repetitions, resulting in closer and closer approximations of the words attempted, until a normal response was obtained. For example, *tea* was *teak*, then *tea; milk* was *mild; chair* was *gor, cor*, then after three more stimulations became *chair*.

With most aphasic patients, new words are added to replace the words that are learned, while the words that are not mastered are retained for further practice. Bill, however, frequently perseverated on the same error, and these reiterated errors seemed to resist modification. For this reason, the first time through the entire set of Language Master vocabulary cards, he was given 10 completely new cards every day. Later in treatment, he reviewed the single words again, and was allowed to drop each word only when he could name the picture correctly without help. *Farmer* was a most difficult word for Bill, and he persisted in saying *firming*. One day, after about 25 stimulations, he looked at the therapist, and said, "We going to argue about this?" We decided it was better not to argue about it. Bill enjoyed the Language Master practice, and often spent three or more hours a day working with it.

Intensive phonetic training was used for about a month for ear training and as an aid to repetition, reading, and spelling. Easy-to-see sounds were started first: *b, p,* and *m,* followed by lingual–dental sounds, and so on. These consonants were combined with vowels to make words: *me, may, my, mow,* etc., and Bill was asked to point to these words when they were named in random order by the clinician. Phonemic discrimination became very good, and gradually third-grade spelling words were substituted. By this time Bill was able to repeat almost any word easily after the clinician, then write it. He sometimes made association errors when the word didn't seem to get in, such as the word *cob* for *corn,* and occasionally he needed many repetitions before he could comprehend the word. Each day brought some improvement, and as less time was required for spelling we gradually worked up to 10 words a day. It can be seen that the phonetic drills and later the spelling words helped train the patient in auditory discrimination and recognition as well as in sounding words and writing them. All modalities were being used, but the patient was being stimulated through the auditory channels primarily. This was reflected in improved speech perception both inside and outside the clinic.

The clinician planned to have the patient move to formulating sentences using spelling words, but Bill's responses made a formal introduction to this unnecessary. One day the therapist gave Bill the word *story;* Bill repeated it a few times until he began to get the meaning of the word, then, still not sure, he said, "You mean like say a story?" . . . "Not say . . . tell?" . . . "Yes, tell a story!" The clinician had Bill write the sentence down, and another therapeutic tool was initiated. Later in treatment he was able to write longer sentences spontaneously and to dictation.

When Bill could not perceive a stimulus by ear, the word or sentence was written for him. He was never allowed to struggle for a response. Often in the therapeutic process, the clinician and the patient have such a good working relationship that the patient indicates very subtly when he wants help and when he doesn't, and the clinician becomes sensitive to these cues.

It was recognized early that techniques that help many aphasic patients did not help Bill because of the auditory imperception. Most patients are able to say the word *door*, for example, if the therapist says, "There is someone at the ___" With Bill and other patients with intermittent auditory imperception, the best stimulus is simply to say *door* over and over, until he can hear, recognize, and organize the word to say it correctly. If Bill was allowed to struggle to say the word, frustration was prolonged. Over and over, early in therapy especially, the therapist would have to ask, "Are you listening?" Bill nearly always admitted he wasn't. Later he would occasionally ask to have something repeated with the apology, "I wasn't listening."

Bill was able to begin outside reading assignments two months after treatment was started. By this time, intensive phonetic drill was replaced by spelling, and less time was spent on this each day as he became better at retrieval of letters and words. Sentences providing systematic practice with common syntactic structures were used for reading practice in therapy sessions. Bill read aloud with the therapist, and then repeated the sentence. Outside reading assignments consisted of articles from the *Reader's Digest Reading Skill Builder Series* (1951), starting at the second-grade level. These articles are very good for adult interest, while sentence length and word frequencies are controlled. At the end of each article there is a multiple-choice questionnaire. At first Bill missed two or three out of five questions, but gradually errors were eliminated and another higher grade-level book was started. Bill was at the fifth-grade level by July, and eventually went through the adult-level books three times. The first time he was given the easiest set of questions at the end of each article. The second time through the set of three adult books he read the article only once before answering the questions. The third time he completed the most difficult exercises. It was concluded that there was little practice effect, since he did not seem to recall seeing the articles before, or remembered them only vaguely. The most difficult questions were those that required the patient to fill in blanks, or asked for synonyms, since these required the reader to generate precise responses. At first Bill had to read an article several times to grasp the principal ideas. Next he was able to answer multiple-response questions on content. Later he did this with only one reading. The next step was to remember details and fill in the answers to questions that required him to generate rather than merely select the correct responses. As he progressed he was able to read the article once and answer questions requiring him to formulate a correct response. Both retention span and vocabulary were increased by these drills.

The therapeutic program, then, was planned to begin on a level on which the patient could respond. Materials were made progressively longer, and the required responses were gradually made more difficult. Bill's spelling words, reading assignments, and materials on Language Master Cards used for repetition all gradually increased in length.

On initial testing the patient was unable to write any words to dictation. By final testing a year later he scored on the eighth-grade level on the *Wide Range Spelling Test.**Initially he was able to repeat only 10 of the 32 monosyllabic words presented, and none of the phrases; at time of retest he made no errors on these tests. He could not repeat any but the shortest sentences word for word, but he was able to understand the sentence and paraphrase it to express the same idea.

When Bill left the hospital one year and one month after he was admitted, his speech was so fluent that most people would not have caught his few errors. He heard errors in speech that others would make, as well as his own. Once when his clinician was overtired and stumbled over a sentence, Bill said, "You having a little trouble?" He admitted that he didn't always understand what was said to him, and this became apparent in long conversations. He handled this well,and did not try to cover up the fact that he had not understood. He scored in the 99th percentile on the Ammons *Full-Range Picture Vocabulary Test.* Writing was still slow, but he was able to write good sentences. He was able to write short sentences to dictation, but sentences like *"What do they pay for the job?* became *What do they have to do the job?* Reading was on an adult level, and comprehension was excellent.

Bill was still aphasic, but he had the tools to use to practice on his own in order to continue to make gains. He was able to read at an adult level and practice retention by telling his wife what he had read. He was able to recognize when he did not hear something correctly, and ask to have it repeated. He was able to write an acceptable letter slowly, but needed more practice on this. His speech sounded normal, but occasionally he made mistakes, which he was usually able to recognize and correct by himself. Most of his errors in speech were association errors (substitution of another word in the same semantic category) such as most people make occasionally. Word-finding difficulty was still present, but not often apparent to the uninitiated listener. Bill made excellent gains, arriving at good functional language.

Everyone was sorry to see Bill leave the hospital. He was not only a pleasant person to have around, but he was helpful to the nurses on the ward. He gently teased the members of the staff. One day when the audiologist was cutting out pictures for a test she was developing, Bill asked her, "Don't you have anything better to do?"

*Part of the Wide Range Achievement Test, developed by J. Jastak and S. Bijou, Psychological Corporation, 304 East 45 Street, New York, New York 10017.

After he was presented to a class of psychology students, his clinician complimented him on his performance and laughingly told him he had been so good that it was difficult for her to demonstrate his aphasia. A few weeks later at another demonstration for students, the clinician was shocked when he performed at lower levels than he was able to before. He later admitted that he had purposely seemed more aphasic in order to make a better demonstration and to please his teacher!

After discharge, Bill worked part-time in a grocery store, where he was able to perform his job well. It remains to be seen whether he will be able to return to his former employment as a sales representative. This does not seem an unrealistic goal in this instance, although we have not yet seen a patient in this diagnostic category achieve employment with such high demands on language.

FURTHER OBSERVATION

Patients with intermittent auditory imperception often behaved as though they did not hear. They were sometimes referred as deaf, even when pure-tone audiometry revealed no hearing loss. We have seen some of these patients shortly after onset of aphasia who either did not speak at all or who produced only jargon. This is not a constant finding, however.

Even when functional speech was present, patients with auditory imperception usually had difficulty pointing to common objects named by the examiner, following simple directions, repeating words, phrases, and sentences, and naming common objects. They also had difficulty reading and writing the names of objects, even when visual rather than auditory stimulation was used, and when they were able to match pictures, geometric forms, and printed letters with no difficulty. They could sometimes match printed words to pictures when they could not match printed to spoken words. The discrepancy between test performance and flow of language was often startling. Patients sometimes failed tests because they did not understand the directions, but they also failed when it was clear from partial responses that they understood the task but could not perform it.

Patients with intermittent auditory imperception understandably appeared bewildered and anxious when anyone tried to communicate with them. We often had the feeling that auditory signals were not transmitted to the language system, or that transmission was too feeble or distorted for pattern perception to occur.

When we used combined visual and auditory stimulation, usually a picture combined with the printed and the spoken words, and presented them simultaneously over and over, day after day, patients began to respond to words. Usually they first began to point to the pictures correctly, when they were named by the examiner. Next they began to repeat, and finally were able to name pictures and objects. At this stage patients sometimes repeated words without recognition. Sometimes recognition came in a flash, after the patient or the examiner had repeated a word several times. Sometimes patients even named objects or pictures correctly but reported they did not know if the response was right or wrong. This was not a persisting phenomenon, however.

When reactive speech began to occur, it was often possible to elicit precise responses by presenting a complex stimulus, such as a picture containing a variety of detail. What was interesting about this was that words elicited from the patient were subsequently easier for the patient to recognize and produce voluntarily than words presented first by the clinician.

One patient with transient auditory imperception was an art student. When he was first shown a picture of a man he could not point to or name any parts of the body or articles of clothing. Neither could he draw a man when the picture was removed, but he began to block out the figure. As he did this, he verbalized something as follows: "Something goes here . . . I used to know this . . . man, man? . . . Is it a man? . . . What goes here? . . . I used to know it . . . arm . . . arm. Does an arm go here . . . Is this right? . . . Does an arm go here? . . . Is this an arm? . . . Is this right . . . arm?" Following this performance, he pointed to the arm on request, and named it when asked what it was. This technique was almost always successful, and we used it until it was no longer necessary.

The clinician observed that the patient talked more when she did not watch him, but was merely there to supply or reinforce a word now and then. Growing bored, she began to draw with him. This amused the patient, and he began to assume the role of instructor and to encourage the clinician. He was an excellent teacher, and the clinician began to show improvement. She would probably have learned to draw fairly well if the imperception had lasted longer, but as the patient became able to deal directly with language, he no longer wanted to spend time drawing.

We interpreted these observations to mean that for such patients, language patterns were more accessible to complex patterns of internal and external stimuli than to more direct sensory channels, and more accessible to visual than to auditory stimulation.

These patients were seriously handicapped in communication, even when they had considerable language. This will be clear from a sample of a conversation with a patient encountered by chance when he was readmitted to the hospital after several months at home:

Clinician: It's nice to see you, Mr. Seller. When did you come back?
Patient: I'm fine. I get along very good. Everything is very good now.
Clinician: Are you going to be here for a while?
Patient: The wife is fine and the children are fine. Everything is very good.
Clinician: I'm glad. Did your wife come with you?
Patient: It's all very good but the job. The job is no good now. That is no good. Everything else is very good.

We think observations such as these have led to the assumption that the patient was deaf, or alternatively, a case of "pure word deafness." In our experience the latter inference has been as unfounded as the former. We have always found a relatively severe deficit in all language modalities on testing. Moreover, the auditory imperception was never complete. Patients responded to spoken language occasionally even at first, and then with gradually increasing adequacy. One patient used to confide happily several times a day, "I can read you now. Used to be I couldn't read you."

We have observed that even after marked recovery, these patients sometimes failed to recognize a common word. They appeared as perplexed as if the word belonged to a language long vanished from the earth. Fortunately, the frequency of these occurrences gradually decreased. We know of no other aphasic phenomenon, however, with this marked on–off effect, as if the signal were or were not received. When recognition occurred after many repetitions, the whole attitude of the patient seemed to ask why we hadn't said what we meant the first time.

While patients in this category sometimes had a high verbal output, it tended to consist largely of generalities and to convey a relatively small amount of information. As recovery occurred, responses became both more appropriate and more specific. That some of them continue to improve over long periods is unquestionable. One of the patients in our series turned his hobby into a gainful occupation and found part-time employment for a period of several years. He continued to show improvement until death intervened from an unrelated cause.

APHASIC IMPAIRMENT IN INTERMITTENT AUDITORY IMPERCEPTION

The most obvious clinical difference between Auditory patients and the other two severe groups of aphasics, Sensorimotor and Irreversible, is the early occurrence of some connected speech, phrases, and sentences, that sound completely normal.

A relevant observation is that normal-sounding utterances seem to occur in Auditory patients when language patterns are readily available. This sometimes occurrs on naming common objects, on highly overlearned tasks such as counting, and on conventional social responses. In contrast, on more difficult tasks, one observes groping movements, struggle behavior, and unintelligible or defective utterances which are similar to the struggle behavior of Sensorimotor patients. It is as though the Auditory patients attempt to force the articulators to organize a response without adequate information or instructions. Sometimes the patient may "know" what he wants to say, as some patients have reported. In such cases semantic but not phonemic information may be available, a deficit which might affect writing as well as speech.

A second observation is that as available language increases, the labored speech, articulatory inaccuracies, and jargon responses gradually decrease and disappear. In intermediate stages of recovery, utterances tend to show restricted vocabulary and little variety of syntactic structure, but usually sound normal. At no time in the course of recovery is spontaneous speech limited to single-word utterances; nor do "telegraphic" utterances, in which words without referents are characteristically omitted, occur in spontaneous speech.

It seems reasonable to postulate that the input to the restructuring device that plans and interprets speech output contains both somatosensory and acoustic information. If somatosensory information were reduced, one would predict a speech deficit characterized principally by lack of spatial differentiation of phonemes, as in the Sensorimotor patients (MacNeilage *et al.*, 1967). If, on the other hand, auditory information were inadequate, the deficit might well simulate a somatosensory (or somesthetic) deficit in the beginning, but as more language became available, tend to follow the course we have described, since spatial differentiation would be intact.

The patient with sensorimotor deficits, at the point of maximal recovery, does not speak like a patient with deficient acoustic information at any point in the latter's clinical course. In the course of the two disorders, there is at no time any overlap. A patient with deficient acoustic information, when his utterances are almost completely unintelligible, only superficially resembles a patient with impaired somatosensory or sensorimotor control. The groping movements are similar, but the sounds that result are not.

Clinical signs that impaired control for the auditory group derives from reduced auditory input are: (1) the presence of well-inflected and articulated jargon responses (such as *whiffer* for *razor, ubalo* for *radio, somaty* for *soup,* and *shotcase* for *salt*); (2) clang responses, such as *beat* for *meat, roush* for *house,* and *batch* for *match;* (3) semantically related responses, such as *candle* for *lamp, pen* for *pencil, bath* for *bed;* (4) occasional occurrence of connected speech that sounds normal. It is sometimes difficult to make such a differential diagnosis initially if almost no verbal responses can be elicited. However, our observations lead us to believe that one should suspect the speech deficit reflects reduction of auditory rather than somatosensory information whenever auditory imperception is present. The decision is of importance, since it has implications for treatment.

TEST FINDINGS

Total test scores by modalities show that the Auditory patients are the most severe aphasics, except for the Irreversible patients. There were exceptions to this in a few subtest scores: Scattered Findings and Visual patients' error scores in matching letters and matching words to pictures slightly exceeded Auditory patients' scores. Sensorimotor patients made 96% error in producing sentences, while Auditory patients made 91% error. Scattered Findings patients made higher error scores than Auditory patients in copying Greek letters, writing numbers to 20, and reproducing a wheel, and Sensorimotor patients' errors exceeded the Auditory patients' errors in written arithmetic problems.

Auditory imperceptives' scores were all above the mean error scores for a large unselected sample of aphasic patients on Schuell's *Minnesota Test.* This does not indicate that the scores for an individual patient must be higher than the group mean in order to be classified in this group.

NEUROLOGICAL BACKGROUND

The mean age of patients with intermittent auditory imperception was 52.6. Auditory patients averaged 13 years of school. Occupational levels for this group ranged from day laborer to professional, with the median at skilled. Etiology was cerebral vascular accident in 50% of the group, 19% trauma, and 31% other etiologies such as endarterectomy, hypertensive crises, and emboli. Thirty-eight percent of the cerebrovascular accidents were confirmed complete thrombosis of the left middle cerebral artery. This was a larger percentage than the total sample.

Auditory patients had a significantly lower percentage of involvement of the extremities than Scattered Findings, Sensorimotor, and Irreversible patients. Paralysis of the extremities was present in 50% of the Auditory patients. The Auditory patients had the lowest percentage of sensory loss, at 42%.

Auditory patients had a high incidence of focal EEG findings.

The most interesting finding for the Auditory patients was that 45% of them showed bilateral neurological signs in the complete absence of bilateral weakness. The author who reviewed all the neurological data (J-P) cautioned that these conclusions were based on the data available, which for many reasons were sometimes scanty. The indications are that careful, more complete neurological data may reveal an even higher percentage of Auditory patients showing bilateral signs.

Visual field defects were reported for 53% of the Auditory patients, which was higher than for any other group except the Visual patients.

Thirty-seven percent of these patients had abnormal mental states, which was higher than for any of the milder groups but not as high as for Scattered Findings and Irreversible patients.

Eighty-one percent of the Auditory subjects were able to perform self-care activities. Those that could not perform initially did not improve. Fifty percent were able to ambulate initially, 62% at final evaluation. Eighteen percent were reported to have an adverse outcome, and 6% (two patients) were able to resume employment.

A FUNCTIONAL SCHEMA FOR APHASIA WITH INTERMITTENT AUDITORY IMPERCEPTION

Aphasic patients with intermittent auditory imperception are often found to have bilateral hemispheric involvement. The aphasia may be severe to relatively mild. For some patients perceptually discriminating speech may be more difficult than understanding the meaning of what is said, while for other patients the reverse may be true. For instance, some patients seem not to hear words correctly, while others hear well enough to repeat words accurately, but are still puzzled as to the meaning. These facts suggest that more than one level of analytic speech processes in the auditory modality are differentially disturbed. Consequently, for some patients the *receptor synergism* component is more severely impaired than the *interpreter* component, while for others the reverse is true.

Initially many of the auditory patients seem to have a sensorimotor deficit. This is due to the fact that for both Auditory and Sensorimotor patients the functioning of the *planner–interpreter* is impaired. For the Auditory patients, however, the *interpreter* function of this component seems more severely impaired than the *planner* function, although both are involved sufficiently to resemble the sensorimotor deficit. Figure 15–1 indicates the three components involved in this form of aphasia.

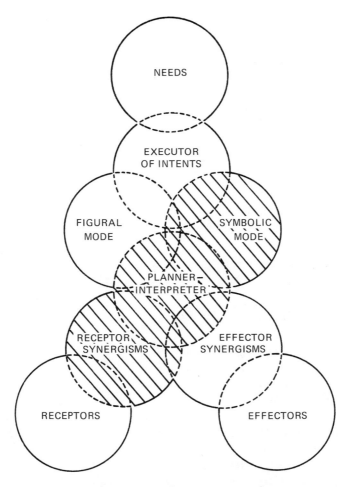

NEEDS

EXECUTOR
OF INTENTS

FIGURAL
MODE

SYMBOLIC
MODE

PLANNER-
INTERPRETER

RECEPTOR
SYNERGISMS

EFFECTOR
SYNERGISMS

RECEPTORS

EFFECTORS

Fig. 15–1. Functional schema for aphasia with intermittent auditory imperception.

chapter 16

AN IRREVERSIBLE APHASIA
SYNDROME

Reed Saunders was a man of physical and intellectual stature who held a responsible administrative position. He had a kindly manner and an air of decision and quiet integrity.

On a hunting trip in November after his 55th birthday, Mr. Saunders observed some weakness in his right hand. By the next morning the entire upper extremity was involved, and his speech was dysarthric. He was taken to the nearest large hospital, and there, two days later, he had a focal seizure that started in the right upper extremity. After this, he gradually lapsed into a coma. At the end of a week, medical records described his condition as profoundly comotose, febrile, aphasic, and hemiplegic, and he was taken to surgery.

Surgical notes reported a large multilocular abscess in a central position in the left hemisphere. It was treated by decompression afforded by removal of a frontoparietal craniotomy flap, and by catheter drainage. Antibiotics were administered both locally, into the abscess cavity, and parenterally. The postsurgical course was one of gradual improvement.

In January, Mr. Saunders was transferred to a second hospital for rehabilitation. Admission findings included flaccid paralysis of the right arm and leg, a positive right Babinski, and right lower facial paralysis. The right pupil was dilated, but reacted to light. Mr. Saunders received daily physiotherapy but was not treated for aphasia. At the end of April he was transferred to the Minneapolis VA Hospital for the aphasia program.

Examination revealed a well-developed, well-nourished man with a skull defect in the left parietal area. Physical examination was essentially normal. Neurological examination showed right hemiplegia with aphasia, right lower facial paralysis, and reduction of sensation on the right. The EEG showed five cycle per second irregular high-amplitude activity in the left hemisphere, most marked in the central areas.

Mrs. Saunders, who accompanied her husband, prepared to spend as much time at the hospital as she could, to learn how to care for him. She had had courses in speech pathology in college and wanted to learn more about aphasia in order to help him. Knowing that her husband would be miserable if he had to be indoors all summer, she also rented a cottage on a nearby lake where he could spend weekends. Mr. Saunders was more than six-feet tall, and big-boned, while Mrs. Saunders was slight, and stood five-feet two. No one ever knew how they got Mr. Saunders in and out of the car those first weekends at the lake, but between the two of them, they managed it. No one ever doubted the healing value of those interludes, or that Mr. Saunders came back relaxed and refreshed on Monday mornings.

INITIAL FINDINGS

On tests for auditory comprehension, Mr. Saunders made errors pointing to common objects named by the examiner. He scored below the first percentile on the Ammons test. He had less than chance success pointing to letters and numbers named by the examiner. He made errors following short simple directions. In earlier medical charts a physician had noted that "He understands well, but cannot talk." We interpret this to mean that his behavior was appropriate, and his facial expression intelligent. In the light of test findings and all subsequent observations, it could mean nothing else.

On reading tests, Mr. Saunders made errors matching letters and matching common words to pictures. On a standardized vocabulary test, he matched words to pictures to Grade Level 3.8. This was his best test performance. He could read no simple sentences with comprehension.

Speech attempts produced jargon, although the patient said *yes, well* anc *now* responsively during examination. He had no difficulty imitating gross movements of the speech musculature, but he could not repeat common monosyllabic words, count to five, or name the days of the week with the examiner, even after repeated stimulation. The best performance that could be elicited was imitation of a few syllables, such as *ah, ma, pa,* and *la.*

Tracing and copying were poor, and Mr. Saunders sometimes attempted to write with the eraser end of the pencil. He could write no letters or words to dictation, nor could he write his name.

He could make change, but made errors selecting correct responses to simple numerical combinations, such as $6 + 7$ and $5 + 3$. On performance tests he seemed to get an idea of what was required and could usually perform part of the task, but never succeeded in completing the test.

He was alert, cooperative, and highly motivated, and he worked with concentration and directed effort.

The picture was one of severe impairment, amounting to almost complete loss of functional skills in all language modalities. The clinician told Mrs. Saunders that the prognosis was extremely poor, but that we would try to get the mechanism working better in order to obtain more intelligible speech. The clinician added that even if this were possible, there was little probability of getting voluntary functional speech, and that she must not hope for too much.

This was a shock to Mrs. Saunders, who had been told by a physician somewhere along the way that her husband would achieve full recovery within two years.

Sometimes professional counselors are critical of people whose expectations are unrealistic. They forget that many people have had no experience with chronic conditions, or tend to associate them only with elderly relatives, and not with someone who has always been active, vital, and dynamic, and who has never had a serious illness before. Most people are conditioned to the idea that recovery follows illness. It is what experience has taught them.

The clinician said: "We will do everything we can, and I will tell you all I know, but it will be slow and hard and the gains will be limited. You must begin to think and to plan in these terms."

It is important, and kinder in the end, to give people the information they need to enable them to make the adjustments that have to be made. Mrs. Saunders sat in on therapy every day, and worked with her husband to give him additional practice, and gradually began to understand the extent of the problem. She began to think, too, in terms of conserving their resources, and implementing them through her own abilities.

THE COURSE OF TREATMENT

By the end of the first month, Mr. Saunders could count, say the alphabet, and the days of the week in unison with the clinician, and complete the series if the clinician dropped out. He could repeat most common words. He could produce short phrases, if simultaneous visual and auditory stimulation were presented, but he could read no words aloud independently. He was more accurate pointing to objects and pictures named by the examiner, although he still made errors with words as common as *table* or *window*. He could name no objects or pictures, and jargon persisted, although there was more reactive speech that was clear. He said things like *Where? Let it go, I don't know, Yes, I know, Pill, Bye, Hi,* and *Fine,* responsively.

At the end of two months, Mr. Saunders' overall progress was reviewed at a neurology staff conference. The corrective therapists reported good progress in ambulation and self-care. The occupational therapists reported improvement in the use of his hands and in using tools. The speech pathologist said Mr. Saunders would not recover functional speech, but that she would like to work with him as long as he was in the hospital to improve comprehension, facilitate movement patterns, and increase reactive responses. The latter are unpredictable, and the patient has little control over them, but they contribute to social adequacy, and this is an important value. The consensus was that

Mr. Saunders should remain in the hospital until he had made maximal gains in self-care and ambulation.

By the end of the third month Mr. Saunders could repeat short phrases, and occasionally read a few single words that had been well-practiced. He was able to read short paragraphs in unison with the clinician, with about 90% of the words intelligible. Words could be elicited by association techniques, which had not been possible earlier. Auditory comprehension had increased to the extent that Mr. Saunders followed directions, followed conversation more readily, and often got the point of a short joke. He could usually tell his name. Reactive speech continued to increase. It was very limited, but occasionally a sentence appeared. His wife reported that he said, "I want to eat," once when lunch had been delayed by a visitor. One day he said, "the water's all gone," to a nurse, when his carafe was empty.

In the meantime, Mrs. Saunders had become a skilled clinician. She had written to the university in the town where they lived, and obtained a position as housemother in a small residential unit for women. Living quarters were provided for both her and her husband while her duties allowed her free time during the day to work with him. When the authorities studied her credentials they offered to increase the salary if she were willing to do a little "deaning" on the side.

THE OUTCOME

Mrs. Saunders' plan worked out very well, although there was little or no further recovery of speech. They came back to Minneapolis when school was out in June, for reevaluation and further consultation. Mrs. Saunders was discouraged but unwilling to give up. The clinician assured her that there were many values in what they were doing. Both she and Mr. Saunders enjoyed their daily lessons, which facilitated communication between them. They helped Mr. Saunders fill his time and gave him something to look forward to. Best of all probably, they stimulated him to become a communicating individual despite severe limitations of language.

The clinician said: "There is nothing else I can tell you to do, but I don't think you should take my word as final. I don't want you to spend your lives running from place to place hoping for a cure, but it's always a good idea to get more than one opinion. I can give you the names of some very competent people, and you can go wherever you like. They are all good."

The Saunders went to one of the recommended clinics, and received some encouragement. Additional techniques were suggested, and group therapy was recommended. The Saunders spent the second year in the east. Mr. Saunders was enrolled for group therapy in a university clinic, and Mrs. Saunders faithfully followed the instructions she had received. Mr. Saunders disliked the group therapy sessions because he could not do most of the things that other members of the group could do. He was always discouraged and depressed, afterwards. Mrs. Saunders was skillful enough to counteract this, however, when he was at home. The clinician saw them in the spring, and Mr. Saunders looked contented and well, although there was no observable change in his speech.

In the fall, Mrs. Saunders obtained a teaching position in a pleasant community where the climate permitted Mr. Saunders to be out-of-doors a large part of the year. She found a house with open country around them, on the outskirts of town. Mr. Saunders began to do more about the house and the yard. Mrs. Saunders found a likable young woman who came in every morning, prepared Mr. Saunder's breakfast and lunch, and helped him with his lessons. By this time it was often possible to elicit a response by asking a question. One day the girl asked him if he knew Marlene Dietrich. Mr. Saunders said "yes," and she asked him what Marlene Dietrich was famous for. He answered succinctly, "Legs."

Mrs. Saunders reported that Reed enjoyed listening to the radio more than he had previously, and that he read the paper and magazines with at least partial comprehension. She said that he frequently pointed out items about people they knew, or events with which he had previous associations. He wanted to work on arithmetic, and he learned to add and subtract. Mrs. Saunders commented that if he made an error, he could usually correct it when she pointed it out.

Five years after the initial onset, Mr. Saunders spent two weeks in a large rehabilitation clinic. Mrs. Saunders wrote that she wanted to be sure they had overlooked nothing that would help. She added: "However, the real reason I wanted Reed to go was to be away from me, and on his own, but with informed supervision. This we accomplished. I suspect Reed was miserable while I was gone, but it gave him the needed jolt away from me, and laid the foundation for his present independence. He still manages better and is happier if I am at hand, but he can do very well if I am not."

She added that the doctors were amazed at how well he walked. Her own comment was, "Reed always walked with dignity, and he still does." She said he walked slowly and had fallen on a few occasions. A few days before he had lost his balance, but shifted his weight and righted himself, which was new.

A year later she wrote that she was sure he was reading more. He had done a history quiz in a magazine, with multiple choice answers, and made no errors. One night at dinner he tried to tell her something, and kept pointing to the radio. She asked, "Was there someone on the radio we know?" He said "yes," and went and found a paper that was four days old, turned through it until he found the little article he wanted, and brought it to her. An old friend had talked to a local group that day, and Reed had heard a broadcast of his speech.

She added: "Now speech. That is our slowest department. . . . Reed does better with individual instruction. He has been a leader so long that he gets confused when he is at the bottom of the class. . . . I don't really think the lessons do much good at this stage, but they keep him talking and are good morale builders." He never learned to write more than his name.

The eighth year after onset found the Saunders again in a community where individual and group therapy were available from a trained speech pathologist. This was supportive but did not materially alter the general picture. Ten years have passed since the Saunders left Minneapolis. The situation is essentially unchanged as far as recovery of language is concerned, but with intelligence, persistence, and devotion the Saunders have done as well as anyone could do in a most difficult situation.

People usually deal with problems as well as they are able to, and often the ways they choose turn out to be the best ones for them. Helen and Reed Saunders kept the relationship between them intact, and continued to enjoy many of the things they had always enjoyed together. They made new friends wherever they went. The latter included another couple in which the husband was aphasic. Mrs. Saunders wrote loyally that he could talk more than Reed but he couldn't read as much, and that he did not have Reed's sweetness or his fine social assets.

For the Saunders, it was right to seek additional professional help from time to time, when it was possible or available. This was supportive to Mrs. Saunders and provided additional stimulation for Mr. Saunders, and made him less dependent upon his wife. We wish that he might miraculously recover, and write the story of these 10 years himself.

FURTHER OBSERVATIONS

It is the hardest thing in the world to accept the fact that a patient like Mr. Saunders will not recover functional language.

More than 1000 aphasic patients have been studied at the Minneapolis VA Hospital, and from 1948 until 1954 all patients who made any test responses at all received at least a trial period of intensive treatment. Early criteria for exclusion or termination of treatment were the following:

1. Inability to participate in treatment, as evidenced by inability to respond to any test items or test materials
2. Consistent inability to retain learned responses for 24 hours, in spite of intensive reinforcement
3. Plateaus maintained over periods of weeks, with no gains or only minimal improvement
4. Agreement that the patient could get along as well or better outside the hospital, and continue to make improvement. This agreement was usually between the clinician, the patient, and immediate family, because maximal benefits had usually been reached earlier in other areas of rehabilitation. Discharge involved careful planning, however, with all the professional staff, including the physician, the social worker, the vocational counsellor, and sometimes others.

These criteria worked fairly well. The only real objection is the amount of clinical time required to reach conclusions that are now predictable as soon as patients are neurologically stable. This is an important economic and social consideration. A bed occupied by a patient who cannot benefit from treatment cannot be occupied by any other patient. The time a clinician spends with a patient who is making no significant gains cannot be spent with another who might. These are important determinants.

Dr. Schuell went on ward rounds in a rehabilitation unit in a state institution for the aged. She was asked to see an aphasic patient to determine whether he was a good candidate for the limited therapy offered by a neighboring university. The patient was an educated man with a delightful personality, but he had all the signs of extensive generalized brain damage. He would undoubtedly enjoy therapy because he loved attention, but it was extremely doubtful than any changes could be effected. All the neurologists agreed except a young resident, who conceded only because the consensus was against him. Before they drove back to the city, he asked to show Dr. Schuell another building.

There they saw an antiseptically clean ward with 100 beds. There was a chair beside each bed. Lying on each bed, or sitting on the chair in an attitude of complete withdrawal, was an elderly man. No one moved, looked up, or spoke. The doctor said, "This is what he will go back to."

People should care about conditions like this. They should care enough to change them. Everyone should care—doctors, nurses, psychologists, social scientists, legislators, and each of us in our capacity as a responsible human being. These patients had lost communication with the world. It was a kind of living death.

One suspects that what was needed was a program, perhaps one with professional directors and volunteer help. These men needed someone to call them by their names, to know who they were, to sit down and talk to them. They needed something to do, to look forward to, to talk about, to get up for in the morning. Volunteer groups in communities and colleges working under professional direction, can do a great deal to change our institutions into something better than prisons with no escape for the human spirit.

There are not enough trained speech pathologists to take care of all the patients in public institutions who need palliative therapy. There are not enough, unfortunately, to provide services for all the aphasic patients who might regain functional language skills. Since selection must operate, it should be informed selection.

Patient responsibility requires that the speech pathologist evaluate the status of every aphasic patient referred, interpret obtained findings, and make recommendations consistente with the best interests of the patient. It is also important to recognize the limitations of human ability. A great neurologist once said compassionately, upon the death of a patient, "I am sorry. I am not God." We should not confuse our roles.

In the interests of humanity, we should take enough time to work through the difficulties of acceptance with the patient and the family. Sometimes a limited period of treatment helps to reestablish communication and to avert tendencies toward withdrawal and depression. Some counseling is always necessary to help the family understand the problem of aphasia, and to support the patient and the family through the early stages of adjustment. It is not sound procedure, however, to treat Irreversible patients for months or years with the expectancy that functional language skills will be regained.

The characteristic of Irreversible patients in treatment is not that they make no gains, but that gains do not become functional. Almost all can learn to repeat, and most of them can learn to copy. They can learn to count, say the alphabet, name the days of the week and the months of the year in serial order, if someone starts them. They can produce associative responses of high strength, and some reactive speech appears, but it is not predictable and never becomes voluntary. It is elicited randomly by outside stimuli.

These responses are often deceptive. They sometimes appear to be of such a high order that observers forget the patient has no control over them. One patient who was fond of music, said, "Stokowski," one evening, while listening to a recording of a symphony Stokowski was conducting. The patient and his wife had once heard Stokowski conduct the same symphony on a concert program, and had subsequently purchased the record. On another occasion, he said to his wife, "Helene, I love you." Such utterances occur as responses to a strong and meaningful pattern of stimulation. The patient remains unable to tell where he lives, where he went to school, or what he wants from the drugstore. He is never, in fact, able to use language to help him carry out any plan or intention of his own.

Experimental techniques developed to provide maximal stimulation and reinforcement of language were successful with severely impaired patients in all other diagnostic categories, but did not produce functional results in this group.

The clinician could almost always get repetition and copying, and highly overlearned serial responses. Some patients could count to 100, when the clinician started them. They could sing words to familiar songs, with practice. With stimulation, they could often repeat a nursery rhyme, or the Lord's Prayer, when someone started them. It is possible to elicit more than 100 different responses in one clinical period by using a completion technique based on well-established associations. In the following examples, the elicited response is italicized.

You get up early in the *morning*.
You go to bed at *night*.
Turn out the *light*.
Please close the *door*.
I like to drive a *car*.
I want a cup of *coffee*.
I would like to go *fishing*.
The sun is *shining*.
The wind is *blowing*.
The birds are *singing*.
Up and *down*.
East and *west*.
Bread and *butter*.
Meat and *potatoes*.
Coat and *hat*.

With some patients, it has been possible to go a step beyond this and sometimes elicit a one-word response by a question such as:

What do you write with?
What do you sit on?
What do you sleep in?
What do you do with a pencil?
What do you do with a knife?

No Irreversible patient, however, has been able to name a set of common pictures, and retain the names from one day to another, with as intensive stimulation as could be devised.

TEST FINDINGS

The profiles in Chapter 9, as well as the ensuing test findings, were based on performances of the only four Irreversible subjects who received intensive treatment for aphasia in the present study. As we pointed out earlier, these patients received treatment because they exceeded the average performance of Irreversible subjects in some respect on initial testing. They represent the top 17% of the group.

On tests for auditory comprehension, they exceeded the mean number of errors for all diagnostic groups on all tests on both initial and final testing, and made the lowest percentage of improvement. When percentages of error were averaged over the nine tests, Irreversible patients made more than twice as many errors as any other group, initially and finally. On final testing, success was below chance level on all tests except pointing to common objects named by the examiner. Ammons test scores were below the first percentile on initial and final testing.

The direction of test–retest differences was positive on all nine tests, indicating that improvement in comprehension occurred. Retests from patients reexamined on later admissions, however, tend to indicate that these gains were lost when intensive treatment was discontinued. When patients were alert and responsive, the extent of auditory impairment was commonly underestimated by professionals and laymen alike.

On visual and reading tests, these subjects also had the highest percentage of error initially and finally, and showed the lowest percentage of improvement. Improvement occurred on matching tests. No performance above chance level was obtained on any reading tests more difficult than matching common words to pictures, and matching printed to spoken words. In no case did reading become a functional skill. Some patients, however, continued to enjoy looking at picture magazines and at newspapers. It is assumed that some recognition took place, but that reading comprehension was extremely limited. Mr. Saunders' performance on the history quiz was remarkably good, but one should probably not assume that he did more than match significant words in the questions to associated words in the multiple-choice responses. At the same time, it is significant that such associations, undoubtedly based on previous learning, occurred.

On speech and language tests Irreversible patients had the highest percentage of error on initial and final examination, and made the lowest percentage of improvement of all diagnostic groups. There was no performance on 8 of the 14 language tests initially, and on 4 tests finally. Best performance was a few highly overlearned serial or associative responses on the easiest test items, made on retest. In no case did speech become functional.

On copying and drawing tests, they performed below all other diagnostic groups initially, but averaged more improvement than did Scattered Findings subjects, who showed more specific involvement of visual processes. Irreversible subjects performed twice as well initially, and three times as well finally, on copying and drawing tests as on writing tests that involved language. There was no improvement on the latter. This suggests that language factors, rather than perceptual or motor ones, are usually responsible for the severe writing impairment found in this group. Many patients learned to copy beautifully, but they did not acquire functional writing any more than they acquired functional speech. Some subjects learned to write their names, and one patient wrote the word *boy* correctly to dictation on final testing. This was the highest success achieved. Irreversible patients performed below all other groups on tests for numerical relations and arithmetic processes on initial testing. This was true on final testing also, except on one test. These subjects made more improvement than Scattered Findings patients on setting a clock, and obtained the same mean number of errors on retest. On this test patients were asked to set the clock to show the time they got up, went to bed, and to other designated times. Most subjects performed the first two tasks on final testing, but could not set the clock to specified times. This seems to indicate that the chief difficulty was in comprehension of language, rather than in visual and spatial relations or in orientation for time. Irreversible patients kept appointments independently and accurately, when sufficient care was taken to insure that they understood the appointment time.

There was no performance on initial or final examination on arithemetic tests. Tests were fourth-grade level and below, except for long division, which was fifth-grade.

Arithemetic tests involve both language and visual and spatial skills. Most aphasic patients make errors because they do not know the names of individual numbers, although they may be able to recite or write them serially, or because they have lost the learned combinations, such as $6+5=11$, or $7\times6=42$. Sometimes steps of a process, such as carrying or borrowing, are forgotten. Patients with visual involvement may confuse numbers such as 6 and 9, or 3 and 8. They may reverse digits in combinations, or omit numerals they do not see. When spatial disorientation is present, the patient may begin at the wrong side of the page and proceed in the wrong direction, or set partial answers down in positions that make it impossible to deal with the array correctly.

These subjects scored below all diagnostic groups on all tests for body parts, on initial and final testing. However, they made more improvement in pointing to body parts named by the examiner and in drawing a man than either the Visual or Scattered Findings groups. These were the groups with specific involvement of visual processes. This is not, at least, a general finding in Irreversible patients, although it is probably present in some. Neither visual or spatial impariement nor disturbance of body image are excluded by the diagnostic criteria, which are essentially loss of functional language skills.

In summary, Irreversible subjects performed below all other groups on all sections of the Minnesota Test on both initial and final testing. They tended to show improvement on only the easiest tests, and did not achieve functional language skills in any modality.

Many patients were alert, well-oriented, responsive, highly motivated, and capable of sustained effort. Their appreciation of any help they received sometimes made it difficult for the clinician to terminate intensive treatment, even when no significant results were achieved. Often, however, when the clinician had extended treatment, unable to admit failure, she found the patient had already accepted it. When she finally said reluctantly, "I don't think we should go on with this. I think it's too hard, and you're not getting enough out of it," the patient concurred with something very like relief. The clinician often had the distinct impression that he wanted to console and reassure her, and to let her know that it would be all right.

NEUROLOGICAL BACKGROUND

Scattered Findings and Irreversible patients were the oldest of the diagnostic groups studied. The mean age for Scattered Findings patients was 59.4 in this sample, and 59.6 for Irreversible patients. No Irreversible subjects were under 40 years of age, and 87% were over 50. Seventy percent were also over 60, and 35% over 65.

Education ranged from less than six years schooling through professional degrees, with the average falling between 10 and 12 years. The occupational level was slightly higher than in other diagnostic categories, although these differences were not statistically significant.

Etiology was cerebrovascular accident in 96% and trauma in 4%. This was the highest incidence of cerebrovascular accidents.

Irreversible patients were the oldest of all clinical groups. With the Sensorimotor patients, they had the highest incidence of cerebrovascular accidents, and the highest incidence of complete thrombosis of the internal carotid and middle cerebral arteries, and of the middle cerebral artery alone. They had the highest incidence of involvement of extremities, and of paralysis with paresis excluded, of lower facial paralysis, reduction of sensation, and focal EEG findings. Although the Irreversible patients exceeded the Sensorimotor group in all measures of severity, the differences between these two groups lacked statistical significance. The two groups do differ from other groups in severity of neurological involvement according to all measures employed, and all of these differences were statistically significant.

Generally, Irreversible patients resembled Sensorimotor patients in severity of neurological involvement, suggesting massive lesions in both these groups. In the high incidence of complicating conditions, however, Irreversible patients resembled Scattered Findings patients. These patients uniformly exceeded all other groups in severity of neurological involvement and showed a relatively high incidence of complicating conditions, as well.

There were so many Irreversible patients like Mr. Saunders, who were highly motivated, stable, and socially adequate, that we tended to think of these patients in this way. The halo tendency was undoubtedly reinforced by the fact that most of the Irreversible patients who received treatment were responsive. This is an example of the unreliability of clinical impressions not supported by data.

These patients scored below all other groups in self-care and ambulation, on both initial and final evaluation. The incidence of commitment, further episodes, and known deaths was the highest incidence of adverse sequelae in any diagnostic group. No patient in this group received educational or occupational training, and none returned to gainful employment.

Some patients returned to their homes, and were comfortable and contented. Understandably, the best adjustments were made by patients whose families accepted them matter-of-factly, and to whom the patient was still *just dad*, whether he could talk or not. The patients got along best when members of the family did the things that had to be done for them as a matter of course, but expected the patient to be as independent as possible.

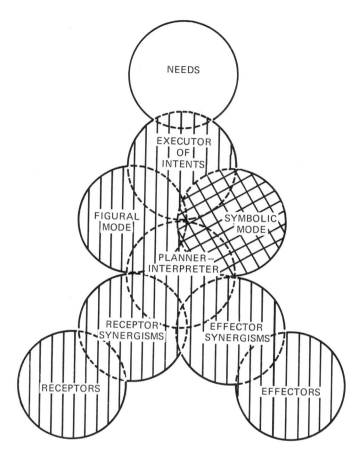

Fig. 16–1. Functional schema for irreversible aphasia.

The wife of one patient reported: "The first time I left Dad alone in the house, I told him I was going over to the neighbors for a cup of coffee. I knew the way he looked at me he was afraid, but I just told him I'd be back in 15 minutes and ran. I made myself stay 15 minutes, too. I knew if I didn't we'd both be living in fear all our lives. Now I can leave him for two or three hours,and he putters around, and I think he kind of enjoys it."

Another wife wrote that her husband went to the barber shop alone, and found his way all over town. At Christmas, he purchased stockings for his wife and three daughters, and managed to get all the right sizes.

It is important for these patients to live as normally as possible. Relevant problems will be discussed in more detail in a later chapter.

The background data presented in the last seven chapters are summarized in Tables 1–4 of Appendix 2.

A FUNCTIONAL SCHEMA FOR AN IRREVERSIBLE APHASIA SYNDROME

Irreversible patients can have such severe aphasia that it is sometimes difficult to tell what components other than the *symbolic mode* might be involved. Some patients clearly have all the complicating conditions, which would involve most of the components to some extent, while other patients seem to have only a subset of the components involved. But for all patients the symbolic system does not seem to function at all. When any residual speech is present, the utterances tend to be automatic or reactive, involving no planning and serving little purpose in communication. Consequently, Figure 16–1 shows the components typically implicated by this aphasic disorder.

part five

THE THERAPEUTIC
PROCESS

chapter 17

PSYCHOLOGICAL PROBLEMS IN
APHASIA

To say a clinician must be aware of psychological problems in aphasia is to say he must be aware that he is dealing with people. Sometimes we are so intimidated by labels, such as emotional lability, catastrophic reactions, anxiety, depression, euphoria, etc., that we forget this first principle. We talk trade jargon with a glibness that betrays our dearth of insights. We speak as though aphasic patients were different from everyone else, and we had to have a different set of rules for dealing with them.

A clinician has a special relationship with a patient or client, and so in a sense he does operate with a conscious set of rules. He is a specialist who acts as a consultant and a counselor in his field. One of the clinician's rules is to recognize the limits of his area of competence. A speech pathologist does not, however, treat aphasia or stuttering or articulation disorders, and leave the patient in the waiting room. He deals with human, not mechanical, problems.

The first requirement is that the clinician communicate with the patient in a meaningful way. In order to do this effectively, he trains himself to become a sensitive receiving instrument. He tries to understand who the patient is, what has happened to him, and what the aphasia, the stuttering, the cleft palate, or the laryngectomy means to the patient.

In addition, the clinician trains himself to behave purposefully toward his patients and clients. They have come with needs and expectancies and sometimes with hope, and the clinician is committed to serve their best interests insofar as he can. He must find out what needs to be done and set about doing it as directly as possible.

The finding out is an essential part of the clinical process. It is senseless to rush in with random noise and futile motion. Until there is a surgical procedure, a drug, an electrode, or a teaching machine that will benefit all patients equally, uninformed activity will continue to do more harm than good. In the meantime we must have information in order to serve the patient. We must be concerned both with the symptomatology of aphasia and with the patient's ability to channel his energies toward recovery.

ALTERATIONS OF BEHAVIOR IN APHASIA

In the present study, only 35% of the patients showed any abnormal mental states. Emotional lability was reported for 19%, confusion for 9%, confusion and lability for 3%, and regressive behavior or organic psychoses occurred in 4% of the population. Seventy-nine percent of the abnormalities observed were in the Scattered Findings group and 20% in the Irreversible group, but 32% of subjects in the first group and 50% in the second showed no observable alterations in behavior. The majority were alert, responsive, and highly motivated individuals who behaved sensibly, used good judgment, and interacted appropriately with others. They often displayed impressive fortitude, perseverance, and ability to withstand frustration and discouragement. This is not to say that 65% of the aphasic patients we saw did not react to what had happened to them, which would have been abnormal in itself. It is rather to say that they made generally creditable adjustments to difficult circumstances.

EMOTIONAL LIABILITY

Almost all aphasic patients show some emotional lability during the acute period of the illness, as, in fact, do many other convalescents. Emotional lability is sometimes defined as inappropriate laughing or crying, or laughing or crying without emotional significance. This observation does not seem to be strictly true.

Labile patients do laugh or cry excessively. They laugh and cry when they do not wish to, in the sense that loss of control is often a source of painful embarrassment. However, this behavior does not tend to occur out of context, and it is inappropriate only in the sense that it is an overreaction. It is as though the patient had a lowered emotional threshold, and abnormal duration and spread of emotional excitation. His laughter and tears are triggered more easily and tend to overflow. Tears, as a matter of fact, are more common than laughter, although laughter may turn into tears. These responses may result from tension or embarrassment. They frequently arise in relation to something the patient has deep feelings or acute anxiety about. A reference to the patient's home, his family, or his job may result in tears the patient is helpless to inhibit. Emotional lability commonly decreases as physiological and neurological conditions improve. When it persists, as it sometimes does, it is usually considered a symptom of bilateral brain damage.

A lifelong friend of one of the authors was a warm and gracious woman with a great deal of natural reserve. She adjusted to the limitations imposed by a series of cerebrovascular accidents with quiet heroism and dignity. The earliest symptoms were scotomas resulting from hemorrhages of the retina. Reduction of vision made it impossible for her to read for pleasure, drive a car, or carry on numerous other accustomed activities. She compensated by deliberately seeking occupations that were satisfying to her, and brought enjoyment to others. After the second episode, there was mild weakness on the left side of her body, and some laryngeal involvement, although there was never any aphasia. She exercised patiently and reported her progress pleasantly when friends inquired. After the third clinical episode, emotional lability was present, and gradually increased until her death. She confessed that she found this the most humiliating and difficult to bear of all the limitations her long illness had imposed upon her.

What seems to help the emotionally labile patient most is to explain that this heightened susceptibility is part of the illness, and that it tends to improve as recovery takes place. This is true, unless there is steady progression of disease or recurring episodes. Partial remission is probably more psychological than physiological. Confidence increases as the patient gets better, and ordinary encounters become less threatening as his own sense of adequacy increases.

It also helps to reassure the patient matter-of-factly that it is all right when he cries. Ignoring his embarrassment may be construed as disapproval, and increase tension. It is better to give quiet reassurance, allow time for recovery, then go on as though the behavior were of no great importance. This attitude measurably decreases the frequency and severity of the episodes. The patient who cried regularly four or five times during the clinical hour breaks down only once, then misses a day. Soon three of four days pass with no recurrence. Eventually it happens only rarely, or may not happen at all in the clinic. This behavior is under the patient's control only indirectly and to a limited degree, but minimizing its importance and helping the patient to tolerate it seems to have a therapeutic effect.

CATASTROPHIC REACTIONS

In his classical monograph Goldstein (1942) described catastrophic reactions so brilliantly and effectively that there has been a tendency to regard all emotional behavior of aphasic patients as catastrophic ever since. This was not Dr. Goldstein's meaning. He described catastrophic reactions as responses that were disordered, inconsistent, and inadequate. He considered catastrophic reactions to be behavior imbedded in physical and mental shock, characterized by disorganization and disintegration of defenses. This behavior occurs when the patient is unable to cope with demands made upon him. Needless to say, threatening situations should be prevented insofar as possible.

A competent nurse once precipitated a catastrophic reaction by telling a patient just beginning to talk that he could not have his breakfast until he asked for it. The patient seized the tray and hurled it across the room. He liked the nurse and was ashamed and embarrassed afterwards. She told him it was a stupid thing for her to say, and she didn't blame him for getting mad. Later, teaching nurses, she used this as an example of how not to treat aphasic patients. She recognized that she had asked the patient to do something he desperately wanted to be able to do, and could not, and had unthinkingly spoken to him as though he were a child who was not very bright.

Catastrophic reactions rarely occur in a clinical situation when the clinician is supportive and alert to signs of incipient stress. There are innumerable ways to intervene to relieve tension. The clinician may change to easier materials or to a more familiar task. She may interrupt an activity with casual conversation, or suggest a break for a cigarette or stopping work for the day. Sometimes she may tell the patient directly to relax, and not push so hard, since this is something many aphasic patients have to learn to do. It does not matter what she does, so long as she reduces the mounting tension and gives the patient a chance to recover his equanimity. She should stay with him, however, until she is sure he is all right. Failure to resolve the situation may increase the patient's discomfort, result in a disturbance he carries with him all day, and make him reluctant to return to the clinic.

Once on ward rounds a staff neurologist demonstrated an aphasic patient to a group of residents. When the neurologist observed that the patient was becoming agitated, he terminated the interview as the only effective way to remove the audience. It might have left the patient anxious and humiliated, however, had not one of the group remained behind, offered the patient a cigarette, and talked to him quietly until he was comfortable.

In 15 years of working with aphasic patients, we have seen so few catastrophic reactions that it is difficult to think of good examples. We have demonstrated patients in medical conferences, in seminars, and in large professional meetings. The patients cooperated willingly and wholeheartedly. They demonstrated what they could do as well as what they could not do, and often stopped to explain difficulties they were having, because they thought it was important that people should know more about aphasia. On one occasion a patient gave an effective impromptu lecture to a group of physicians, telling them why they should understand aphasia better. He was a professional man, although not a physician. He told his audience he used to think that aphasics were mentally deficient, and that nothing could be done for them, and that doctors, at least, should be better informed. Since he ended his remarks with a testimonial to the Aphasia Section, no one ever believed we had not rehearsed him. It is nevertheless a good example of the ability of an aphasic patient to respond adequately in a situation that is often stressful for individuals who have never experienced brain injury.

In general, one does not need to fear catastrophic reactions when a relation of confidence has been firmly established between patient and clinician. The clinician can and should demand a great deal from the aphasic patient, within the limits of his capacities, in order to insure maximal recovery. Nothing restores confidence as much as consistent improvement.

DEPENDENCY NEEDS

In a hospital clinic, at least, the speech pathologist usually spends more hours than anyone else in direct communication with aphasic patients. If he is not the only person the patient can communicate with, he is usually the most available one. The patient feels the clinician knows him, understands his problems, and is concerned about them. For these reasons and out of his need he brings them to the clinic.

The clinician accepts this role. Treating aphasic subjects is relationship therapy from beginning to end. The patient must know that he can depend on the clinician for the help he requires. The clinician knows that the aphasic patient is dependent because he must be, and for this reason accepts the dependency. His objective, however, is to increase the patient's adequacy, restore his confidence, and thus gradually reduce his dependency needs.

At the beginning of treatment, the patient's only security may be the clinician's unfailing acceptance, understanding, and support. This cannot be withdrawn, but over a period of time it should become of decreasing importance. It is the clinician's responsibility to insure that this happens, and to take deliberate steps to this end.

One of the first steps is to interpret the patient's problems and needs to his own family, and to facilitate the reestablishment of communication between them. The family need to know what the patient cannot do, and why, but they also need to know the limitations of the disability. Sometimes a wife needs to be told that her husband's judgment is sound, although his speech is limited, and that she can talk things over with him and ask his advice. This probably will be supportive to her, as well as good therapy for the patient.

Another initial step is to interpret the patient's problems to members of hospital staff. This is usually a matter of exchanging information, because nurses and attendants make important observations about patients. Sometimes an aphasic patient appears confused or uncooperative because he does not understand what he is told. If the ward personnel know that he will understand if they make instructions short, repeat them, and take time to be sure the patient has grasped them, they are glad to do this. This makes the patient feel more secure and contributes to his recovery.

Sometimes a patient who is spatially disoriented and gets lost in the hospital is considered generally confused, although he is an intelligent and responsible person. He senses that he is regarded as mentally incompetent. He may conclude that he is, and react catastrophically. If staff personnel know that the principal source of difficulty is a poor sense of direction, they can react more appropriately. The patient will know they understand his problems, and this will help him learn to adjust to them.

One young aphasic patient appeared so sullen and hostile that he was rejected by patients and staff alike. His intelligence was above average, and he had a record of substantial achievement. When the clinician talked to him about the interesting work he had done, his response showed how deep was his need for recognition and approval. It took an active campaign to make people understand this need, because he was extremely defensive, but it worked. He was given responsibilities that gave him a somewhat privileged position on the ward, and his eagerness to be of service was apparent to everyone. His critics soon became his friends, and he responded warmly. In this case, the speech pathologist did nothing but toss the stone that started the ripples.

This is to say that the speech pathologist accomplishes many of his objectives better through other people, and so does not remain the significant person in the aphasic patient's world. He tries rather to extend the boundaries of that world. Each success that the patient has beyond the protective walls of the clinic works to this end, increases the patient's security and confidence, and decreases his dependency needs.

Another effective method of making the aphasic patient less isolated and dependent on the clinic is purposeful referral. The clinician listens understandingly to the problems the patient presents, but he does not try to solve them all. Instead, he says, in effect: "This is something you should talk to your doctor (or the social worker, vocational counselor, physical therapist, or some other staff member) about. He can help you better than I can. Would you like me to tell him about it, and ask him to stop by and see you?" Often the aphasic patient is unable to take the responsibility of making the appointment, or communicating his concern to someone he does not know well. With only minimal liaison, however, successful communication often results. The patient receives competent help, and he makes another friend.

One aphasic patient had been a league bowler. There was some weakness in his right arm, although it was stronger than the left. One of the recreational therapists persuaded him to try bowling to strengthen his right arm and improve his coordination. This was threatening to the patient, and it required a great deal of initial encouragement to keep him from giving up. However, the patient liked the instructor, and was soon acting as his general assistant. He improved enough to help other patients, and to go bowling with his family when he went home. He also made friends in the hospital. As a result he became less and less dependent upon the clinician, and increasingly willing to venture forth on his own.

It is the responsibility of the clinician to give the aphasic patient strong enough support to provide initial security, and then to implement the basis of this security in such a manner that the patient becomes increasingly independent. Facilitating successful interactions with other people is the most effective way to accomplish this. It is not enough, however, simply to transfer the dependency to another person. The point is rather to extend communication, and give the patient as many successful experiences as possible to increase his confidence in his own adequacy.

PROTECTIVE MECHANISMS

Ciardi (1963) observed that people have certain assumptions upon which they act in what seems to them to be "the natural way." These assumptions and expectations seem natural to us because of a long process of conditioning. We feel threatened if they fail us, and react defensively. The nervous system has extremely complicated protective mechanisms.

The aphasic patient needs strong defenses. Like anyone who suddenly in the midst of the journey of his life has found himself alone in a dark wood where the straight way is lost, the aphasic patient knows despair. Surely anyone partially paralyzed and unable to communicate must feel himself in a dark wood, indeed, and surely the straight road he took for the natural way must seem lost to him in his helplessness. Survival depends on his ability to organize his defenses.

Goldstein stated clearly that the value of defense mechanisms is survival, and that interference can only produce disaster. It is important that every clinician know this truth. He should realize that the patient with frequent catastrophic reactions does not have adequate defenses, and try to structure his regime to afford greater protection. Milisen (1963) has frequently stressed this need. He has suggested more extensive use of sedation to protect the patient from trauma in the early stages of recovery, as one advantageous measure. The idea has merit, although it must be considered in relation to overall medication, and sometimes in relation to the patient's need for environmental stimulation.

Most aphasic patients need a place of retreat from the constant demands of a social environment. We have referred to the patients' library at the Minneapolis VA Hospital. These inviting rooms have been a refuge to many aphasic patients, who have found them a congenial atmosphere and a quiet place in which their minds could function.

Some attention should be given to the patient's tolerance level when he goes home on pass or is discharged. Too much activity going on about him or the presence of too many people may cause him acute distress and impede recovery. Often all that is necessary is an understanding that he should excuse himself and retire for a while, when he feels himself becoming tense. All he usually needs is to be alone for a little while. One patient used to take his little girl and go for a walk. Her prattle made no demands upon him, and he found her presence relaxing. Another, who lived in the country, tramped with his dog. A third retired to his room and played a game of solitaire.

These independent activities have another value. They tend to lessen the fear of being alone that many stroke patients have. This fear can make a patient dependent and demanding, sometimes to the extent that his wife's health cannot stand the strain. If there is any reason the patient should not be alone, the doctor will make this clear. Then arrangements should be made to divide the responsibility of attendance.

Aphasic patients frequently discover defensive activities for themselves. One patient sat for hours with an open book in front of him, which he could not read. Another copied pages of meaningless material out of any book he found at hand. In these cases it was easy enough to substitute more meaningful activity by giving the patients materials they could work with productively. Another aphasic patient wove rugs endlessly throughout his long hospitalization, and bought a loom to take home with him when he left. On a later admission, however, for a different medical problem, he spent most of his time playing cards, and stopped everyone who came by to talk to him. Usually when the need for defensive activity no longer exists, it will be discontinued. When there is something more rewarding to do, it will be preferred.

Sometimes an aphasic patient develops a defensive mannerism as a cloak for embarrassment. This may be a silly laugh, or excessive use of a stereotyped expression, such as, "Like the man said," or, "Sure, sure." These reactions not only are inappropriate in many situations, but may be interpreted as regressive behavior. If they are defensive mannerisms, they drop out as the patient develops confidence and a more adequate repertory of responses is available. In short, they disappear when they are no longer necessary.

Persisting euphoria is more serious since it may indicate regression or depression. The patient denies his problems because he is not intact enough to appreciate them, or because they are so threatening he dares not admit them. When mental deterioration is present, little change can be expected. Sometimes euphoria is a mask for deep depression and suicidal impulses. This is a case for a psychiatrist, although the speech pathologist may continue to work with the patient under his direction.

PSYCHOTIC CONDITIONS

Aphasic patients sometimes present or develop psychotic conditions. It is important that these be differentiated from aphasia. Aphasic impairment is confined to language processes, and is systematic and orderly. There is a consistent reduction of vocabulary and of verbal retention span. Errors tend to increase as words decrease in frequency of general usage in the language, and as stimuli or required responses increase in length. Confusions may appear between words that sound alike, look alike, or are linked by strong semantic associations. Aphasic patients respond appropriately to situations and to people, even when comprehension of language is impaired. Their behavior is reasonable, and their responses are predictable within the framework of what is known about the organization of language. They do not present bizarre responses or behavior.

On the Weigl–Goldstein–Scheerer *Color–Form Test* (Goldstein and Scheerer, 1941), for example, where subjects are required to sort blocks for color and for form, severe aphasics who do not grasp the instructions completely usually arrange all the pieces carefully with colors matched in rows and forms in columns, or vice versa. Aphasics with more language perform as normals do, proceeding casually from form to color, or from color to form. One schizoid patient, on the other hand, arranged the pieces in a circle, placed one in the center, and remarked with a gleam in his eye, "That's the king!"

A young aphasic patient made good recovery from aphasia resulting from a self-inflicted gunshot wound. He has had intermittent schizoid episodes over a period of years, when he suffers strange fears and delusions, loses contact with reality, and requires hospital care. During one episode he believed that the EEG was a brainwashing machine and that the hospital had been taken over by Communists. Between episodes, however, he has gone to school, and been reasonably happy and productive.

Another patient was also making a good recovery from aphasia when he incurred an involutional depression. During this period he was inaccessible to treatment for aphasia. He sat endlessly reiterating, "Dark, dark, dark, it's all dark, dark, dark; black, black, black, everything is black, black, black." He made no response to the clinician, who visited him daily. He ignored the beautifully illustrated books in his field that she brought to the psychiatric ward, and over which he spent many hours when he was better. He responded to shock therapy and eventually returned to the Aphasic Clinic. He performed better than on initial testing, but a little below the level he had achieved before the onset of depression. He soon regained the lost ground, however, continued to improve, and returned to his former profession.

Sometimes an aphasic patient is a person whose general adjustment was precarious before he became aphasic. In our experience, aphasia does not alter basic behavior patterns. Some patients with marked pathological traits respond well to treatment for aphasia, and make the same kind of borderline adjustments when they leave the hospital as they have made before. One such patient was a severe aphasic. He had worked hard all his life, and he worked hard to recover from aphasia. He had paranoid tendencies, and a fanatic attachment to a dependent relative, about whose welfare he periodically became violently agitated. A psychiatric consultant advised the clinician that paranoid patients need the security of authoritarian attitudes and well-structured situations. One day during a long outburst of unusual violence, the clinician said firmly, "Mr. Haldon, I cannot work with you when you are so upset. Go back to your ward." He subsided immediately, but the clinician said only, "You may come back tomorrow, if you feel like working." Although he occasionally came in disturbed after this, it was never necessary to say more than, "Mr. Haldon, do you feel like working today?" to quiet him. When he left the hospital he continued to live by himself, as he had done before admission. The social worker had planned very carefully with him, however, to insure that his environment was supportive. She persuaded him to take an apartment near friends, to have his dinner in a convenient boarding house, and to let his bank administer his financial affairs. She arranged transportation to a community rehabilitation center for outpatient treatment two or three times a week. Problems occasionally arose, which she was called upon to mediate over a period of several years. This was to be expected, since he had always had difficulty relating to people. It was nevertheless encouraging that a patient with his psychological history should be able to get along outside an institution after the additional trauma of severe aphasia and hemiplegia.

Some patients have developed unremitting organic psychoses, not amenable to treatment, that tend to become more severe as a result of progressive and irreversible changes in the brain. These patients were often delusional and sometimes subject to outbursts of violence. They usually could not be cared for except in a mental hospital.

MEMORY LOSS

It is sometimes necessary to differentiate aphasia from general loss of memory. Aphasic patients sometimes report memory failure when they mean inability to evoke words. One patient who reported loss of memory was asked to give an example. He said, "I couldn't remember the men I work with. I had to describe each one, and ask my brother to tell me his name."

Another said, "I couldn't even remember my wife. Well, I knew who she was, of course. I knew she was my wife, but I couldn't remember her name."

Another reported that he tried to remember his office and the details of his work. He said he could see the office, and the orders that he handled, but he could not remember the names of the cities to which they had to be routed.

Aphasic patients keep appointments and appear on time, even when the regular hour is changed, if they understand the instructions in the first place. They remember assignments, and bring the correct materials with them. They return library books when they are due. If they have to go to the dentist when they are scheduled for the clinic, they stop by and report the change of program.

This is quite different from the behavior of a patient with generalized loss of memory. In this condition, the patient who has just received medication forgets he has had it, and asks for it over and over. He forgets that his wife has just left the hospital, and asks again and again if she is coming to see him. This behavior goes on repetitiously all day long, day after day. When the condition is severe, the patient may not remember he has met the clinician before, although he has spent several hours in his office.

It is apparent that such cases represent very different instances with reference to our schema of the communication functions. The aphasic is troubled by his inability to retrieve the symbolic material. He remembers the people and events in his life but has difficulty with their names and difficulty talking about them. In addition, he may have difficulty staying "on the track" because he lacks the organizing support of language. The patient with memory loss, on the other hand, is suffering from a figural rather than a symbolic deficit. In the most common case, it is as if the patient is no longer "laying down traces" in the figural system or has difficulty accessing and integrating information of a figural sort. Even this is not complete loss of memory, for the patient may talk interestingly and well about experience or knowledge drawn from the past. It is rather as though no new experiences were being registered in the brain. This again is not aphasia, but is a condition indicative of severe generalized brain damage. It is usually irreversible.

EMOTIONAL REACTIONS

Aphasic patients have feelings like everyone else, which is their human right. They have problems other than aphasia, and problems aphasia brings in its train. Sometimes they suffer from depression and anxiety, which is usually realistic and which may be acute. Most psychiatrists consider reasonably that treating aphasia is the most effective way to deal with the patient's anxieties, rebuild his confidence, and help him to achieve whatever readjustments are necessary. Psychiatrists usually advise clinicians to encourage patients to express their feelings when occasions arise.

Often the aphasic patient has repressed his feelings about his condition for a long time because he could not communicate them, or perhaps because the people close to him could not tolerate them or believed they should try to keep him in a cheerful frame of mind. Perhaps the patient himself believes he should not inflict his troubles upon others. Awareness and permissiveness on the part of the clinician may enable the patient to give expression to deep feelings and experience relief from tension and from isolation.

It is necessary first to reach the patient, to somehow get where he is and deal with him with respect and integrity. The clinician needs to be a perceptive listener and observer, with awareness of patient's situation. Pity is a morass, but recognition of the patient's reactions to his altered circumstances is solid ground beneath his feet. Superficial optimism is often difficult for a patient to endure, but quiet understanding and acceptance restores his shaken confidence. Nothing is so bad if he can talk about it without evasion. Panic comes when the patient feels that no one will tell him the truth.

One aphasic patient suffered occasional mild seizures. They were accompanied by such great fear that he usually collapsed afterwards and spent the rest of the day in bed. A neurologist had discussed seizures with him. The patient understood what was happening and knew the episodes were not dangerous or harmful, but panic persisted.

One day, in the clinic, he stopped in the middle of a sentence and said, "I can't go on. I think I'm going to have a seizure." The clinician said quietly, "It is all right. It will be over in a minute or two. Try to tell me exactly what is happening. What do you feel, now?"

He said he felt as though something were fluttering in his head, and then as though everything were slipping away. The clinician stood behind his chair with hands on his shoulders for support, but continued to ask questions and he continued to answer steadily. The storm gradually subsided, and in a few minutes the interrupted activity was resumed. Years later the patient wrote that he had never had any fear of seizures since that day in the clinic. Probably putting the experience into words dispelled some of the formless terror, while the matter-of-fact acceptance by the clinician reduced the humiliation the patient had suffered over the episodes.

Sometimes an aphasic patient is unable to talk outside the clinic, because he is afraid someone will think he is mentally defective, laugh at him, or feel sorry for him. Sometimes, in such cases, the clinician can manipulate the situation to produce a desirable result. One patient, who was an intelligent man with extremely adequate speech, was told that his assignment was to initiate a conversation with five patients on his ward. He was told it would be all right if he said nothing more than, "How are you, today?" The only requirement was that he should say it first, and wait for a reply. The following day he came back and said enthusiastically, "I have met some of the most interesting people. There is a man, here, who comes from Hibbing. You know I lived up there for a while. This fellow knows everyone on the Range. He knows a lot of my friends up there, and we talked all evening."

Another patient, a lawyer, had a similar experience. He met a fellow who told him all about coon hunting. They became friends and planned to get together when they left the hospital. The patient said, "I want to get him up in my country to go hunting."

The assignment was trivial enough, but it was another example of a pebble cast into a pool. Both aphasic patients were men who had always taken pride in doing things extremely well. Moreover, they had both assumed that when you had a stroke, you were finished. They had been gradually learning that this was not true, but had not accepted the new concept entirely. The assignment was double-barreled. It forced them to observe that people who had had strokes were often interesting and intelligent men, with whom they could find common interests. In addition, they learned that they could communicate with people and enjoy it.

Proving these things for one's self is part of the process of recovery from aphasia. However, one should not generalize too much about it, for the experience of aphasia cannot be the same for any two people, nor for one person, perhaps, from one time to another.

In general, aphasic patients are adjusting. They assimilate their losses, somehow, and go on. They experience grief and despair and anxiety for the future. They also experience love and friendship and hours of pleasure and contentment. In short, they are very human.

Time brings changes to them as to other people. A friend and colleague of one of the authors for many years, who was aphasic as a result of penetration of exploding missile fragments into the brain during World War II, recently wrote:

I've been experiencing something to which I think you have often alluded in your letters. . . . I believe you were trying to help me place recovery and rehabilitation into a broader perspective, and thus make it a more comfortable experience . . . you wrote, 'You know there is such a thing as being comfortable with yourself.' . . . I had not the slightest notion of what you were really trying to tell me. Throughout the whole effort, I had but one philosophy, if you can give it such a dignified name. . . . The only method of dealing with the effects of brain injury was to fight and fight hard. . . . It seems to me, as I search back that I withheld feelings. . . . I could afford to have only those feelings which would keep me fighting. . . . I had to keep genuine feelings under wraps . . . but the wraps are beginning to come off . . .

This is the voice of experience speaking, but like the searching student he is, the writer leaves us with questions, not answers. He asked himself if the insights he continued to gain were perhaps a result of his own increasing maturity, and had nothing to do with aphasia. He left other questions unanswered. Could he have achieved so significantly had his drive toward recovery been less? Had he been able to accept himself, when he returned from the war as a young hemiplegic and aphasic who had sacrificed so much that nothing more would be required of him? Finally, was any compromise possible? Could the wraps have come off sooner, or did he have to wait until the need was reduced through his own experiences, his own searching, and the slow accrual of insights and increasing maturity? We are inclined to think the latter is the process of becoming.

FAMILY COUNSELING

We know that good clinical results can be reinforced or negated by the behavior of the important people in the patient's environment. Ordinarily these are the members of the immediate family. The usual procedure is to arrange a series of interviews to interpret the patient's language disabilities to a responsible member of the family and to prepare the family to assist, not impede, the patient's recovery. This, however, is not how one begins in most cases.

Relatives of patients sometimes endure a good deal in hospitals and clinics. Even clinicians who are sensitive to patient needs may regard a relative as an instrument for achieving their ends. The clinician may appear impatient with the layman's lack of specialized knowledge and skills. He may give so many instructions and precautions that the relative is confused or goes away with the feeling that whatever he does will be wrong.

In a VA Hospital, the responsible relative is usually the patient's wife. She has been shocked and frightened by her husband's illness and has spent long anxious hours at the hospital. At first, she was afraid he was going to die. Perhaps he still seems so helpless and altered that she cannot help thinking that death would be easier, even though the thought distresses her.

She has had to keep things going at home, somehow, and perhaps to deal with upset children. She has had to make arrangements and decisions when she did not know what to do. She was accustomed to depend on her husband, not only in emergencies, but in many little ways she took for granted and misses every day.

She probably has not been able to eat or sleep very well. She doesn't know what is going to happen or how they are going to manage, and she is often bone weary. She sometimes feels that she cannot carry on much longer, but she is ashamed of this for she feels she should not be thinking about herself. The hospital is frightening to her. She is anxious about this interview and afraid to hear what she thinks she may be told.

It makes no sense at all to talk to this woman in technical language. It makes even less to demand that she do more than she is doing. What can a clinician say that will help her? The answer is nothing. It is not the clinician who needs to talk. It is necessary to listen first, to find out what the situation is, and what the immediate needs are. Surely the focus of the first interview should be the person who has carried so much of the burden, the person who will continue to live with it, and upon whom success or failure will ultimately depend.

One young wife said gratefully at the end of the hour, with tears still in her eyes, "I cannot tell you how much you have helped me." The clinician had seen the signs of stress that were all too obvious, and said, "This has been hard on you." Except for an occasional murmur, she had said nothing else during the interview.

Although the social worker is the person trained to deal with family problems and give skilled professional direction and assistance, the clinician can reinforce the support the social worker has given. This is a necessary preparation for what the clinician must demand of the wife later, when she is ready to play her role in the rehabilitation process. The clinician can support the wife by telling her it is not only natural for her to think about herself, but necessary, because so much will depend on her. Some way can usually be found for an exhausted person to get sleep. There is usually some competent person in the family or community who can advise her about decisions that worry her. When she is rested and less desperate, she will probably come back and say, "Now tell me what I can do to help my husband."

Next, she needs information about what has happened. This information should both describe and delimit the practical problems. She needs to know that her husband will not always understand what people say, for example, although he will understand well enough if they use short sentences, do not say too much at a time, and give him time to grasp one idea before they go on to another. She needs to know that aphasia affects reading and writing and the use of numbers as well as speech. She needs to know what will change and what will not. Above all, she needs to know that her husband is responsible and dependable, and that he has not lost his mind although he cannot talk or his speech sometimes sounds confused.

It is important to take a good deal of time about this, and to be sure that the client understands what she has been told, knows what to expect, and what to do. Once a clinician explained to an elderly woman that her husband would have trouble finding his way about. She looked at him and said comfortingly, "It will be all right, John, when you get home. I can find my way around the whole house in the dark, and you will be able to, too." The clinician explained gently that it was just this sense that her husband did not have. She looked at him for confirmation, and he nodded slowly. Nothing, however, daunted her long. She drew herself up and said, "Well, John, I've depended on you for 48 years, and I guess it's your turn now. You'll just have to depend on me, for a change." John held out his hands to her, and it was obvious that they would make whatever adjustments had to be made.

If emotional lability is present, the wife needs to learn how to deal with it. It will be disturbing to her to see her husband cry, but if she knows this is part of the illness and that it embarrasses him, she will be less vulnerable and less prone to respond emotionally when his control breaks down.

The family as well as the patient need to understand that the patient may have limited tolerance for noise and confusion and prolonged social demands upon him. The chances are better that this tolerance will increase if there is a generally understood arrangement that the patient should be encouraged to excuse himself when he wishes. This procedure prevents outbursts of irritability that are difficult for everyone, especially the patient who often feels bitterly ashamed later.

In giving information to the family, it is essential that the speech pathologist be honest about limitations. A young clinician once told the wife of a severely impaired patient that no further significant changes in her husband's condition could be expected. The wife met the clinic director as she left the office, and stopped to say, "I want to tell you that no one has ever helped me as much as Miss S. I understand the tragedy as I never have before, but I can go on, now. I know what I have to do."

Acceptance is not always as immediate as this, nor should one expect it to be. In this case, the patient had been treated in one institution after another, over a period of years. The wife's own observations had prepared her, although not consciously, for what she had to be told. Relief followed, because she no longer had to try to accomplish the impossible. Her husband wanted to go home, and she wanted him there. She could use her energies and her considerable strength and resources for rebuilding a family life for them and for their children.

In many cases, we train the wife to work with the patient when he goes home. We ask her to write at regular intervals and report problems and progress. Before setting up such a plan, it is necessary to ascertain if the wife can function in the role of clinician, and if the patient can accept her in this role. People are not always able to assume this relationship to each other, even when mutual devotion is present. On the other hand, it often works very well and has strong positive values. It usually works out in practice that the activities the patient and his clinician like and enjoy are continued, sometimes for years, and others are dropped. This is not only acceptable but should be encouraged.

The most understanding counseling sometimes fails, however. The clinician should remember that when the family rejects the patient, there is usually some deep underlying reason. Sometimes it lies in past relationships and is imbedded in betrayals and hostilities that have grown up over many years. Sometimes the rejection can be traced to the immaturity of the marriage partner, who may never have been able to accept responsibility. Some patients show personality changes that are disruptive to family life, and make care of the patient in the home untenable. None of these situations are occasions for judgment, but the clinician must take them into account in assessing the part the family can take in rehabilitation, and what can realistically be asked of them.

chapter 18

SOME UNDERLYING PRINCIPLES OF TREATMENT OF APHASIA

First, we want to make it clear that what we are going to say about treatment of aphasia refers only to adults. Some of the same principles may be valid for children, to an unknown degree, but there are tremendous differences to be taken into account. The most obvious difference is that language patterns were organized in the adult brains before the onset of aphasia. We must assume that a brain so structured is different from a brain in which language events have not occurred. This fact alone would make a considerable difference in treatment, but we shall not elaborate the point further.*

A PHILOSOPHY OF TREATMENT

Methods of treatment are usually determined by ideas about the nature of the disability being treated, and consequently are subject to prejudices of one kind or another. We shall try to state our prejudices clearly.

First, we believe in a general philosophy of treatment, but not in an arbitrary method. There is no room for rigidity in clinical practice. Both patient and clinician are a part of the therapeutic process, and interact in a complex manner. If the method leaves the patient behind, or if a patient outstrips the method, the method must be altered. When

*Readers interested in the relation between childhood and adult aphasia should see Schuell (1966).

an urgent problem arises, the method must be put aside. The clinician must have room to explore, to adapt, to adjust, to search, to feel out a need, and to use a moment.

A supervisor in a university clinic once told a story about two clinicians she observed working with one small boy. The first clinician spent an hour trying to make him keep his hands out of his pockets, sit still, and pay attention, while she conscientiously went through all the steps of a detailed lesson plan. The second one said, "What have you got in your pockets today?" and made an articulation lesson out of the collection of spark plug, rusty nail, caterpillar, gum wrapper, and licorice stick that emerged. After the pockets were empty, their treasures exhausted, and the clinician had gravely accepted the gift of a moribund caterpillar, she brought out her materials. The moral is that there are ten thousand roads that lead to paradise, and some roads that lead nowhere at all. It takes flexibility to avoid cul-de-sacs, as anyone who has watched rats in mazes knows.

A clinical technique is only a device for accomplishing an end. A good clinician needs a repertory of techniques, but should never be caught unaware by the question, "Why do you do this?" It is the why that matters, and the why should not be a secret. The patient should understand the purpose of what he is asked to do. In other words, patient and the clinician work together for one purpose, and techniques are secondary.

Undoubtedly some techniques are more effective than others. Some techniques work well for one patient, but not for another. Some work well at one time in the recovery process, but not at another time. It is part of the clinician's job to evaluate the techniques he uses, to try to improve them, and to develop new ones to accomplish his ends. There is no technique that cannot be improved by a continuous process of evaluation and revision. Probably the most important thing to be said about a technique is that one should always be ready to discard it when it doesn't work. These, incidentally, are some of the reasons that a clinician needs to be more than a technician.

We believe that the primary objective in treatment of aphasia is to increase communication. What the aphasic patient wants is to recover enough language to get on with his life. One man is content to be able to ask for what he wants, and is ready to go home when he has achieved a basic vocabulary. He will tell you he was never much of a reader or a talker, and that writing is his wife's department. He wants to go home and get the crops in, or get on with some jobs he has lined up. Another man has speech that sounds normal, but he is afraid he will make a mistake talking to a client or a customer, and that someone will conclude he is not equal to his job. A third is a scholar who expects to continue to lecture and to publish in his field. This has been achieved, but probably not often.

We believe that the clinician should accept the patient's goals when they are realistic. It is a fine when a patient does not feel handicapped by a residual disability. Some people enjoy being dub golfers, and some like to sing off-key. Perfectionism is not a requisite for happiness or usefulness.

Usually when a patient is accepted for treatment, he should be told that it is going to take a long time, and that he is going to have to plan one step at a time. He should be told that recovery will be hard and slow, and that he will have to be patient with it, and give it time. This is about all that should be said at the beginning in most cases. It is enough to give the patient something to hang on to, and to be supportive while he is making initial adjustments. It gives him time to come to terms with his situation. He soon observes that he is making progress, and this is encouraging.

Several important things happen during the initial adjustment period. The patient sees other aphasic patients, and gets to know them and to know about them. He makes comparisons. He lives with his limitations, finds that he gets along fairly well in spite of them, and gradually they become less threatening. Acceptance comes, and he begins to make his own plans.

The time comes when he thinks he could go home and his wife could help him with his speech, or he decides he knows what to do and could work just as well at home if we gave him some materials. Sometimes he has ideas about kinds of work he could do, and we refer him to the vocational psychologist. The psychologist begins to explore possibilities with him, and perhaps tries him out on various jobs around the hospital.

Sometimes the patient thinks he is ready to go back to his own job, at least on a part-time basis. Usually the clinician reviews the requirements with him, and asks what he thinks he could do now, what he could not do, and what he would expect to have trouble with. This patient, also, will be referred for vocational counseling. For the most part, aphasic patients have been honest and realistic. A man with a small business of his own has been thinking about getting someone to handle the books. A salesman has decided to serve an established clientele, but not to take on new territory or new products. A foreman in the factory may reach the conclusion that it would be better for him to go back to a bench job.

In most cases, and with certain safeguards, we are more inclined to accept the patient's judgment than the results of standardized tests. There is no intelligence or performance test that does not reflect aphasia. Tests tend not to reveal the patient's competence, judgment, and ability to function in a familiar situation, and in an area in which he has the authority of long experience.

Sometimes it is not medically desirable for a patient to return to a former position because of the stress involved. Sometimes it is not physically possible for a patient to go back to his previous work. In these cases most of the counseling is done by the physician or the vocational counselor. It is when the question revolves around aphasic impairment that the speech pathologist cannot evade responsibility.

Sometimes the decision is clear, but there are times when some measure of calculated risk is involved. Possible failure must be considered, and weighed against the effects on a man of loss of confidence and incentive. The positive value of stimulation from the work itself cannot be overlooked. We have frequently counseled patients against trying to return too soon, in order to give themselves as much time for recovery as possible. Patients who are extremely determined rarely take this advice, and as far as we can judge, the results have usually been good. Some patients have to be held back a little and others encouraged to attempt tasks within their capabilities, but, in spite of this, we have learned to respect the convictions aphasic patients have about what they are ready to attempt. Probably what this means is that there are competencies tests do not measure, particularly when residuals of a language disability are present. The aphasic patient can often do more than he can explain, and he often knows more than he can tell you. This is particularly true in the areas of his strongest interests. It is important that the clinician should tap these in therapy. In order to do this, he must select materials and structure a program individually for each patient.

This brings us to the last point. It is unthinkable to work with an aphasic patient without knowing the level at which he is able to perform in each language modality, and why performance breaks down when it does. Nothing fails so surely as missing the patient with the program. This is like a film strip we once saw made by a novice with a new camera. The photographer went around the track at the Olympic races just ahead of the horses that never got into the show. Similarly, a clinician sometimes misses a patient and concludes he is uncooperative or not motivated.

What this means is that the first principle is to work on what needs working on, and at the level where performance breaks down. A good rule is find the level at which the patient has some success, but has to work a little for it, and then keep moving with the patient.

A THEORETICAL BACKGROUND OF TREATMENT

It is our basic premise that an aphasic patient is aphasic because there is a lesion in his brain that interferes with processing symbolic messages. Our evidence indicates that the nature and severity of aphasia, and prognosis for recovery as well, depend on the locus and extent of the lesion and the physiological condition of the rest of the brain. In other words, we do not attribute persisting aphasia to psychological trauma or to personality structure. Please note that we have not said that aphasic patients do not incur psychological trauma or that they do not show a wide range of behavior. We have not said one should ignore these events or these differences. We believe, however, that it is unrealistic to minimize organic trauma.

We regard aphasia primarily as an interference with language processes resulting from brain injury. We have defined aphasia symptomatically as a reduction of available language affecting all language modalities, and pointed out that it may or may not be accompanied by other specific perceptual or sensorimotor deficits compatible with brain damage.

We believe that the interference that produces aphasia disrupts both analysis and integration of symbolic communiques. Analysis and integration of language require continuous and dynamic discriminatory and feedback activity. If we accept the idea that feedback plays an essential role in communication, we cannot talk about aphasia primarily in terms of destruction of images or word memories. Gooddy (1956) has pointed out in another context that we miss the point of modern neurophysiology if we merely substitute one term for another without revising our thinking about the nature of the process in question.

The clinical evidence in aphasia indicates that the language storage system is at least relatively intact. Irreversible patients repeat, count, name the days of the week, finish a nursery rhyme, or say the Lord's Prayer, if someone starts them. They supply popular associations to common words, and occasionally respond to strong nonverbal stimuli with appropriate language. They can usually point to some pictures and objects named by the examiner, and match some printed words to pictures. It is almost always possible to demonstrate some residual language in an aphasic patient. This can be attributed to the redundancy of verbal encoding, and to the fact that extensive cerebral areas undoubtedly participate in storage.

The point is that the integrity of previously stored patterns is not a sufficient condition for complex discriminatory and selective behavior. Most of us, for example, could produce a fairly accurate map of a route we drive regularly, and indicate landmarks, turns, stop signs, and traffic lights from memory. Nevertheless, none of us would attempt to drive the route blindfolded. We need a continuous stream of incoming information from receptors in the retina, the cochlea, the joints, the tendons, the fascia, and the skin to guide our movements from moment to moment, and carry out our plans.

Admittedly, neither neurophysiology nor cybernetics can yet give us a neural model for recovery from aphasia. They can point directions at best. Converging evidence from many lines of research indicates, however, that repeated sensory stimulation is essential for organization, storage, and retrieval of patterns in the brain, and it would be strange if language patterns operated according to some other principle. We would argue that it is more reasonable to formulate principles of treatment for aphasia that are compatible with what is known about language and what is known about cerebral function, and to try to implement these principles with clinical techniques, than to continue to use techniques based on vaguely defined principles and no tenable neurophysiological theory.

Any principles we can formulate must undoubtedly undergo successive revision as more information becomes available, but that is no reason against setting up experimental procedures now and subjecting them to clinical test.

SOME PRINCIPLES OF TREATMENT

Before discussing principles of treatment, it is necessary to define the essential task. In our opinion, the clinician's role is not that of a teacher. He has nothing to do with teaching the adult aphasic to talk or to read or to write. He does not teach the patient sounds or words or rules for combining words. Rather he tries to communicate with the patient and to stimulate disrupted processes to function maximally.

It would seem that sensory stimulation is the only method we have for making complex events happen in the brain. All the evidence suggests that auditory stimulation is crucial in control of language processes. However, since feedback from more than one sensory modality may contribute to behavior, there is no reason for using this mode exclusively. This suggests that the first principle of treatment for aphasia should be the use of intensive auditory stimulation, although not necessarily stimulation through auditory channels alone. We have mentioned before that patients who could neither repeat nor read a word responded correctly when they could look at the word while it was spoken by the examiner. Subsequently, either stimulus could evoke the correct response. From a series of studies using simultaneous stimulation, Bender (1952) concluded that the influence of one stimulus upon the percept evoked by another seems to be a fundamental principle in all perception, and reported that extinction did not occur in combined visual and auditory tests. Harris (1953) considered intersensory facilitation related to summation. In aphasia, combined auditory and visual stimulation is effective in eliciting language on progressive levels of complexity. It should be continued until the patient can respond to each modality alone on any given level. Skills become functional if this procedure is followed.

This brings us to the second principle, which is that of the adequate stimulus. In other words, we must insure that the stimuli we use get into the brain. Auditory processes are always impaired in aphasia. As a result, the aphasic patient receives reduced verbal stimulation from his environment, and it is probable that signals that get in are often distorted.

People talk too fast and say too much at a time for the aphasic patient to follow. Patients sometimes tell us that people do not seem to be talking right. To some patients it often seems they are not even talking a language he knows. Therefore, the clinician must manipulate the stimulus so that the patient can perceive it. Using combined auditory and visual stimulation is one way to do this. As soon as the patient can respond without such assistance, either stimulus mode can be used alone. The objective is always to enable the patient to communicate as normally as possible.

There are other ways to increase the probability that the aphasic patient can respond to auditory stimuli. First, there is considerable evidence that meaningful patterns of stimuli are recognized more readily than nonmeaningful ones, so the clinician will get the best response if he uses meaningful units of language. We know, also, from studies of perception that recognition occurs more readily with high-frequency than with low-frequency words. Language is highly organized in the brain, and words have strong associational linkages with other words, so that one word elicits other words in the same semantic category. It seems reasonable to assume that more associational linkages exist with words like *car*, *dog*, and *house* than with words like *shallop*, *leveret*, and *kiva*. Both from a linguistic and a neurophysiological standpoint, we should expect that more would happen in the brain in response to the frequently used words in the first series than in response to the rarely used words in the second. Although there is more interference from competing responses when words with high associational probabilities are used, the evidence indicates that both short-term and long-term retention are better.

This does not mean that a clinician must limit himself to the thousand most commonly used words in the language in dealing with aphasic patients, but he should be aware that he can make a task easier or harder for the patient by controling this dimension. One should begin with material the patient can respond to, but gradually progress from one level of difficulty to another.

We know that auditory retention span is always reduced in aphasia. This means that length of stimulus should be controlled. The clinician may begin with short words and phrases, and over a period of time progress to words and sentences of gradually increasing length. The patient will hear words like *house, car,* and *dog* before his auditory analyzer can deal with sound sequences such as *Methodist Episcopal,* a phrase still loved by medical examiners, if not by Methodists.

Sometimes it is effective to increase the loudness of an auditory signal until an optimal level is found. In our experience this level varies from patient to patient. Most aphasic patients prefer speech at ordinary conversational level, adjusted to the size of the room and extraneous noise. They do not want people to shout at them. They usually prefer direct reception to listening through earphones, probably because they rely on more than auditory cues. It may also be that the earphones produce additional distortions to which they are sensitive. Patients with clear-cut perceptual problems, however, sometimes appear less perplexed and seem to respond more readily when the clinician raises his voice moderately, although not enough to produce reverberatory effects.

We need more systematic investigation in this area. We reproduced the Birch and Lee (1955) study with masking tones in Minneapolis but did not get the same results. Our patients showed a small increment on naming tasks on the first trial, which disappeared on successive trials. There was no carry over on immediate repetition of the task, or on repetition after 24 hours. Using materials equated for difficulty, we found it possible to get equal increments by varying presentation in other ways. On one set of trials naming pictures of common objects, the patient turned over the card and named each picture as he exposed it. On the test presentation the examiner presented each card, saying abruptly, "What is this?" There was no carry over of the obtained increment on this task. We concluded that both techniques merely served as distracting devices. Some patients reacted catastrophically to masking tones, and no patient was comfortable with them.

It is also possible to manipulate the duration of an auditory stimulus. We have found that patients with perceptual problems are often able to respond more adequately when a word or phrase is spoken a little more slowly than in ordinary conversational speech. However, inflection should be natural, and the slowing should not fragment or distort the language unit. Like increasing loudness, slowing down rate seems to help severely impaired patients initially, then to make no difference. It should be discontinued when no longer necessary, since the objective is to enable patients to respond to natural conversational usage as soon as possible.

The third important principle involves the use of repetitive sensory stimulation. Over and over, aphasic patients who looked perplexed and bewildered when a word, for example, was spoken once, showed instantaneous recognition when they heard it the fourth or fifth time. This seemed to be an all-or-none reaction. Moreover, the patient whose attempted repetition was jargon on the first try, gave closer and closer approximations as he continued to listen, until reproduction was normal. Finally, the patient who could name five or six out of 20 pictures after 24 hours when he had received 10 successive auditory stimulations for each word, was able to recall from 15 to 20 words the next day, when he received 20 successive stimulations on each word. Someone who has not seen this process in operation may well believe 20 successive repetitions of a single word to involve unbearable monotony, but this is not true. Certainly it is not true for the patient who wants to acquire a functional vocabulary. We shall describe this technique in more detail in the next chapter.

The fourth principle for intensive controlled auditory stimulation is that each stimulus presented should elicit a response. There are two reasons for this. In the first place the response permits the clinician to determine when the stimulus was adequate. But equally important for recovery is the feedback activity that results from the response itself. When a patient listens and makes an appropriate response, a whole cycle of activity is set in motion. This cycle involves discrimination, selection, integration, and facilitation of ensuing responses. A very relevant observation is the one we have made before, that when aphasic patients first begin to produce associations to given words or sounds they respond with a single word. *Building,* for example, may produce *barn.* With continued stimulation the response to the same word may be *house, church, school, bank, barn.* There is obviously an increase in the number of responses available as recovery occurs.

The fifth principle that we insist upon is that the clinician should elicit, not force, responses. If stimulation is adequate, responses follow. If a response is not available, more stimulation is needed. It is as simple as this. Obviously, the kinds of responses that can be elicited vary with severity of aphasia. The first response that can usually be secured is pointing to a picture or a word when it is spoken by the examiner. This is better than no response. Discrimination and selection are taking place. Usually, some time during the process, the patient begins to repeat stimulus words effortlessly and almost unconsciously, as he makes his selection. Pointing, as a response, can then be discontinued.

When repetition becomes easy, the clinician can usually elicit the response by supplying a frame for it. For example, she may elicit house by saying, "You live in a_____." Next perhaps, she can elicit the same response by a question, such as, "What do you live in?" Finally, the patient is able to name the picture or read the word without any auditory cues. The important factor is that the clinician has enabled the patient to respond successfully at each level of recovery. The patient has moved from easy to successively more difficult tasks. He has had a far different experience of language from that of a patient required to spend the clinical hour watching the shape of his mouth in a mirror while he imitated phonemes, or trying to name four or five pictures of objects that begin with *b,* and repeatedly failing.

The sixth principle follows the fifth one rather closely. It is that the clinician should in general stimulate rather than correct. The idea which we have repeatedly proven clinically is that defective responses drop out as language functions increase. Errors decrease as available language increases. Clinical time should be spent in stimulation and in eliciting language, not in forcing patients to struggle for responses or in correcting erroneous ones. The objective is to get language processes working, not to teach the patient that whatever he says is wrong. This does not happen when adequate stimulation is given.

It is sound procedure to use one language modality to facilitate another throughout the course of treatment. Spelling words aloud helps the patient to write them, hear them, and recall them. Writing sentences to dictation helps him to hear and retain longer language sequences. Reading aloud in unison with the clinician reactivates language patterns, and facilitates speech and reading.

Finally, we should like to close with the idea that the clinician's objective is maximal recovery of language functions for each patient, within the framework of the patient's needs, his overall condition, and the extent of the irreversible damage that is present. We believe that the clinician should work systematically and intensively with the aphasic patient towards this objective. When limitations are so great that the goal of functional language must be abandoned or greatly modified, the clinician should define the limitation precisely and specifically. If any question exists in his mind, he should give the patient the benefit of doubt. A trial period of treatment will usually resolve the uncertainty. Probably this procedure should always be used when patients are seen in the first three or four months after onset of aphasia. An alternative for the patient who is too ill or unresponsive to cooperate is to ask to see him again if there is any change in his condition. One should never sell a patient short, but one should recognize the obligation to use clinical time productively and purposively.

GROUP THERAPY

We would argue that individual therapy and group therapy are two entirely different classes of events, serve different purposes, and should not be confused.

Adult aphasics have only one thing in common, which is a disturbance of communication processes. They present a wide range of individual differences in such significant dimensions as age, intelligence, education, occupation, family background, general interests, physiological and neurological conditions, mental status, and nature and severity of aphasia, as well as other variables.

We consider it of primary importance to work intensively with each patient, with the problems he presents, at the level at which he needs to work in each language modality. One patient will fail where another succeeds, and vice versa, and the cause of each failure is critical and should be taken into account in attacking the aphasic problem. The clinician needs to judge when and how to facilitate a response, and when to give the patient time to produce one independently. He needs to adapt materials to individual needs and interests at successive stages of recovery. In short, treatment for aphasia must constantly be dovetailed to patient response. There are no mass methods, and none are possible. What reaches or helps one patient at one point in time loses another. For these reasons, we are unable to have confidence in group therapy as a basic method of treatment for aphasia.

In this age of instruments and laboratories there is no longer even economic justification for mass treatment of aphasic patients. It is now comparatively simple to give each patient individually selected materials with which he can practice independently. Taped materials are available which enable severely impaired aphasic patients to see and hear short language units, and repeat them as many times as necessary, until auditory stimulation is no longer required to elicit the correct response. Other instruments and materials are being developed and used experimentally in various centers, and more of these will be available in the future. These clinical tools do not replace the clinician, but they implement his task effectively.

The aphasic patient needs a clinician who will help him understand and deal with the problem of aphasia as he experiences it from day to day, throughout the recovery period. The patient needs materials and methods selected for him, for his individual problems, and his rate of progress, at each step of the way. He should never practice with materials that present no challenge to him, nor should he experience daily failure where other patients succeed. He should measure his progress in terms of gains he has made, and not against the performance of patients with a dissimilar clinical picture. These are some of the reasons that group therapy is wasteful and sometimes deleterious, if used as a substitute for individual treatment.

Group activity may, however, be a good adjunct to individual treatment. The most positive value is probably that it helps the aphasic patient to feel less isolated. Another is that it gives him an opportunity to observe other aphasic patients. He may observe that there are people with more difficult problems than his, or be encouraged by the progress he sees others making. Increased awareness of other people and their problems is always a significant step towards recovery.

The extent to which a group can plan and carry out its own program varies with the constituency of the group and how long it has been together. Certainly an effort should be made for the members to know and to appreciate each other, and secondly to provide activities in which everyone can participate. No one should feel that he is always at the bottom of the class. The patient should feel that he is with people who like him and who understand his problems. The accent should be on general rather than individual problems.

Most aphasic patients enjoy group singing. If old familiar songs are used, patients frequently develop great favorites. Sometimes these become individual theme songs, and the good-natured ribbing that results gives the patient a solid feeling of inclusion. If all patients are encouraged to join in and sing the tune when they cannot sing the words, words usually begin to come in. Sometimes patients with little or no functional speech love to sing, and can participate in quartets or duets or even do a solo turn, to the pleasure of everyone. It meant a great deal to one patient to be able to sing Christmas carols with his family when he went home for the holidays. The previous Christmas he had cried whenever he heard them.

We do not have group meetings of aphasic patients in Minneapolis because this function is performed by other hospital services. Patients work in groups within other departments, and share a planned program of recreational activities with other patients. They make their own friends on the wards. Sometimes two aphasic patients become friends, but more often than not the closest relationships develop between aphasic and nonaphasic patients. This is obviously desirable. It often draws the aphasic patient into groups and activities he would not attempt on his own or even with another aphasic patient. It gives the other patients on the ward some understanding of aphasia, which makes a better climate for the aphasic patients. In turn, the aphasics come to understand that other patients have problems also, and find ways to help them.

There is usually a good deal of camaraderie among the patients who come to the Aphasia Clinic, but we feel that it is preferable not to isolate them and make this a closed society. Most of us, after all, like to choose our own friends. This reminds us of the experience of a foreign doctor who studied in this country for several years. People generally assumed she would find anyone congenial who came from her native country, in spite of differences in age, interests, or points of view. She found this extremely exasperating. Aphasia is no one's native country, and does not insure compatibility any more than nationality does.

Outpatient clinics operate under conditions different from clinics in hospitals where there is an established rehabilitation program. Patients are relatively isolated in their homes, and coming to the clinic may constitute their only opportunity for wider social experiences. Then it becomes a necessity to structure a program that provides for interaction with other people. There can be no question about the importance of group dynamics in rehabilitation.

It is not unusual in a hospital to find individuals who do a good deal of complaining. They are anxious and uncomfortable and homesick, and they sometimes feel sorry for themselves. They complain because they feel like complaining. This behavior usually does not last very long. They see other patients working persistently towards recovery, and they begin to feel ashamed of self-pity and to try to help themselves. This happens again and again, and in general it is the other patients who make it happen. Once in a while there is a chronic complainer who does not respond to the gentle nudging and encouragement of the others. One day an aphasic patient turned upon one of these, who was grumbling about the excellent food in the dining room. The aphasic patient said, "Cut it out. You get better meals here than you get at home. You never had it so good, and you know it." The bystanders said, "You tell him, Joe," and it was hard to tell which patient derived more benefit from the episode. The point is that one should not underestimate the influence that a group may have on its members, or the members upon each other. This is an important part of the therapeutic process.

Where group programs exist, the clinician's responsibility is only to insure that patients participate to the extent that this is desirable. Some patients need rest and privacy more than additional activities, while others need companionship and wider interests. We try to achieve an optimal milieu for each patient, through individual and group conferences of hospital staff, to call attention to special needs and enlist expert help in dealing with them.

Special assistance may involve encouragement to participate in recreational activities or utilization of other hospital facilities. We once secured permission for a former judge to use the legal library to track down a court decision. Members of the legal staff courteously offered him the freedom of the library, took time to talk to him when they could, and generally treated him as a colleague. This meant more to the judge than anything that had happened to him since his stroke. An accountant worked a part of the day in the auditing department. He found an error the department had been trying to locate for two days. Everyone congratulated him, and the head of the department suggested they go into business together. A priest with severe aphasia undoubtedly received the deepest and most meaningful support anyone in the hospital could give him from the Catholic chaplain. Hospital volunteers took a woman patient shopping and sightseeing, and invited her to their homes, because the patient was so far from her home that relatives and friends could not visit her. In all these instances, the clinician served as a liaison in the utilization of available resources to meet a patient need. We realize that we are fortunate in the resources that are available to us. Within the framework of another situation it would be necessary to function in a different manner.

In summary, we wish to reemphasize that individual treatment of aphasia and group therapy for aphasic patients have different values. Neither is a substitute for the other. Maximal recovery of language skills requires individual diagnosis and treatment. Total rehabilitation is a function of a widening circle of meaningful social relations. Both are a part of the communication and the recovery process. However, they should not be confused.

CONCLUSION

There has always been a good deal of discussion about the art and the science of professions that include clinical practice as well as laboratory research. If by art one means appreciation of the fact that one is dealing with human life, and by science one means precise information, both are necessary and must go hand in hand. In a sense they have always done so. This is to say that asking questions and making observations is not the exclusive domain of either art or science, of the clinic or the laboratory. The dichotomy seems to reflect the either–orishness Aristotelian language habits have tended to impose on our thinking.

What the clinician cannot get along without, and what great artists and scientists alike have always had, is a kind of reverence for human life. The inexpressibly moving thing about the Elgin marbles is their tenderness for the human form. The important thing about Brahms's Requiem is its compassion for human suffering. The great literature of all times and places has had something to say about the human condition as searching and as probing as the questions scientists have asked about the nature of the universe and the nature of man. Scientists have learned that one cannot leave the observer out of the equation, and clinicians know that one cannot leave the laboratory out of the clinic.

It is irresponsible to treat a patient without comprehensive information about the problem he presents. But the clinician must also deal directly with a human individual, and often with one upon whom suffering, physical weakness, anxiety, and other sequelae of incapacitating illness have imposed their inexorable indignities and humiliations. This is the hard fact the clinician cannot turn away from if he is to help the patient assimilate traumatic experiences so that healing can occur. In addition, the clinician requires a hard core of scientific knowledge, if he is to help the patient more than any kind, well-meaning, but untrained person can. Professional competence is never an absolute achievement but is, rather, something in the nature of a lasting commitment.

chapter 19

TECHNIQUES AND MATERIALS FOR TREATMENT OF APHASIA

We believe so strongly that clinical techniques should be adapted to individual patients and immediate problems that we are somewhat reluctant to detail procedures. We have no magic formulas, and no materials better than those any experienced clinician can devise. However, since it usually takes a considerable period of time to develop an adequate clinical armamentarium to tussle with aphasic difficulties, we shall describe techniques we have found effective. We hope the reader will regard our suggestions as tentative and as points of departure from which he may follow his own perceptions and insights. We tend to feel that all techniques should be stored in bottles marked: *Poison: Use only for good reason,* since any technique is ineffectual if used indiscriminately.

In our experience there are several common errors beginning clinicians make working with aphasic patients. First, they tend to talk around the patient, instead of to him, simply and directly. Second, they fail to appreciate the patient's need for strong stimulation to compensate for his own defective feedback processes, and so do not control stimulation effectively. Third, they use too much material at a time, and do not succeed in making materials meaningful to the patient. Fourth, they do not make adequate use of the principle of repeated stimulation. Fifth, they do not elicit an adequate number of responses from the aphasic patient. Hundreds of patient responses should occur during every clinical hour. Sixth, they tend to overcorrect and overexplain.

In general, the clinician should restimulate until a maximal response is obtained rather than try to elucidate errors. Seventh, they tend not to be evaluative enough of what happens in therapy. Probably the best way to acquire this facility is to record and study patient responses consistently.

From these common observations, we can formulate seven positive rules for increasing clinical effectiveness.

1. Talk simply and directly to the patient, eliminating extraneous noise that has no communicative value.
2. Control stimulation to elicit maximal response.
3. Control amount of material used and make it meaningful.
4. Use the principle of repeated stimulations to facilitate discrimination and recall.
5. Work to elicit a maximal number of responses. The patient should be responding continuously throughout the clinical period.
6. In general, restimulate rather than explain or correct.
7. Evaluate the effectiveness of each procedure with each patient.

If these rules sound mechanical, they should be reexamined. Each one directs the clinician to be more sensitive to the patient, and to what he as a clinician is doing.

TECHNIQUES FOR GETTING THE MUSCULATURE WORKING

Here the caution should read: *Do not use if the patient can repeat any words, if he has any speech that sounds normal or even an expressive flow of jargon.* These patients require intensive controlled auditory stimulation, rather than practice of movement patterns.

The techniques in this section were developed for the initial period of treatment of severe sensorimotor impairment. The patients with whom they were used often seemed literally not to know what to do to make the speech musculature work. They had difficulty initiating movements and often produced the wrong movement, or no movement at all, when they attempted to imitate the examiner. They could not repeat.

These are all facilitating techniques, to be used sparingly and abandoned as soon as the ear will take over and repetition is possible.

TO FACILITATE PHONATION

Some patients with severe sensorimotor involvement are unable to produce phonation voluntarily, although there is no observable paralysis or paresis of the musculature. Phonation is physiologically possible, but the patient cannot initiate it. The patient coughs when he wishes to clear his throat, and involuntary phonation occurs when he laughs or cries. He does not talk, however, and he cannot open his mouth and say *ah* at the physician's request.

Now economy of effort is a very sound principle. We want to get voice simply and easily. We try imitation, and it doesn't work. The patient sitting in front of us in a wheel chair tries to talk, but no sound comes.

First the clinician should tell the patient that his voice is all right, because he can cough, or he makes sounds when he laughs, or whatever is true. The clinician should explain that the trouble is only that the patient cannot produce a sound when he wants to, but this will come with practice.

Next, the clinician should stand beside the patient, place his hand firmly over the patient's larynx, and say, "Press here. Push hard. Say *ah* with me. Now." Phonation does not always come on the first two or three attempts, but the clinician repeats the procedure, encouraging the patient to try again, and always producing the sound himself. Both the auditory and the tactual stimulation are important. The clinician may say, "Let's try it 10 times, and see what happens," then rest and try again.

Phonation can almost always be secured in one clinical session by this method. However, it is always permissible to say, "Shall we stop now, and try again tomorrow?" if the patient appears fatigued or discouraged. The clinician should not give up too soon lest the patient infer that the clinician does not expect the method to work or does not expect him to succeed. Aphasic patients need the confidence of the clinician at all times.

The first attempt should be approved, no matter how feeble it is. The only objective is to get the patient to produce a sound voluntarily. He should be told immediately, "That was good. You made a sound, and that means you will be able to make it again. It gets easier each time."

The next objective is to enable the patient to produce the sound at will. Here, again, a practical procedure is to make 10 attempts, then stop to rest. This time the patient is told: "We are going to try again 10 times. If you get a sound once in 10 tries, that is good for now. It is something like learning to play basketball. If you make one basket out of 10 in the beginning, that is good enough. Your score will improve with practice."

When the patient can produce a tone at will, the clinician proceeds to manipulate the sound. On successive blocks of trials he works to get the patient to prolong the sound, timing duration with a stop watch. Next he works to increase loudness. There is no particular benefit to be derived from pushing either of these dimensions to limits, because the patient has normal voice. When he can prolong phonation for 10 or 15 seconds and produce a clearly audible tone, one can ask the patient first to open his mouth and say *ah*, then close his lips and hum. With the humming tone one can work for variations in pitch, going up and down the scale, then humming a familiar song. This is about all one needs to do with voice in sensorimotor impairment.

TONGUE MOVEMENTS

Facilitating techniques for tongue movements are designed for patients who are unable to imitate tongue movements voluntarily and who cannot repeat due to paralysis or paresis of the speech musculature. (Patients who have difficulty repeating because the auditory system is impaired need auditory stimulation, and not practice with movements of the speech musculature.) Facilitating techniques can be started as soon as the patient can hum a familiar tune.

The clinician tells the patient to hum the tune with him again, but this time to move his tongue, and to try to keep it moving all through the song. The clinician adds that it doesn't matter how it sounds. The only important thing is that the tongue should move. The clinician illustrates by singing the song with the syllable *la*, and showing the patient that his tongue is moving. The clinician should sing with the patient, but stop to say, "Keep the tongue going," when necessary. Approval should be given when the tongue moves at all. This is just following the general principle that the patient should know what he is working for, and when he achieves what he is attempting.

It is a good idea to instruct the patient to practice moving his tongue around in his mouth whenever he thinks about it during the day. One patient who could get little movement on Friday came in early Monday morning and triumphantly stuck his tongue out at the clinician. He had practiced all weekend and mastered the trick.

When the patient is able to move the tongue, other exercises can be used to help him acquire more specific control. The patient may sometimes be able to secure protrusion by holding a tongue blade an inch or so in front of his lips, and trying to touch the tongue blade and then retracting his tongue to a rhythmic command of *In–out*. The height of the tongue blade may then be manipulated to assist the patient to elevate and lower the tongue tip. Lateral movements may be similarly induced.

These exercises should be discontinued as soon as relatively controlled movement is obtained.

SPEECH MOVEMENTS

As soon as the patient can initiate phonation and move the tongue voluntarily, one should attempt to get articulated speech patterns. When easy repetition can be secured through auditory stimulation, it is not necessary to use mirrors, tongue blades, or other artificial devices to obtain good speech. These patterns are organized in the brain of the adult aphasic and need only to be reactivated. There is no need to work for individual sounds and then try to combine them into words. For the adult aphasic, this is an artificial procedure, and a good way to delay recovery of speech and insure that it will be labored and unnatural.

These again are facilitating techniques. They rely on highly overlearned language patterns for their effectiveness, and on strong auditory stimulation. The objective is to make the ear take over as early as possible. These techniques can be used as soon as there is voice and the tongue will move.

One effective technique is singing. When the patient can sing a familiar tune with *la*, or an approximation thereof, the clinician can ask him to try to sing the words. He should instruct the patient again that the way it sounds is immaterial, but to sing the words with the clinician when he can. We have found *Happy Birthday* and *I've Been Working on the Railroad* good songs to begin with, but any familiar song will do. The clinician must sing louder than the patient until the patient has the words. Words usually begin to come in almost immediately and increase on successive repetitions. The repertory can gradually be increased also.

Another technique is to ask the patient to count to five with the clinician. The patient is told it doesn't matter what the words sound like, but that he should keep going. The clinician should make the auditory pattern strong and rhythmic. On the first attempt the patient may not produce an intelligible word, but he will probably get the rhythmic pattern. On successive trials approximations of words begin to appear, perhaps only the vowel sounds. Next words begin to resemble the stimulus more and more closely. The clinician may then begin to drop out, and finally the patient can count to five intelligibly and without assistance. Then one may go on to 10, then 15, 20, 30, and so on, successively.

The same technique may be used with the days of the week, and then with letters of the alphabet. Usually during this process, all the consonants begin to appear.

We usually do not use the months of the year at the beginning. They are much more difficult. The patient is able to repeat words and phrases long before he is successful with words with such long and complex auditory and articulatory patterns.

As soon as repetition is possible, the facilitating techniques should be discontinued. Repetition is a much more versatile method and will take the patient much further.

TECHNIQUES FOR STIMULATION OF LANGUAGE

Techniques for stimulating language are the backbone of aphasia therapy. They depend upon a barrage of controlled auditory stimulation and upon feedback processes from obtained responses. We shall describe techniques for various levels of severity of aphasia.

It is always necessary to begin at the level where language breaks down for each patient, and to proceed systematically from easier to more difficult tasks. A good method may fail if materials are too easy or too difficult at a given time. The patient should build from success to success at gradually increasing levels of complexity.

INTENSIVE CONTROLLED AUDITORY STIMULATION

The first method we are going to describe is most effective for patients with little or no functional speech. It is the method of choice for patients with severe sensorimotor impairment and should be initiated as soon as the patient can produce phonation.

Materials consist of a set of cards, each picturing a common object or action, and a printed word. The word should be placed where it can be readily covered, and should appear alone on the back of the card. All speech pathologists have made sets of cards like this, cutting pictures from magazines and catalogues, and mounting them on cardboard. It is a good idea for the clinician to take time to make a set of 200–300 basic vocabulary cards for adults, with clear pictures and heavy print. Most printers will cut heavy poster board to any desired size, and the finished cards can be sprayed with plastic, becoming almost permanent clinical properties.

If commercial sets are used, childish pictures should be removed before the cards are used with adult patients. Commercially available sets are useful adjuncts to the clinician's basic series and serve a number of useful purposes. We have used the Dolch *Picture-Word Cards* (1949), the Bryngelson and Glaspey *Speech Improvement Cards*

(1941), the Taylor and Marks *Aphasia Rehabilitation and Therapy Kit* (1959), the Longerich *Aphasia Therapy Sets* (1959), and a set of cards developed for articulation published by Word Making Productions. When we use sets developed for articulation problems, we shuffle the cards to avoid series of words beginning with the same sound.

The first procedure is to select 20 cards from the series. We use this subset every day for a week, then go on to a new one, keeping the ones used earlier for review.

We use the principles of controlled auditory stimulation described in the last chapter. The objective is to enable the patient to hear and to think the word. The instructions are: "Look at the picture, and look at the word, as I say it. Try to hear it, and try to think it. When you have it, let it come out, but do not force it." These instructions should be repeated as often as needed until the clinician is certain the patient understands and is actively listening during the exercises.

The clinician points first to the picture, then to the printed word, saying the word strongly and clearly each time, and using about 20 repetitions. The interval between repetitions should be long enough for the patient to rehearse or say the words. Usually the patient begins to repeat effortlessly during this process. The patient should be stopped, however, if struggle behavior occurs, and told just to listen until his ear will do it for him and the word comes easily.

If the patient does not repeat, the clinician should stop when four words have been presented, and spread out the four cards, asking the patient to point to the card he names. The clinician names the cards in random order, until the patient is able to select the appropriate card rapidly and with confidence.

If the patient has no trouble pointing to the designated card, the clinician may vary the procedure by asking a short question to elicit a differential response. If, for example, the given words are *house, coffee, knife,* and *car,* the clinician might ask questions such as: *What do you live in? What do you have for breakfast? What do you cut with? What do you drive?* Patients frequently begin to answer the questions orally as they point to the pictures.

If the patient produces an approximation of the word, he should not be corrected, although he may be told again to listen and try to hear it. As repetition becomes more fluent, the clinician may vary the presentation of the stimulus. Duration, rate, and inflection may be altered as the word is repeated.

At first patients tend to want to say the word simultaneously with the clinician, and in fact sometimes can produce it only in this way. They should be encouraged to try to listen, then say it. Next the patient may be asked to say each word twice, which requires more control. He may also be asked to wait a few seconds, and produce it at a given signal from the examiner, such as a pencil tap.

As soon as the patient is repeating words readily, he can be asked to repeat short phrases that supply common frames for the word, after the 20 repetitions. For example, for the words above he might be given:

In the house.
Go in the house.
Build a house.
Drink coffee.
A cup of coffee.

I want a cup of coffee.
Knife and fork.
Cut with a knife.
I have a knife.
Drive a car.
Park the car.
Get in the car.

After the phrases are practiced a few times, the clinician should return to the card, and ask "What is this?" as he points to the picture and again as he points to the word, to again elicit the response.

When the set has been completed, the clinician should go through it again. This time, he asks the patient to say the word if he can, and adds, "If it does not come, listen, and say it after me."

The same set of cards is used every day for five days. Usually at the end of the week the patient is able to name all the cards independently, and 80–100% of the cards from previous weeks. Percentages may not be this high the first week, but usually they increase rapidly from one week to another until complete recall becomes the rule.

It is interesting to record the latency of responses when patients are naming pictures. We usually gave the patient 60 seconds before supplying a clue. When latencies were recorded, it was found that they decreased progressively as the proportion of correct responses increased. It is possible that the proportion of correct responses would show a higher increase if the clinician waited longer than 60 seconds, but this is not as productive as using the time for stimulation. Once the clinician was called out of the office to take a long-distance telephone call almost 60 seconds after presentation of the stimulus. Five minutes later, when the clinician returned, the patient produced the correct word.

We use the same words for writing. The patient is given five words from the list each day to practice writing. He is told to copy each word until he can write it correctly without looking at the copy. Each word is spelled aloud several times in unison with the clinician. On the following day the patient is asked to write all the words he has had during the week to dictation. On Friday review words are added from previous weeks.

When the patient is naming the cards easily, he is asked to perform the task with the words covered, relying on the picture alone, and then to turn the cards over, and read the words without the picture.

As soon as repetition is easy, the patient is given the *Picture–Word Series* for the Language Master (Moore and Schuell, 1954) and assigned 20 new cards a week for independent instrumental practice. Almost all Sensorimotor patients acquire a functional basic vocabulary for speech, reading, and writing within a few weeks in this manner, if stimulation is adequate. It is interesting that not only is this vocabulary functional from the beginning, but words that have never been rehearsed appear in the patient's speech with increasing frequency. Supplying frames for the words by using them in common phrases and short sentences accelerates the rate at which connected utterances appear in spontaneous speech.

When the patient is writing words successfully to dictation, one or two of the short phrases or sentences may be assigned each day for practice, and the patient subsequently asked to write these to dictation and to read them aloud.

At this stage, we usually place short sentences on cards. The patient reads each sentence four or five times in unison with the clinician. Then he is asked to read it alone and, finally, to repeat it without looking at it. In this way auditory retention span is gradually increased. The patient is also given phrases and short sentences to practice on the Language Master. He is instructed to follow the same procedures for practice, then to try to read the sentence before he hears it, and listen to correct his errors.

It should be noted that all of these techniques—repeating, reading in unison, and writing to dictation—involve auditory stimulation, and all of them elicit responses that provide feedback. At first, however, the patient's responses are too defective to provide adequate feedback, and he is dependent upon the clinician's voice or the machine playback for control.

ELICITING RESPONSES

Techniques for eliciting responses may also be used from the beginning of treatment. The easiest one supplies a frequently-used frame for the word and provides a popular association. The patient is asked to complete phrases or short sentences, such as:

A cup of *coffee*.
Bread and *butter*.
Turn off the *light*.
Wind the *clock*.

This technique gives the patient early success and stimulates language. It should be remembered that it is successful even with Irreversible subjects who do not acquire functional speech. One should not, therefore, attach prognostic importance to results achieved by this means.

A more productive technique can be used as soon as the patient can name pictures or read words. When he produces the word, the clinician says, "Tell me something about it." The response may be one word at first, but gradually series of words, phrases, and even short sentences appear.

When this happens the clinician may alter the instructions to, "Use it in a sentence," when the patient produces the word. At this time the patient may begin to write two or three original sentences a day using selected spelling words, and to read sentences aloud.

Another technique to elicit responses is free association. The clinician supplies a word, and the patient responds with whatever he thinks of. This is particularly productive when the clinician supplies words that are closely related to the patient's major interests. If words are well-chosen, they tap more than language experience. This undoubtedly facilitates responses, and extremely interesting responses occur. One patient, for example, with very little functional speech triumphantly produced *Stratford-on-the-Avon* and *All's Well That Ends Well* as responses to *Shakespeare*. Later, asked who wrote *Hamlet*, he said with a twinkle in his eye, "Bacon," but added, "I don't think so." A judge, also severely aphasic, produced *first-degree homicide* in response to *murder,* and then proceeded to outline and define degrees and penalties. A young patient produced song titles in response to almost everything, and then went on to sing parts of the songs.

Sentences can be read aloud with the patient and one-word questions can be asked to elicit an elliptical response from the sentence. For example, the clinician and patient can read together, *The boy played in the park.* Then the clinician asks, *Who?* and tries to elicit, *The boy.*

Situational pictures may also be used to elicit responses. We do not like this technique, however, until enough language is available for the patient to produce connected responses freely. Until this is possible, it is better to use techniques that supply verbal stimulation.

An excellent technique that does this is reading sentences or short factual paragraphs aloud, with clinician and patient reading in unison. The paragraph is read five times in this manner.

There is an art to this reading. On the first trial the clinician leads strongly. He reads slowly, but with normal phrasing and inflection, and with pauses between phrases. The patient is instructed to pay no attention to how he sounds, but to try to keep going. Usually the percentage of correct words increases on each trial. As the patient's reading improves, the clinician may increase rate gradually, and begin to let the patient lead. Eventually the clinician drops out when the patient is going well, but comes in again when he falters. Finally the patient is reading paragraphs aloud independently.

After the oral trials are finished, the clinician should permit the patient to read the paragraph silently for meaning, and then ask specific questions about content. At first the patient is allowed to look at the paragraph as he answers the questions. If he responds by pointing to the appropriate answer, this is accepted, but the clinician repeats the answer. Patients usually give single-word responses at first, but responses gradually increase in length, and eventually the patient is able to retell the paragraph without being prompted by questions.

ON HIGHER LEVELS

Some mildly aphasic patients have no difficulty naming common objects or writing common words to dictation. They do have trouble finding words, however, and expressing connected ideas, and they encounter difficulties on a similar level in reading and writing. The two most useful measures for determining the materials to be used are spelling grade level, and the length of sentence which the patient can repeat correctly.

If the patient's spelling tests at fifth-grade level, for example, the clinician should use 8 or 10 words a day from a fifth-grade spelling list for general word study.

The clinician writes the first word syllabically, and pronounces it, asking the patient to listen, and repeat it after him, until repetition is correct and fluent. Next, the clinician and patient spell the word in unison four or five times. The clinician leads strongly at first, but allows the patient to take the lead when he can.

Next the clinician uses the word in a series of sentences adjusted to the patient's verbal retention span, asking the patient to listen and then repeat.

Finally, the clinician asks the patient what the word means. Defining words is a difficult task for aphasic patients, and the clinician should assist the patient to achieve a functional definition when necessary. If the patient gives a meaningful example or illustration, this should be accepted. The object is to elicit language and gradually encourage more precise expression of ideas through usage. Stimulation rather than correction is the rule, however, and literary definitions should not be required.

Patients with this amount of language are usually given a sentence illustrating the use of each spelling word to practice reading and writing, and to write to dictation the next day. They are also asked to write sentences using selected words as part of their preparation, and to formulate sentences orally using spelling words.

We usually use short articles for reading material at this level. We may begin with paragraphs from graded reading materials, such as the *Reader's Digest Reading Skill Builder Series* (1951), or other factual material with controlled vocabulary and sentence length. When this is no longer necessary, we use adult materials, with selection determined by the interests of the patient. Patients are asked to read and retell consecutive paragraphs. They are soon able to summarize the article at the end and to express opinions about it.

We ask patients to read the daily paper as soon as possible, and to report on news items that interested them. We also ask them to do some daily reading for practice or pleasure. They select books or magazines from the library independently, or with the help of the librarian or the clinician, and read for content only. Usually we ask the patient to read for 15 minutes, half an hour, or an hour a day, and report the number of pages read and any difficulties encountered.

Oral reading and retelling provides more stimulation and more feedback than silent reading, and consequently the immediate gains in language facility are greater. This technique gives the patient a variety of interesting things to talk about, and stimulates language as well as the patient's own ideas. Independent silent reading is much less effective for these purposes, but it has other values. It facilitates reading for continuity, gradually increases reading rate, and helps to make reading functional. With daily practice, reading gradually becomes rewarding. This is especially important for patients who love books or who have a good deal of time to fill.

Another good technique is to ask the patient to listen to a radio newscast once a day and report an item that interested him. The principle value of this assignment is that it forces the patient to listen, and to get information through the ear. Reports usually become much more precise with practice. At first the patient may be able to say little more than, "He said something about France—de Gaulle," but two or three weeks later he may present a good resume of the principal events of the day. This assignment also stimulates the patient's interest in what is going on in the world and often reactivates previous knowledge and previous interests. Television serves the latter purpose for patients who cannot follow a radio program. Patients tend to be conscientious about using the radio, however, when they understand the reason for the assignment. We also encourage patients to attend movies shown in the hospital. They often report such observations as, "Last night was the first time I followed the story all the way through," or, "I am beginning to get more and more of what they say."

We use systematic repetition of sentences, in addition to the sentences used with vocabulary and spelling words, as soon as patients are able to repeat sentences consistently. For patients with a severe language deficit, we use common words in familiar phrases and short sentences. Mimeographed sheets can be used for this. Later we use a set of sentences illustrating the usage of a common structural word, or structural form. The patient reads a sentence at a time in unison with the clinician, if he cannot read it alone, and then repeats the sentence without looking at the copy. When all of the sentences have been practiced in this manner, the clinician reads each sentence and asks the patient to repeat it, depending on the auditory stimulus alone. When the set has been completed, the clinician asks the patient to give three or four sentences using the given form. The patient is permitted to keep the sheet for practice and review.

With patients who have more available language we use longer sentences that emphasize verbal retention span rather than structural usage. Sentences that contain series of items are effective for this purpose. The same technique as above is employed.

TECHNIQUES FOR SPECIAL PURPOSES

THE ALPHABET

Almost all aphasic patients require some practice with letters of the alphabet. Many patients with mild aphasia can recite or write the alphabet in serial order, but have difficulty pointing to letters named in random order and writing letters dictated in random order. This is usually because they cannot make the fine auditory discriminations required to differentiate between letters whose names sound alike. If specific visual involvement is present, there is also difficulty discriminating between letters with similar visual configurations, and if proprioceptive cues are reduced, difficulty discriminating between phonemes with similar articulatory patterns.

We have found it most effective to practice saying and writing the alphabet in serial order until the patient is able to produce it spontaneously in either mode. This supplies a frame or a context for reference, which facilitates perception and recall.

Next, using a group of letters at a time, we stimulate the patient with each letter, giving the name, the sound, and a common word that begins with the sound. For patients with severe aphasia we use the grouping *abc, def, ghi, jkl, mno, pq, rst, uvw, xyz.* With milder impairment we use *abc, defg, hijk, lmnop, qrst, uvw, xyz.*

We say the name of the letter, repeat the sound rapidly several times, say the word, and ask the patient to repeat the entire series. We have found we get better initial responses, and easier transitions into words, if we add a short neutral vowel to each consonant. Presentation is something like this:

A (āāā) ate	N (nnn) night
B (bbb) boy	O (ōōō) open
C (kkk) cat	P (ppp) pie
D (ddd) dog	Q (kw,kw,kw) queen
E (ēēē) east	R (rrr) radio
F (fff) fish	S (sss) Sunday
G (ggg) gun	T (ttt) table
H (hhh) house	U (ūūū) union

I ($\overline{\text{iii}}$) ice cream	V (vvv) vote
J (jjj) job	W (www) watch
K (kkk) key	X (ks,ks,ks) taxi
L (lll) lamp	Y (yyy) yellow
M (mmm) man	Z (zzz) zone

Materials are a set of cards, each one containing a letter, with the word on the back, and one large card containing the alphabet in serial order, but with letters grouped as they were given to the patient. After the stimulation procedures, we ask the patient to respond in some manner. Usually responses appear in a hierarchical order, as follows:

1. Pointing to letter named by examiner
2. Producing word to auditory stimulus, when letter is named or sounded
3. Writing letters dictated in random order
4. Using shuffled deck of alphabet cards, naming letter, producing sound, and giving examples of the sound in words
5. Sounding words
6. Spelling words orally, unassisted

After the patient can perform step 4 above, we begin to add new phonemes, such as the short vowels, the s–sound for c, ch, sh, th, wh, ing, and various dipthongs. Before sounding words, we point out that many English words are not sounded as they are spelled, that there are silent letters, letters that have several sounds, combinations of letters with different sounds, and so on. Knowing the common sounds simply helps the patient to hear words better, and provides helpful clues for reading and writing. This has never seemed to bother patients particularly.

During later stimulation, we may use several words for each sound, and finally words using given sounds in various positions, providing more phonic drill. For example, we might use *at, bat, cat, hat, sat,* for ă, or *day, may, pay, play, say* for ā. We do more of this with Sensorimotor patients than with patients in the Simple Aphasic and Visual groups, who usually need less practice because auditory and proprioceptive discrimination is less impaired. When Sensorimotor patients learn to associate through sound, there is usually a marked spread of vocabulary in all modalities. We wish to repeat the caution, however, that patients should not be required to discriminate sounds before a basic functional vocabulary is acquired. The task is too hard, and results in frustration, defeat, and inhibition of language if attempted too soon. The time to begin is when the patient needs these tools to make further progress in reading and writing.

DYSFLUENCY

For aphasic patients who show a mild aphasia accompanied by persisting dysfluency, we use the techniques for language stimulation that we have described earlier, because there is reduction of available vocabulary and of verbal retention span reflected in all language modalities. Usually rapid gains in all language modalities follow. It was one of these patients who found the error in the accounting department we referred to previously. However, treatment for the language deficit must be accompanied by treatment directed specifically towards reducing the dysfluency from the beginning.

First, we begin to work on the phonemes that are defective. These are often found to be *s*, *sh*, *ch*, *j*, sometimes *r* and *l*, and consonant blends. The consistency with which we have found this group of sounds defective suggests difficulty with fine muscle coordination due to an impairment of proprioceptive feedback. We use intensive practice on each defective sound.

One effective technique is to practice the consonant or consonant combination followed first by long vowel sounds, then by short vowel sounds, with a list of words using each combination, and phrases containing these words. This might go something like this:

sā—sē—sī—sō—sū
sā, sail, same, save, safe, sane
sail—go for a sail
same—the same time
save—a penny saved
safe—a safe driver
sane—a sane Fourth

This is all strong rhythmic practice, which forces the patient to produce hundreds of repetitions in a short time.

Another technique is to give the patient a list of phonetically edited sentences to read aloud and then repeat without looking at the copy. The clinician monitors the performance by interrupting with, "Repeat," whenever a defective sound is produced. The same technique can be used with reading and retelling a paragraph. This helps the patient to utilize the auditory feedback in order to monitor and correct himself.

A third technique is to give the patient a list of words containing the sound, and ask him to use each word in a sentence, and monitor as above.

Usually patients with this form of dysfluency master all the consonants and consonant blends within a relatively short period, but speech remains slow and halting, and articulation breaks down when they attempt to increase rate and when constant control is not exerted.

There are techniques that help this somewhat. One is drill with polysyllabic words. Each word is divided into syllables with the accented syllable underlined. The patient repeats the word after the clinician, first slowly, but with natural inflection, then at more normal rate. It sometimes helps to tell the patient that the accented syllable is given more time as well as more stress in English, and that sounds are often elided in unstressed syllables. When the patient can pronounce the word acceptably, he is asked to use it in a sentence.

Another technique that helps is repetition of phrases, emphasizing important words, and subordinating the others. For example: in the *house*, around the *block*, to the *store*, with a *smile*, on the *table*, an *apple*, an *orange*, an *umbrella*, the *car*, the *letter*, the *bicycle*, a *stamp*, a *dollar*, etc. The patient may then be asked to use each phrase in a sentence. Short sentences may be practiced in the same way, such as, "It is *raining*, It is *snowing*, How are *you?* I am *fine*, Where are you *going? What* did you say?" and so on.

The purpose of this kind of drill is to facilitate natural inflection and fluency, and to make frequently used conversational units somewhat more automatic. This much can usually be achieved, but beyond conventional responses conscious control seems to be required, or articulation patterns disintegrate. Patients report consistently that they must rehearse what they are going to say silently or it comes out jumbled. Auditory stimulation increases vocabulary and verbal retention span, but articulation never becomes wholly automatic. This was one of the reasons we first postulated that this syndrome might result from a frontal lesion, or at least from interference in the control of higher over lower motor centers. Conscious control can be achieved, but not complete automaticity.

DYSARTHRIA

Other aphasic patients present a form of dysarthria characterized by general slurring of consonants and a tendency not to use or maintain sufficient vocal intensity for audibility. With these patients we also work to stimulate language and simultaneously to improve intelligibility. We usually begin by trying to increase loudness and duration of phonation. We want first to be sure that the patient can achieve and sustain an adequate tone. When he achieves strong phonation, we ask him to count to three, then to five, then to 10, stopping him whenever voice begins to fade. The alphabet and the days of the week can be used similarly. After this we use repetition of phrases and sentences, oral reading of sentences, then of short connected materials, interrupting with, "Repeat," whenever a word is unintelligible.

To get carryover into spontaneous speech, we ask the patient to formulate sentences using given words, and to retell what he has read, monitoring his speech as above. We sometimes use a tape recorder, encouraging the patient to listen to his own speech and evaluate intelligibility.

There is a tendency to mumble the end of the word, the end of the phrase, or the end of the sentence, and to talk in a monotone. Articulation is good and inflection is within normal limits, however, when the patient makes a strong effort. One should remember that there is usually some paresis throughout all the musculature, and the amount of effort required to achieve a good result may be considerable. For this reason spaced practice throughout the day is better than massed practice.

Some increase of general intelligibility usually results from directed spaced practice, although the quality of speech usually continues to vary from one situation to another and appears to be contingent upon the amount of effort the patient is able to put forth at a given time. There is undoubtedly a relation between the general neurophysiological condition of the patient and his ability to maintain and utilize the improvement he makes in the clinic. Sometimes the chief value of treatment seems to be that the patient acquires a tool he can use to reduce the frustration of not being understood when he wishes to do so. When there is something he wants to say, he talks clearly instead of breaking into helpless tears, which is something gained.

Sometimes varying degrees of paralysis or spastic paresis are found throughout all the musculature, including the muscles of respiration. When the paralysis is severe, the speech pathologist should work with the physical therapist for synchronization of breathing and control of expiration, and with the nursing service for control of swallowing, chewing, and sucking movements. Language stimulation can sometimes be carried on before phonation or articulatory movements are possible, if the patient is aphasic. The latter is sometimes difficult to determine if the patient is paraplegic and has visual involvement also, for he has no way to respond. Initial patience and persistence may be rewarded, however, for sometimes language abilities are obscured by the initial gross motor impairment, and functional communication can be achieved.

Another form of dysarthria that sometimes occurs results from partial or unilateral paralysis of the tongue or soft palate. With specific involvement of this kind, we work to strengthen movements and to improve articulation through the use of compensatory techniques. This usually involves working with the patient to secure the best approximations of sounds that he can, through monitoring by ear. In other words, he learns a new way to produce a sound so that it appears within normal limits, and he is most successful when he discovers this way by listening to himself. The clinician may guide him by giving a minimal placement clue when necessary. For example, just saying, "Can you pull your tongue back a little? Don't let it touch your teeth," may improve a defective sibilant, or asking the patient to say *ah*, and to try to raise the tongue a little as he prolongs it, may help him to get an *r*. Practicing sounds in syllables, words, and short units of connected speech has produced better results, in our experience, than practicing sounds in isolation in most cases.

All of the dysarthrias may exist in the presence or in the absence of aphasia. If aphasia is present, it is important that it, as well as the dysarthric impairment, should be treated from the beginning.

VISUAL PROBLEMS

Since patients with visual problems have a language deficit also, and since this tends to respond readily to treatment, initial treatment begins with auditory stimulation to increase vocabulary and retention span. Oral spelling may be substituted for written spelling.

If the patient does not recognize or recall letters at all, work relearning the visual forms should be initiated immediately. The best technique we have found is copying and naming a letter simultaneously, until the patient can produce it without looking at the copy. We use the letters in alphabetical order, a small group at a time. Subsequently the patient is asked to point to letters named in random order, name them when they are presented in random order, and write them to dictation in the same manner.

As we have observed before, patients with cerebral involvement of visual processes often must learn each visual form of the letter, upper case, lower case, print, and script, separately. In our opinion it is most productive to begin with lower-case print. There are two reasons for this: First, print facilitates reading, and reading in turn facilitates recall of forms. Second, print is easier for the patient than script at the beginning, contrary to general expectation. Our guess is that this is because there is less individual variation in the forms of letters, and the problem of connecting letters does not arise.

Besides individual letters, we use words of two or three letters from the beginning, for both reading and writing. In the beginning patients usually have to decipher a word letter by letter and spell it to themselves for recognition to occur. Since they usually do this aloud, the process is easy to follow. Recognition of a word as a unit occurs with short words first, then with words of gradually increasing length. It frequently takes a patient 20 minutes to read 20 common three- or four-letter words on initial trials. Rate also increases gradually, and in a short period patients are able to read phrases and sentences, and print them to dictation.

It is very clear that patients utilize proprioceptive information to aid defective visual recognition and recall. It is not uncommon for a patient to trace a letter in the air when he is trying to name it or recall how to write it.

Capital letters are introduced gradually when lower-case letters are learned. It is not usually necessary to teach script letter by letter. A patient who has been printing his name as *John R. Doe* one day produces a flourishing signature, and from this time on signs himself *J. Richard Doe*, because this is the way he always signed his name. Next, he begins to write the words the clinician printed in his assignment. He rarely needs to do more than practice a few of the least frequently used letters and connections between letters to write as he did before. We print assignments as long as patients are using print, but transfer to script when they do. Patients scarcely seem to observe the change.

Recovery of reading and writing lags behind recovery of language in patients with visual involvement. This makes it advisable to use materials on different levels of difficulty during the early period of treatment. A patient may use fifth-grade words easily for oral spelling and sentence formulation when he has difficulty reading and writing words of two or three letters. The gap closes rapidly, however, as soon as the visual forms of letters are reestablished. Recovery is almost complete, except that reading rate remains retarded and inconsistent errors occasionally occur.

Some patients show only mild visual involvement from the beginning. These patients occasionally confuse letters and words that look alike, misread a word, or guess the end of it from the beginning, and guess wrong. They sometimes write words phonetically, substitute one letter for another with a similar appearance, distort a letter form, or cannot remember what a *q* or a *z* looks like. In such cases we work only on the letters the patient has trouble with, and we work on a higher spelling level from the beginning. Oral spelling is always an effective tool.

Reading and writing rarely become functional skills when severe visuospatial impairment is present. Most aphasic patients compensate readily for visual field defects, but this is not true when the field defect coincides with disturbed spatial perception.

The patient who can only see a constricted portion of space and who cannot perceive spatial relationships or his own relationship to objects in space lives in a distorted and frightening world. He often feels anxious, bewildered, and lost. Frequently the most effective thing the clinician can do is to define his assets and disabilities clearly and repeatedly, until the anxiety is reduced enough for the patient to utilize the information and begin to make adjustments. (Interestingly enough, it is usually the patient who initiates this repetition. He may say, "You tell me I'm not stupid, but I have a poor sense of direction. Well, I ought to be able to get along with that, oughtn't I?") We have sometimes given patients typed statements something like this, after we have worked through their problems with them and reviewed the statements day after day:

Assets
1. Your understanding is good.
2. Your judgment is good.
3. You have a good sense of humor.
4. You have many friends.
5. You have a fine record of achievement.

Limitations
1. You do not see well to the left.
2. You have a poor sense of direction.
3. You do not hear well in noisy places.
4. You cannot stand as much stress as you could when you were young.

The patient begins to understand what he can do and what he cannot do and becomes less anxious because he knows what to expect. He is willing to tell people he has a poor sense of direction, and to ask for help when he gets turned around. He gains confidence and becomes more independent. All of this helps to restore the self-respect that has been so badly shaken by repeated failures he has suffered and could not understand.

MILD APHASIA

Patients with mild aphasia frequently require intensive treatment to enable them to return successfully to their work. These patients are sometimes dismissed too casually because their needs are less obvious. The difference between success and failure can be tragic when the potential for achievement is so high. The period of treatment need not be long, for an intelligent patient can carry out a large part of it on his own. Often the most important aspect is giving the patient an understanding of the aphasic problem, and working through enough procedures for him to know what to do. Formal treatment should be continued until the patient knows what kinds of problems to expect and has experienced enough success to acquire confidence in the reversibility of the difficulties he encounters.

He should receive systematic stimulation to reactivate vocabulary and increase verbal retention span. Materials should be consistent with educational level and occupational needs. Practice reading, writing, defining, and using words commensurate with his cultural background gives the patient confidence in his ability to handle language in ordinary situations. If there is a specialized vocabulary in his field, these words should be reviewed. The patient is often more competent than the clinician in explaining the usage of these terms, and it is a good experience for him to find this out.

Repeating sentences and retelling paragraphs should be practiced to increase verbal retention span. Another good technique is repeating names, addresses, and telephone numbers from the telephone book, and writing them to dictation. Aphasic patients tend to be anxious about their ability to deal with this kind of information because they have suffered frequent embarrassments from the inability to recall a familiar name. One cannot substitute another word for a proper name, so the penalty is inescapable. Practice with unfamiliar names and addresses forces the patient to pay attention to names and numbers when he hears them and restores his confidence in his ability to handle materials of this kind. The experience makes him less defensive and more willing to ask to have a name and an address repeated, and to write it down when it is important.

The clinician should ascertain what the patient needs to do at work, and have him bring in materials for practice. We have used catalogues, price lists, insurance policies, and professional and trade journals as clinical materials. Patients have prepared reports and sales talks, and practiced dictating letters to customers and clients. They have abstracted papers in journals, written sermons, and reviewed changes in laws resulting from current legislative action.

University students have practiced outlining materials in textbooks and encyclopedias and taking notes as the clinician read aloud. At first they tended to try to get down everything the clinician said, which produced a hopeless jumble. Practice abstracting topics and principal ideas produced more meaningful notes, better grasp, and recall of content.

Another good technique is to require patients to write answers to specific questions on reading materials. This is good practice for many patients with mild aphasia; it is particularly important that students learn to answer the question that is asked, and to give specific information.

Many patients have worked successfully with book-length materials, writing summaries of chapters, presenting them orally, and discussing questions that interested them. It is not necessary that the clinician read all the books that patients report on, for the burden of clarity should be placed on the patient. This is usually a pleasant kind of therapy, for the patient becomes the instructor, and the clinician may learn a great deal.

The clinician should obviously never pretend to knowledge or understanding he does not have. It is conceivable that an aphasic patient might need to review materials too technical for the clinician to follow, but at this level he requires a tutor trained in his own field rather than a speech pathologist, and should be so counseled. State Vocational Rehabilitation Services have sometimes provided such assistance in areas such as mathematics, and have financed courses in left-handed typing and improving speed of reading.

Most aphasic patients need some stimulation and practice in the recall of learned numerical combinations and simple arithmetic processes. This is an aphasic problem involving language rather than mathematical concepts. You have to be able to tell yourself that $8 \times 7 = 56$, and what to do next when you perform a series of operations. There may be additional interference resulting from impairment of visual or spatial perception.

In our experience, patients recover competence in mathematics as they recover language, and to comparable degrees. When mathematical skills are important to the patient's work, limitations should be explored thoroughly, and treatment initiated. In the hospital we frequently refer patients to the department of educational therapy for practice in arithmetic, and concentrate on language in the clinic. It is important that the nature of the aphasic problem be explained when a referral is made for tutoring, for failure may result if this is not taken into account.

CONCLUSION

It is hard to avoid sounding didactic when talking about specific things to do in treating aphasic patients. It begins to sound like a prescription, when there are no prescriptions. For this reason, we have chosen to let someone who can speak with the authority of experience say the final words in this chapter. (the italics are ours).

> . . . Of one thing I am quite certain. There has been a spiritual quality in the significant relationships I have had with certain people who have helped me along the way. There was an element of faith. *For none of us had all the answers. We did the best we could, but we did this together. We were united in this effort.* There is a spiritual quality in this kind of a relationship. We customarily use the word 'rapport' to describe such a relationship. This is a good word I suppose, but I don't use it when I describe my feeling about these people who have contributed so significantly toward my 'becoming.' This is a better word than recovery.

This would seem to be the essential nature of the therapeutic process. It is what is remembered when all the techniques are forgotten. Nevertheless, at some time, the techniques play an indispensible role.

This brings us back again to the importance of the clinical relationship. We think Bill Masterson was talking about the same thing when he said that man does not live by bread alone. The clinical techniques are the daily bread and they are essential. One must do something to effect the desired changes. Even more important, however, is the integrity of purpose shared by patient and clinician, and the meaningfulness of the communication that occurs between them.

chapter 20

LONG-TERM PLANNING WITH APHASIC PATIENTS

Aphasia is a complex disorder, and it is necessary to think of recovery in terms of years, rather than weeks or months. Although progress is slow and gradual, needs and capacities alter markedly from one period to another. It is sometimes useful to think of recovery as a series of steps, and to plan one step at a time. A hospital clinic may be the best solution at one time, and working with someone at home a happier situation at another. Attending an outpatient clinic, taking vocational training, or working part-time may be stimulating and challenging, and produce a spurt in recovery later.

Aphasic disorders are usually treated by speech pathologists who work in hospitals, outpatient clinics, university clinics, rehabilitation centers, or in private practice. The professional organization in speech pathology and audiology is the American Speech and Hearing Association, which maintains a national office at 9030 Old Georgetown Road, Washington, D.C. 20014. The association certifies the clinical competence of members and will furnish information concerning qualified clinicians in desired geographical areas.

The responsibility for examining the aphasic patient, evaluating language impairment, determining if treatment is indicated, and setting up a long-range program with realistic goals belongs squarely to the speech pathologist.

Ideally, the patient should be referred by his physician with a request for consultation, a summary of pertinent medical history, and present neurological findings. If referral is made through another source, the speech pathologist should obtain permission for release of information from the patient and call or write the physician.

The speech pathologist needs medical information. He needs to know the etiology of aphasia, how much time has elapsed since onset, if the patient has had previous cerebrovascular episodes, if cardiovascular status is precarious, if he has seizures and if so how well they are controlled, if there are any active or progressive disease processes, if there are limitations on activities, and, in some cases, life expectancy. One would not, for example, keep a homesick patient in a clinic or a hospital for treatment of aphasia if he had only a few months to live. All these factors influence long-term planning.

The physician, in turn, usually wants to know the extent of brain damage indicated by the aphasic findings, and the outlook for recovery of language functions. If the patient is not neurologically stable, the speech pathologist can only report observed findings, and say it is too early to predict the outcome. Symptoms resulting from transitory effects of brain damage are not intrinsically different from those resulting from destruction of tissue, and there is no way of predicting which symptoms will persist and which will subside. Sometimes the medical history combined with clinical experience permits an informed guess. This may be stated, if it is so labeled. There is some value in defining clinical impressions and submitting them to the validation of time. This process forces awareness of the kinds of observations and judgments clinicians make, makes it possible to formulate testable hypotheses, and serves to sharpen and refine the processes of diagnosis and prediction.

If the patient who is not neurologically stable is receiving treatment, he can be watched, reevaluated later, and a report sent to the physician. If immediate treatment is not indicated, the physician will usually refer the patient again when more time has elapsed. Sometimes the speech pathologist can suggest things for the family to do during the waiting period, and ask that a record of observed changes be kept.

A reliable examination cannot be obtained nor can patients benefit from treatment for aphasia when they are too ill to participate in clinical procedures. So much has been written about the advisability of early treatment that this fact is sometimes neglected. We have found it a useful rule to say that generally we do not want to see a patient until he is responding to what is going on about him, and can sit up for two hours without fatigue.

THE HOSPITAL CLINIC

Planning a program of treatment for an aphasic patient must necessarily take into account the institutional or community structure in which the speech pathologist works. Situations vary considerably, and every situation has limitations and advantages. This discussion is confined to the hospital inpatient clinic, because we have had experience with no other kind. We believe, however, that the assets and liabilities of other situations can be assessed in a similar fashion, and the inherent advantages utilized and limitations circumvented to develop a program from which patients can benefit.

The chief limitation in a hospital clinic is that patients cannot be treated for prolonged periods. Even when cost to the patient is not a prohibitive factor, the speech pathologist must be aware of the need to make the best use of hospital beds, and the possible deleterious effects of long hospitalization. As one of our patients commented, "A man shouldn't stay in a hospital too long. He gets to like it too well. He gets afraid to leave, and afraid to go back to work." This patient, with acute insight, was describing what is known in the trade as hospitalitis. Besides this obvious danger, a man misses his home and family, and the stimulation that comes from seeing people he knows, resuming activities he enjoys, and picking up the threads of his life again. These factors must be weighed, and the best solution is usually a compromise. We have tried to circumvent the disadvantages of a limited period of hospitalization by making treatment as intensive as possible, and by doing extremely careful planning with the patient and his family before discharge from the hospital.

The chief advantage of a hospital clinic is the staff of highly trained professional workers in many areas. Medical and psychiatric consultation is readily available, and any observed changes in patient performance can be investigated immediately. Nurses and attendants make invaluable observations about the patient's behavior on the ward, his interactions with other patients, and the kinds of difficulties he encounters. Social workers explore relevant family problems, utilizing an amazing variety of resources to deal with immediate and long-term needs.

Physical therapists work with acutely ill patients to retain range of motion and prevent contractures, and later to strengthen weakened musculature and obtain maximal function. Corrective therapists teach patients to get from bed to chair, from chair to a standing position, to walk, climb stairs, and take care of their personal needs. Occupational therapists provide a series of graded activities to help patients increase manual strength and dexterity, as well as to develop interests and abilities that help them compensate for activities they can no longer pursue. Special Services provides diversions for evenings, weekends, and holidays, and trained recreation leaders consider the special interests and aptitudes of patients who are homesick or depressed and skillfully draw them into congenial activities. A young aphasic patient once won a spelling match that was part of an evening's entertainment. All the patients in his ward were rooting for him, and this was a tremendously reassuring experience. He said, "I didn't expect to win, but you told me to keep trying new things, so I decided I would. I don't think they knew I was aphasic."

Educational counselors sometimes work with aphasic patients to help them recover special skills, such as arithmetic or typing, to help them return to their jobs with more confidence. This, of course, is feasible only for certain patients at certain stages of recovery.

Vocational psychologists evaluate vocational assets, liabilities, interests, and aptitudes, and institute programs of vocational training for patients who cannot return to their former occupations, or give patients additional assets to compensate for disabilities they have incurred. They offer opportunities for patients to test work tolerance and vocational skills through a program carried on in various departments of the hospital, under the supervision of selected hospital personnel. They guide patients to available positions and arrange job interviews for them. Upon the patient's request, they may serve as a liaison between the patient and his former employer.

These services play a role in rehabilitation and enter into discharge planning. This planning is done on an individual basis through a series of interviews with the patient and his family. The planning involves the physician and all the services that have worked with the patient. The speech pathologist may carry the major responsibility in planning with the aphasic patient, or he may not, depending upon the primary needs of the patient at time of discharge.

COUNSELING FOR PATIENTS WHO WILL NOT RECOVER FUNCTIONAL LANGUAGE

The work of the clinician begins, but does not end, with diagnosis. It is our feeling that every patient who can cooperate with test procedures should receive a limited period of treatment, with the general objectives of establishing communication, increasing auditory comprehension, and facilitating verbal responses.

Communication occurs during the examination, with or without language. The examiner conveys that he is interested in the patient, understands what has happened, and wants to know how the patient is getting along. By his cooperation, the patient tells the examiner that he appreciates his concern, and that he is able to do some things but not others. The behavior of the patient often tells the examiner how well he understands his situation, and what he is most troubled about. If the examiner is sensitive enough to these reactions, he can often verbalize them for the patient as they occur, and make it possible for the patient to experience the relief of sharing his feelings about what has happened to him. In turn, the examiner's attitude tells the patient that these feelings are natural and understandable, and that it is important to talk about them. The examiner does not need words to tell the patient he knows this is not easy, but that he is not alone and will have the courage that is required.

What the examiner must tell the severe aphasic is something like this: His speech will not be as it was before. It may be a little better, but recovery will be hard and slow, and nothing will come easily. The first thing he can do is to try to listen as well as he can. This will help more than anything else. While he is in the hospital, we will try to get the speech mechanism working a little better. We will work on listening, and trying to hear words clearly. Is there anyone who can help him when he goes home, if we show them what to do? The most important thing however, will be to try to find things he enjoys doing so that he may live as normally as possible in spite of the difficulty he has talking. This takes courage but is worth doing.

Whenever possible, one should try to get the patient to the point where he can repeat words and phrases, and produce common associations. This increases reactive speech, and makes the patient appear more responsive. This in turn helps people respond more naturally to the patient. One has only to contrast the social responsiveness of a severely aphasic patient like Mr. Saunders with the withdrawn habits of many nonaphasic inmates of our poorer public institutions, to appreciate the importance of maintaining communicative attitudes. Communication is not altogether dependent upon verbal facility.

When it is feasible, one should try to teach the patient to tell time, make change, and sign his name, and encourage him to go to chapel if he is accustomed to attending church services, to watch television, go to movies with other patients, look through magazines, and read the headlines in the newspaper when he can.

FAMILY COUNSELING

The first objective of family counseling is to help the family to understand and accept the limitations imposed by severe aphasia. There are three important facets of this phase of counseling: The first is acceptance of the fact that no dramatic changes can be expected. There is a positive aspect even to such negative information. It means that resources of time and energy and money that might have been fruitlessly expended on treatment for aphasia are released for more potentially productive ends.

The second important facet is the very positive one of making it clear that the aphasic patient is neither feeble-minded nor mentally deranged. This is such a common fear or misapprehension that it should always be dealt with openly. The aphasic disability should be clearly delimited.

The family should understand that the patient will not understand everything people say. They should know that he will understand best if they say something simply, in a short sentence, and give him time to grasp one idea before they go on to another. He will follow most easily when he is talking to only one person at a time. They should know that aphasia affects reading and writing as well as speech. Above all, they should know that the patient is reasonable and dependable and that he needs to be treated as a responsible adult. He should have a voice in family decisions, and should be encouraged to be independent. The best thing that anyone can do for him is to make him feel that he is needed and has an important place in the family.

The third important facet is achieving and maintaining communication. This is usually facilitated if the wife, for example, sits down and works with her husband on his speech for a little while every day when he first goes home. The clinician can teach her what to do with the idea that this stimulation enables him to respond to what is going on around him a little more adequately, and so prevents withdrawal and depression.

The second important overall objective of family counseling is to help the family and the patient make the best possible adjustment to the altered situation. It is essential to stress the importance of living as normally as possible within the limitations imposed by the illness.

Probably the single most effective thing that can be done is to set up a systematic and regular daily routine for the patient. This structures his days, and gives him a feeling of confidence and security, as well as something to get up for and to look forward to.

The wife of one aphasic patient described the routine they established something like this.

> We get up and have breakfast together, then James goes downstairs and exercises for an hour, while I do up the morning work. He has a shower, and rests a little, and then we have coffee, together. After coffee, I help him with his lessons. I give him some words to copy, or sometimes we write a letter to one of the children. I write down what he wants to tell them,

and he copies the letter, and looks through the paper or a magazine while I get our lunch. After lunch he rests for two hours. Usually he sleeps. After that I try to get him out for a while if the weather is at all possible. We do some errands, or some marketing, or go for a little drive. Sometimes, when it is nice we sit out on the lawn. We feed the birds, and James has become quite interested in them. When we come in, I usually read something to him from the paper, or one of the news magazines. He usually watches a news program while I get dinner. Before dinner we always have an old-fashioned, and James smokes one cigarette. This is always a pleasant time, and we both look forward to it. After dinner, we listen to records until James is ready to go to bed.

On Wednesday Annie comes and gets James' lunch, and I try to get out. We do his lessons after breakfast on that day, and then I leave. I do a little shopping, and sometimes go to the club for lunch, and stay for the afternoon program. Sometimes I have luncheon with a friend, or make a few calls. I'm always home early enough to spend some time with James before dinner.

On Friday night, I try to invite one or two people James enjoys to come for dinner. We have our drink before dinner and usually music afterwards, just as usual, and I think he looks forward to this. Usually Jim Junior comes and takes him out for lunch on Saturday. They eat downtown, and James sees people he knows. They come over and talk to him, which he enjoys. We go to church on Sunday, and usually the children come over for a while in the afternoon. They love James and crawl all over him, and he loves it. He talks quite a bit to them, too. We really get along very pleasantly.

This program has all the essential things in it. The days are structured with intervals of rest and activity. The little rites of morning coffee, a drink before dinner, and music afterwards provide pleasant interludes. There are periods of companionship and periods of independent activity, which everyone needs. There are changes of scene, and, of extreme importance, arrangements for continued associations with other people, which are stimulating and help to avert depression and withdrawal. The daily exercise with simple pulley apparatus prescribed by the Corrective Therapy Department is important for maintaining circulation and preventing stiffness and soreness. Periods of working and resting alone help the patient to develop confidence and independence, and gradually overcome the fears that helplessness engenders.

The patient whose program we have described was limited by severe disabilities. A patient with less severe hemiplegia walked around a small lake every morning except in the most inclement weather. Another man, with no functional speech, walked downtown daily, went to the barber shop, and did occasional shopping on his own. Other patients have enjoyed hobbies such as weaving, building bird houses, feeding birds, and indoor and outdoor gardening.

It is not easy for a man who has been busy and active all his life to alter his way of living, and settle for what he sometimes regards as trivial occupations. Adjustments are facilitated, however, if the patient receives enough counseling in the hospital to understand the importance of keeping himself active and stimulated, of having a regular routine, and of developing increasing independence. It is usually easier for a patient to accept a plan that has been set up for him by professional counselors, and one that he has had a part in making, than well-meant suggestions from members of his own family.

With a severely aphasic patient, it is usually desirable to have the clinician gather together the recommendations from all departments and spend as much time as necessary working through the essential parts of the program with the patient. This is simply because the clinician usually knows the patient best and can communicate with him most effectively. On the other hand, it is preferable that the patient's wife, or whoever is responsible for planning, interview the physician and other staff members who have worked with the patient directly. We prefer to talk to the wife alone about any difficulties that can be foreseen, and then to have a final interview with the patient and his wife together, and work through the details again. We usually send home materials and typed instructions, and suggest that they send us reports at regular intervals.

The results are often better than anyone could anticipate. Once a good routine has been established, the days pass quickly and pleasantly. Ten years after her husband incurred severe hemiplegia and aphasia, Mrs. Saunders wrote:

> Reed's greatest progress is in awareness or alertness. He handles himself more like a well man. He takes care of his daily medication entirely. I never have to remind him that it is pill time. I help him wash his hair, and manicure his nails. The rest he does—chooses his clothes, dresses, keeps his shoes shined, et cetera. He always shaves before he comes to breakfast. He does dishes, shovels snow (how, no one can figure!), rakes leaves, puts the trash out for collection—remembering the first Thursday of the month—had a garden, mows the lawn with a hand mower, et cetera. The neighbors are aghast at all he manages. He doesn't seem to mind being on his own all day—I think he rather enjoys it—and we go out some, for dinner, or the evening. This winter we have even managed a restaurant with a revolving door!
>
> I have a few observations—of all the men we have known who had aphasia when Reed did, few are still alive. The ones who are had tender, loving care at home. That may not prove anything. A wife has to reorganize her life, I think, if she is to successfully cope with aphasia —I don't think it can be 'fitted in' to a former routine.

The best results we have seen were all those where a new routine, adapted to the abilities, interests, and limitations of the patient, and to the needs and interests of the rest of the family as well, was thoughtfully planned and systematically adhered to. This adherence, should not, of course, be slavish. Details can be altered according to changes in circumstances. Everything, however, cannot be left to chance.

PATIENTS WITH LIMITED RECOVERY OF LANGUAGE

The patients in this category are largely Sensorimotor patients, those with severe aphasia complicated by sensorimotor impairment. These patients should receive from six months to a year of intensive daily treatment for aphasia. Initially they can do almost nothing to help themselves, and can get very little without intensive controlled auditory stimulation. Formal treatment must be continued until the patient has achieved a firm basis upon which to build. Gains are inevitably lost unless the patient acquires enough language to be able to respond to the verbal stimulation in his environment. This means, in general, that he must have a functional speaking vocabulary, a basic reading and spelling vocabulary, and enough phonetic concepts to give him clues to words he does not know. In short, he must have stable tools to work with.

When a patient cannot be seen by the clinician every day, it is necessary to train someone to practice with him, or make arrangements for him to work with an instrument, such as the Language Master, which provides simultaneous visual and auditory stimulation. It is extremely unrealistic to expect that patients who cannot discriminate and retain auditory patterns can profit from a half hour of treatment once or twice a week.

Sometimes, when circumstances are favorable, we have recommended that patients spend the first six months working systematically with someone at home under the supervision of the clinic, and then come into the hospital. This is only possible when there is someone who can work effectively with the patient, and who can carry out instructions intelligently and sensibly. It permits the patient to come into the hospital when the slow initial gains have been made, and he is ready to handle more complicated materials and procedures, and to move more rapidly from one level to another. This is the period when it is most important to have a highly-trained clinician with enough experience to know how to alter methods to keep pace with favorable changes as they occur, and to utilize them to the best advantage.

It is important that plans be made for treatment to be continued when these patients leave the hospital, since, as we know, significant recovery continues over periods of years. This is the crux of planning for Sensorimotor patients.

The optimal discharge plan is one that permits the patient to live at home and receive treatment at an outpatient clinic. This is usually possible only for patients who live in or near large population centers. Sometimes, particularly with young patients, we have made arrangements for them to attend a university clinic with a full-time program. This also necessitates being away from home, but it provides an atmosphere that is more like a college than a hospital in many ways, so that it is another step towards independence and normalcy.

Very often, we train a member of the family to work with the patient at home, sending home materials and instructions, and making arrangements to follow the patient through correspondence, or through periodic reevaluations in selected cases.

When there is no one in the family who is able to do this, we look for someone in the community. Sometimes there has been a public school speech correctionist who has had experience with aphasia, or, in the absence of such experience, is willing to work with an aphasic patient with guidance from the clinic. Sometimes a retired teacher has been an excellent clinician, when given enough tutelage to understand that stimulation rather than instruction is required.

Vocational psychologists have often contributed most significantly to the discharge planning of patients with limited language, suggesting and arranging vocational or prevocational programs or employment. Vocational counseling is more successful toward the end of the treatment period, when the clinical picture is more promising than at the beginning.

It is most important that patients with limited language understand that there will be improvement as long as they continue to work systematically, although it will not be rapid. They should know also that recovery will take a long time, so that the regime they establish must be comfortable, rewarding, and reasonable. They need to relax and play as well as work, and, again, to live as normally as possible.

FAMILY COUNSELING

Since there are more young patients, with young families, in this group, there are often more family problems to be worked through. Aphasia can be a severe handicap in dealing with children or adolescents, and the aphasic patient often feels more insecure and inadequate in these relationships than in any others.

There are several things that help in most cases. One is for the children to be given complete and honest information about what has happened, and what it means. What the children are told, and the way the information is presented, is different for young people of different ages, but they should all know that their father or mother has been very ill, and what the effects of the illness have been. They should know what he can do, and what he cannot do, and that he will tire more easily than before. Their questions should be answered honestly, and they should have a part in making plans for the parent's homecoming. Children are much more secure when they are given straightforward information than when they sense that something is wrong, and are left with vague and formless fears and anxieties.

Children cannot be expected or required to be always quiet and considerate. Both parents should realize that the aphasic patient, however, may have limited tolerance of noise and confusion, and try to plan a family routine to reconcile the needs of children and adults. Different methods are effective in different families. Sometimes a basement area, for example, can be set aside for active play. Sometimes it is easier to arrange a relatively quiet room to which the parent can retire. In one family the father made a practice of not coming downstairs until the children were off to school; then he and his wife had a leisurely breakfast together. In another family the mother gave the small children an early supper, and they watched a favorite television program while the parents had dinner. After this, the father took over the bedtime rituals, and reversed the usual procedures by letting the children take turns telling stories to him. Another father took one child at a time on a Saturday expedition to a museum, a park, or a movie. He could not manage three active children, but he could have a pleasant time with each one in turn.

It usually works better with older children if the parent with moderately severe aphasia agrees to leave discipline to the other parent. This is sometimes hard for the parent who has to handle all the problems and for the one who has to school himself to keep hands off, but it prevents situations that are frequently catastrophic for the entire family. If problems are talked over by both parents and policies agreed on, most of the evils are averted. The aphasic parent does not feel excluded, and the parent who administers the discipline has the support of the other. In one family where this policy worked very well, a 13-year-old boy often sought his father's approval. He once said seriously to his father, "Dad, Mom doesn't understand that I'm old enough to have a job. Try to make her see that it's all right for me to work after school, will you? If I keep my grades up?" The mother was wise enough to encourage this masculine solidarity, which meant a great deal to both father and son.

One woman who was wise about living used to say that a home should meet the needs of every member of the family. This is a particularly important consideration in post-discharge planning. A plan will not work that overlooks the mother's needs for rest and occasional respite from family care. A program will not work that requires children to behave like adults. A plan will not work that places demands on the aphasic parent that make him feel helpless and defeated.

There are always problems, but problems can be solved more easily when they are anticipated, and when the family receives some preparation for handling them. Aphasia is a new problem for most families, and most families need professional help in adjusting to it. Not to provide such help is to jeopardize all that the best rehabilitation clinics can accomplish. Counseling cannot always be successful. However, in spite of occasional and tragic failures, we are impressed with the ability of the human race to survive disaster and to carry on in the face of difficulties. We have learned a great deal from our clients, and have far more reason to pay tribute to their courage than to be critical of their shortcomings.

PATIENTS WITH MILD APHASIC DISABILITIES

Because the period of hospitalization is usually comparatively short, patients with mild aphasic disabilities usually require an interim plan to enable them to return to full-time employment. The nature of this plan depends upon the patient's ultimate goals.

For young patients who wish to return to college, we usually recommend beginning with a modified academic program. Some patients have started by working in the university speech or reading clinic, and taking one additional course. It is desirable to arrange that the returning student be followed by the university counseling service, so that problems can be solved as they arise and failure prevented. One patient with mild residual aphasia found he could not follow the lectures of an instructor who habitually talked very fast. In another class section where listening was less taxing for him, he did very well.

Several aphasic patients have reported that a course in public speaking helped them to gain facility in expressing ideas, and to recover confidence. English composition, algebra, and foreign languages have been the most difficult courses. Many patients with mild residual aphasia require special tutoring to pass courses that require learning of a new symbol system, and courses like this should probably be deferred as long as possible. The most important considerations seem to be that the course load should not be too heavy, and that understanding counseling should be available.

Sometimes vocational or prevocational courses have served as stepping stones to college, or to returning to a job. Patients have taken remedial courses in arithmetic, English composition, typing, and reading, as well as in other vocational subjects. Patients who were retired have joined a Dale Carnegie Group, a Great Books Club, or taken an evening course in fields that ranged from archeology to current events, for intellectual stimulation.

When the patient should attempt to go back to work is always an individual decision. If he returns too soon, he may become discouraged by difficulties he encounters and jeopardize his chances for eventual success. On the other hand, if he waits too long, he may become increasingly fearful of going back and increase mental hazards to a paralyzing degree. The optimal plan is probably for the patient to begin with a modified schedule and gradually increase the scope of his activities, as his tolerance and confidence return. This plan has the advantage of being stimulating and rewarding without being threatening, but it is not always possible to arrange.

The recommendations of vocational psychologists are invaluable in helping aphasic patients reach vocational decisions. Vocational counselors need information from the speech pathologist, and vice versa, so that cooperative planning is clearly to the best interest of the patient. The vocational counselor is better equipped to evaluate vocational potentials and job requirements, and the speech pathologist to predict and explain difficulties the aphasic patient can be expected to encounter.

The patient with mild residual aphasia should understand that many tasks will be difficult the first time he attempts them but will become easier with practice. If the patient knows this, he will react less catastrophically to the occasional failures he encounters. He will be more willing to try new things if he realizes that this is the way to recovery, and that trying something new can be scored as a victory for his side, regardless of the outcome. An aphasic patient will certainly not succeed in all new undertakings, but like the patient who won the spelling match, he will sometimes win when he did not think he could, and he will gain increasing confidence in his ability to handle the problems aphasia presents. Certainly the realization that one can fail sometimes and go on from there is an important strength for anyone to acquire.

FAMILY COUNSELING

The most important objective in family counseling with patients with mild residual aphasia is usually to enable them to understand the real difficulties under which the patient labors. These are not obvious because he sounds so normal most of the time. When Bill Masterson lectured dogmatically to his wife when she was busy and tired and could brook no interruptions, she did not understand that this behavior resulted from his anxiety that he would forget what he wanted to say and fail to communicate something important to both of them, and that he could not stop to listen to her without losing his own train of thought.

It is sometimes difficult for the family to understand why a man with mild aphasia can talk so well in some situations, and on an important occasion or in a crucial interview say almost nothing. They need to be told that newly regained skills are not stable and tend to disintegrate under tension. They must acquire the insight that the aphasic patient does as well as he can *in a given situation*, so that they do not misjudge him and think that he just decided to make no effort through some kind of obstinacy or perversity. They need to understand that the effort to communicate makes situations stressful to the aphasic patient that were not stressful before, and that his ability to withstand prolonged pressures of this kind is limited. They need to become aware of signs of tension, and to learn how to keep them from mounting to catastrophic proportions.

The patient with mild residual aphasia can make his own plans and decisions, and handle most of his own problems. The important thing is to be able to talk over problems that arise, and work out solutions for them. Problems are not trivial because aphasia is mild. The problems of mild aphasia are often exceedingly critical, because the potential for achievement is so great. To disregard them is comparable to saying we shall not bother about gifted students because they will get along all right anyhow.

THE ROLE OF THE PHYSICIAN IN LONG-RANGE PLANNING WITH APHASIC PATIENTS

The physician's role in long-term planning is of primary importance for all aphasic patients. We have no hesitation in saying that no planning should be done without medical concurrence. The inexorable fact of aphasia is that it is a symptom of cerebral disorder. Involvement may extend throughout the cerebrovascular and the cardiovascular system. The patient who is discharged from the hospital has survived the initial insult, but he must learn to live within new neurophysiological limits.

There are almost always some ongoing medical problems such as prevention or control of seizures, of hypertension, or of arteriosclerotic disease. The physician is responsible for medication and for the entire physiological regime of the patient. He may alter medication from time to time as indications occur. He may prescribe some forms of activity and restrict or prohibit others.

The physician is a source of important psychological support to the patient and his family. His knowledge and familiarity with diverse aspects of disease and trauma relieve the fear, the anxiety, and the apprehension that may attend them. His calm authority reassures the patient, and enables him to develop a confident attitude toward recovery.

More than anyone else, the physician can help the patient accept the residuals of illness, and view them in perspective. One of our patients was a retired executive who incurred a slight stroke with mild aphasia, and made an excellent recovery. Before he left the hospital, he was asked to resume his former position for an interim period. The patient thought he could handle the work, and was inclined to consider it his duty to go back. The physician told him not to do it. He explained that the patient did not have the neurophysiological reserves to sustain the pressures the position involved. He advised the patient to be content with his long record of distinguished service, and the honorable retirement he had earned. The patient commented later, "I liked having them ask me to come back, but I did not know how relieved I would be to have someone take the decision out of my hands."

On the other hand, some patients are afraid to attempt the exercise and activity they need to maintain physical well-being, and to achieve maximal restitution of functions. These patients need the reassurance and encouragement of the physician to enable them to move in the direction of recovery.

The role of the speech pathologist is very different. His job is to stimulate the patient's mind, relieve the isolation of aphasia, and give the patient the tools with which to become a thinking and a communicating individual. Today, however, few people believe that mind and body are divorced from one another. It is important that disciplines work together to the best interest of the aphasic patient.

The problems of aphasia can be understood only through the resources of the many disciplines that deal with theoretical and clinical aspects of human behavior in health and in disease. The problems of recovery from aphasia and the complex in which it occurs can be solved only through individuals trained in the various professional services concerned with rehabilitation processes.

One of our thoughtful informants distilled the following from his experience with aphasia: "Life is good. Through recovery, this is what I have been trying to prove . . . I decided that the greatest contribution I could make would be to demonstrate that we could recover from war. . . ."

It seems appropriate to close this monograph with the recognition that recovery from aphasia, whatever the etiology and whatever the degree of recovery achieved, represents a triumph of the human spirit over adversity. We trust that our patients will know that in a deep sense this book is theirs.

NEUROLOGICAL BACKGROUND FOR
APHASIA

The development of human language is a combined result of anatomical adaptations and unique cerebral integrative mechanisms acquired in man's evolutionary progress. Throughout the book in describing language behavior, we refer repeatedly to the organization of the human brain. This Appendix discusses relevant aspects of cerebral anatomy and physiology to provide some guidance for readers untrained in neurology.

THE GENERAL ORGANIZATION OF THE BRAIN

The brain is the enlarged portion of the central nervous system that lies within the cranial cavity. It is divided into three parts:

1. The *hind brain*, or *rhombencephalon*, which includes the medulla, pons, and cerebellum.
2. The *midbrain*, or *mesencephalon*, which includes the quadrigeminal plate and cerebral peduncles.
3. The *forebrain*, or *prosencephalon*, which is subdivided into an endbrain, or telencephalon, and an interbrain or diencephalon. The *endbrain* consists of the cerebral cortex, corpora striata, rhinencephalon, and the optical part of the hypothalamus. The *interbrain* consists of the epithalamus, thalamus, subthalamus, and hypothalamus.

THE CEREBRAL HEMISPHERES

The longitudinal fissure divides the endbrain into two cerebral hemispheres. These are connected by fiber tracts known as commissural fibers. Each hemisphere has been divided into five major areas known as the frontal, parietal, temporal, occipital, and insular lobes, as shown in Fig. 1. This is not, however, a true anatomical or functional division; it is based on the topographical relation of these areas to the skull, and arbitrary lines determine some of the boundaries. Sulci or fissures on the surface of the brain determine some of the lobes. The term *sulci* originally designated furrows which do not go through the whole thickness of the hemisphere, while *fissures* were considered to have a counterpart on the ventricular side. However, these words have been used interchangeably in the literature. In addition to the five major lobes, the gyrus fornicatus on the medial aspect of the hemisphere is sometimes referred to as the limbic lobe. It includes the cingulate gyrus, the isthmus, the hippocampal gyrus, and uncus.

The boundaries of the cerebral lobes are as follows (Crosby *et al.*, 1962):

1. Dorsolateral aspect (Fig. 1A). The frontal lobe extends from the frontal pole to the central sulcus of Rolando, and the Sylvian fissure defines its inferior border. The parietal lobe is separated from the frontal lobe by the central sulcus, but since its borders with the temporal and occipital lobe are indiscernible, they have been arbitrarily defined. A vertical line from the parietooccipital fissure to the preoccipital notch separates the parietal from the occipital lobe, while a horizontal line from the lateral fissure to the parietooccipital line separates the parietal from the temporal lobe. The insula lies buried beneath the Sylvian fissure.

2. Medial aspect (Fig. 1B). The cingulate gyrus forms the inferior border of the frontal lobe. A line dropped from the tip of the central sulcus to the cingulate sulcus defines its posterior border. From this line the parietal lobe extends posteriorly up to the parietooccipital fissure. Its inferior border is limited by the subparietal sulcus, which is an extension of the cingulate sulcus. The occipital lobe is bounded dorsally and rostrally by the preoccipital fissure, and ventrally by the collateral fissure. The cingulate and subparietal sulci form the dorsal boundary of the limbic lobe. This lobe is limited ventrally by the sulcus of the corpus callosum, posteriorly by the subparietal sulcus, and is separated from the occipital lobe by a line drawn from the anterior calcarine fissure to the preoccipital notch.

3. Ventral aspect (Fig. 1B). The frontal lobe includes the olfactory structures, several orbital gyri, and the gyrus rectus. The anterior border of the temporal lobe overlaps the caudal portion of the orbital gyri; medially it is limited by the collateral fissure. Its caudal border includes the inferior temporal and fusiform gyri.

Each lobe, with its cerebral, central, and peripheral interconnections, contributes to speech and language processes. The frontal lobe is essential to motor activities of the entire body. Thus, it participates in the production of speech, which requires well-coordinated movements of the lips, tongue, soft palate, larynx, and the muscles of respiration. The anterior areas of the frontal lobes appear to maintain the integrity of the personality and intellect. Rylander (1948) demonstrated that lobotomized patients lose many of their interests and may show intellectual deficits. Greenblatt and Solomon

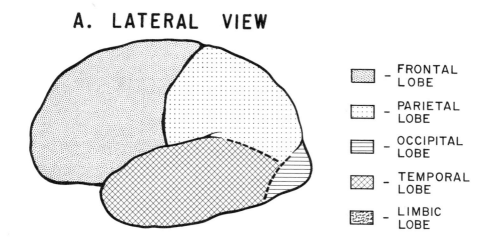

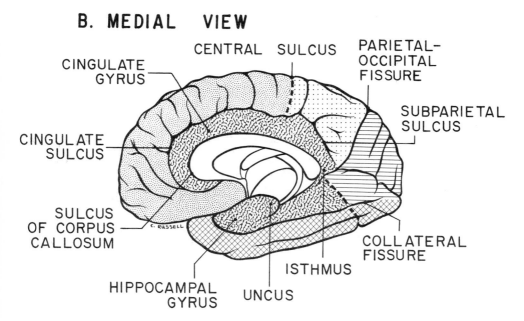

Fig. A–1. The lobes of the cerebral hemisphere.

(1958) characterized the results of total bilateral frontal lobotomy as a reduction of drive and incentive, and added that although anxiety was decreased, the patient led a more shallow life emotionally.

The temporal lobe has an auditory function, and also has been shown to be involved with such complex processes as language, memory, and vision (Penfield and Rasmussen, 1950; Kluver and Bucy, 1939). Movements of the face and jaw have followed stimulation of the temporal tips and the amygdaloid nucleus in man (Baldwin *et al.*, 1954) and monkey (Schneider and Crosby, 1954).

The limbic lobe plays an important role in the retention of recent memory and attention. The amygdala, which is included as part of the limbic lobe by some authors, receives visceral afferent fibers and has direct connections with the hypothalamus and orbitofrontal cortex. These connections allow the amygdala to play an important role in the control of emotions, conditional reflexes, motivation, and reinforcement. Damage to the human medial temporal lobe including the posterior left hippocampus and crus of the left fornix produces loss of recent memory (Smith and Smith, 1966).

The parietal lobe plays a role in the discrimination of size, shape, and texture, and helps maintain awareness of body movements and of the position of the body in space. It has motor functions, also. Complex movements—such as conjugate deviation of the eyes to the opposite side of the body, and flexion and extension movements of the contralateral limbs—have followed parietal stimulation (Peele, 1944; Fleming and Crosby, 1955). In a monkey, these responses have been described as simulating running, turning, and avoidance movements.

The occipital lobe has visual functions. Bilateral destruction of the occipital cortex is followed by cortical blindness. In man, however, the pupillary light reflex is retained, and some visual impressions are probably mediated by the quadrigeminal bodies. Stimulation of the visual cortex produces visual hallucinations of color, light, movement, and elementary forms. Stimulation of the visual cortex in primates has been followed by movements of the face, limbs, and trunk.

The insula is concerned with intraabdominal sensation, gastric motility, and tone (Penfield and Faulk, 1955; Frontera, 1956). Speech functions have been ascribed to it, although conclusive evidence for this is lacking.

The usual indices of physiological maturation of the brain are differentiation of cells, myelinization of nerve fibers, and spontaneous electrical cortical activity (Lindsley, 1938; Smith, 1938). At birth, or shortly thereafter, maturation is most advanced in the primary sensorimotor, visual, auditory, and olfactory areas of the human brain (Vogt, 1898; Langworthy, 1933). Fibers in these areas are the first to become myelinated, while in other areas, such as the prefrontal lobe, the myelin sheath does not develop until several months after birth. The sleeping newborn infant shows rhythmical activity of various frequencies and amplitudes over the sensorimotor complex. By contrast, the prefrontal and occipital areas barely show any electrical activity. By the third month, however, frequencies of 3–4 per second appear in the occipital cortex. It is in this period that the infant begins to respond to objects in his field of vision, and to follow them with eye movements.

THE CEREBRAL CORTEX

The outer superficial gray mantle of the cerebral hemisphere is known as the cerebral cortex. It contains about 14 billion cells and about 200 million incoming and outgoing projection fibers (Kappers *et al.*, 1960). In most of the cortex, six layers, or laminae—based on the arrangement and the density of the cells—are recognized.

Four major cell types are found in these layers. Lorente De Nó (1933) has classified them as cells with descending, cells with short, cells with ascending, and cells with horizontal axons. Cells with descending axons send processes to the lower cortical laminae, or their axons may leave the cortex as projection or association fibers. The giant pyramidal cells of Betz, which contribute fibers to the corticospinal tract, are cells of the first type. Cells with short axons are, in other words, rich in dendrites, as they have many arborizations near the cell body. Cells with ascending axons give off collaterals to one or more of the cortical laminae as they pass upward to Layer I. Both the axons and dendrites of cells with horizontal axons are confined to Layer I of the cortex. On the other hand, cells with short and ascending axons are found in all layers, and interconnect all layers.

The most important information obtained from cytoarchitectonic and myeloarchitectonic studies of the cortex may be summarized as follows:

1. The cells that form Layer I do not send axons outside the cortex. This layer receives nonspecific or sensory fibers.
2. Layers I and II are well developed in man. They receive collaterals from fibers belonging to association, commissural, and nonspecific afferent systems. Layer III may receive collaterals from specific afferent fibers. Therefore, these laminae are involved in receptive and associative processes.
3. Layer IV receives specific afferent fibers from the thalamus, and is chiefly a receptive zone.
4. Layers V and VI give rise to association, commissural, and projection fibers, and receive collaterals from incoming association, commissural, and nonspecific afferent fibers.

Thus, the cortical cells and their fibers constitute a dense mat, or network, that permits tremendously complicated patterns of activity.

ASSOCIATION AND PROJECTION FIBERS

Cortical areas within each hemisphere are interconnected by association fibers of varying length. Short fibers may be cortical or subcortical. The subcortical fibers that connect adjacent gyri are known as arcuate association fibers. These are shown in Fig. 2. Longer fibers, shown in Fig. 3, connect lobes within one cerebral hemisphere. For example, the uncinate fibers connect the anterior aspect of the frontal, limbic, and temporal lobes, and the inferior occipitofrontal fibers connect the frontal and occipital lobes. However, not all cortical areas possess long association fibers (Dusser de Barenne and McCulloch, 1938; Le Gros Clark, 1940–1941; Lashley, 1958).

Lashley (1958) investigated the importance of transcortical fibers in visual performances, maze learning, and retention in rats by excising the cortex in various planes. He found no deficits in the performances he tested that could be attributed to the cuts. Using a similar technique, Sperry (1947, 1958) demonstrated a lack of any significant functional disorganization resulting from severing transcortical connections in cats and monkeys. Penfield and Roberts (1959) have reported similar findings for man.

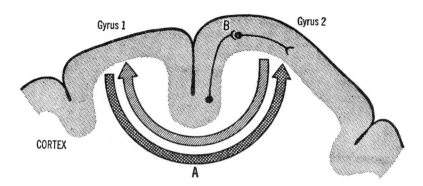

Fig. A-2. Short association fibers. **A,** Arcuate fibers. **B,** Intracortical fiber.

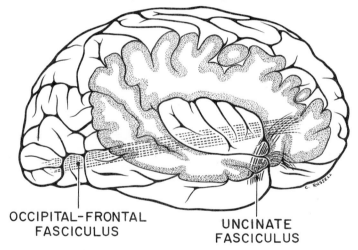

OCCIPITAL-FRONTAL
FASCICULUS

UNCINATE
FASCICULUS

Fig. A-3. Long association fibers in the primate. Ulcinate fibers connect frontal, limbic and temporal lobes. Occipitofrontal fibers connect the frontal and occipital lobes.

Fibers that connect the two hemispheres are known as commissural fibers. These are shown in Fig. 4. The most prominent commissural tracts are the corpus callosum, and the anterior and hippocampal commissures. The corpus callosum is the largest of them all; it is also an avenue for decussating fibers (Locke and Yakovlev, 1965). Many homotopic and heterotopic cortical areas are connected by the corpus callosum. In monkeys, some areas such as the visual cortex (area 17) and those representing the distal segments of the fore and hind limbs in somatosensory cortices I and II do not receive any commissural fibers. Recent studies in animals have confirmed the distribution of corpus callosal fibers to all cortical layers (Heimer et al., 1967; Jones and Powell, 1969). Bremer (1958) showed that impulses in the corpus callosum facilitate the cortical

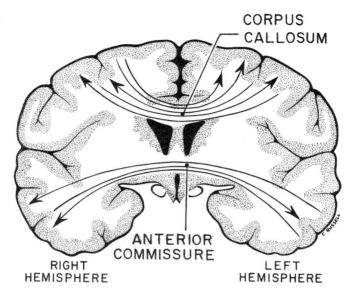

Fig. A–4. Commissural fibers. The commissural fibers connect homologous areas of the cerebral hemispheres.

responses to a thalamocortical volley. He also demonstrated that impulses from specific thalamic somatosensory nuclei are conveyed to the ipsilateral sensory cortex, then relayed to the opposite homologous area by way of the corpus callosum. Myers (1956) demonstrated the importance of the corpus callosum in transferring visual information from one hemisphere to the other. He sectioned the optic chiasm in cats, then, with one eye covered, trained them in visual discrimination tasks. Next he sectioned the corpus callosum, and covered the trained eye. Subsequently the animals could not perform the tasks that had been learned through the opposite eye. Sperry (1958) reported similar results on tasks involving tactile discriminations. Different types of disconnection syndromes follow injury to association fibers (Geshwind, 1965).

Akelaitis (1943, 1944) emphasized the absence of any neurological deficits following transection of the corpus callosum and the anterior commissure in man. Recently Goldstein and Joynt (1969) reported on a 27-year followup of a patient originally studied by Akelaitis. The corpus callosum of the patient had been sectioned, except for some fibers in the splenium. In the followup, this patient showed deficits in transfer of training in manual tasks and in crossed visual tactile identification. These findings were not reported by Akelaitis, but they probably were present at that time.

Additional reports emphasize the functional deficits after disconnection of the cerebral hemispheres. Visual motor coordination between two hemispheres depends on transcallosal delivery of visual information from one hemisphere to the other (Gazzaniga et al., 1965; Lehman, 1968). Smith (1951) concluded that destruction of most interhemispheral fibers in man is followed by inconsistent diminution of ability to transfer motor function to the opposite side of the body, when learned with the preferred side. Maspes (1948) concluded that the corpus callosum transfers information between hemispheres, citing two cases of visual impairment which followed sectioning the posterior third of the corpus callosum. An interesting case studied by Geshwind and Kaplan (1962) supports these observations. Gazzaniga and Sperry (1967) studied language function after section of the cerebral commissures. Their results indicate almost total control of speech, writing, and calculation by the major hemisphere, while comprehension of language—both spoken and written—was found to be represented in the minor as well as the major hemisphere.

The anterior commissure has an anterior and a posterior limb. The anterior limb is associated with the olfactory system, while the posterior limb interconnects the two middle temporal gyri. Whether or not it has any significance in relation to language processes is not known.

The hippocampal commissure connects the hippocampal regions of both hemispheres. The hippocampi have been implicated in memory mechanisms, emotions, visceral activities, and in the general suppressor system of the forebrain.

Projection fibers connect the cerebral cortex with the brain stem and the spinal cord. They are classified as afferent, or incoming fibers, and efferent, or outgoing fibers. Among the afferent projection fibers are the visual, the auditory, and the thalamic radiations. Efferent fibers include the corticothalamic, the corticobulbar, and the corticospinal tracts, which carry impulses from the cortex to the thalamus, the brain stem, and the spinal cord. Afferent and efferent pathways have connections at various levels that permit events in one pathway to modify events in another.

THE DORSAL THALAMUS AND ITS PROJECTIONS

The subcortical connections which relate the cortex to the brain stem are indispensable, and are of major importance in effecting the integrations required for speech. The dorsal thalamus, commonly referred to as the thalamus, plays a key role in the integration of neural systems. This is a large nuclear mass centrally located within the cerebrum. It has been divided into five main groups of nuclei, namely, the anterior, medial, lateral, and posterior nuclei, and the nuclei of the midline. Each major group is subdivided into smaller groups.

The dorsal thalamus receives incoming afferent impulses, and relays them through thalamocortical fibers into the cortex. In return, it probably receives corticothalamic fibers from all cortical areas. Thalamocortical fibers have been classified as belonging to specific or to nonspecific (diffuse) projecting systems (Dempsey and Morison, 1942a,b; Morison and Dempsey, 1942; Jasper, 1949). The specific projecting systems are sometimes classified as follows:

1. Primary afferent relay systems (Fig. 5A). Fibers belonging to the primary afferent relay system originate in the posterior ventral nucleus of the thalamus, and in the medial and lateral geniculate bodies. The posterior ventral nucleus receives somesthetic sensation from the periphery of the body through the medial lemniscus, spinothalamic, and secondary trigeminal tracts, and relays them to the primary somatosensory cortex in the postcentral gyrus. The medial geniculate receives auditory impulses through the lateral lemniscus and relays them to the primary auditory cortex in the supratemporal transverse gyrus. The lateral geniculate body

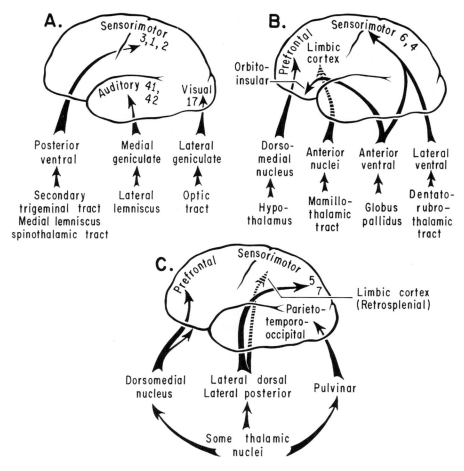

Fig. A–5. Specific thalamocortical projections in man. The diagrams show the main sensory imput to the thalamic relay nuclei and their cortical projections. **A,** Primary afferent relay systems. **B,** Secondary afferent relay systems. **C,** Specific elaborative systems.

receives fibers from the optic tract, and projects them to the primary visual cortex, which is the striate area in the occipital lobe.

2. Secondary afferent relay fibers (Fig. 5B). Secondary afferent fibers arise from the anterior ventral nuclei, the lateral ventral nuclei, the anterior nuclei, and portions of the dorsomedial nuclei in the thalamus. The anterior ventral nuclei receives fibers from the globus pallidus, and projects them to the motor area and orbitoinsular region of the frontal lobe, while the lateral ventral nucleus receives cerebellar impulses through the dentatorubrothalamic tract, and conveys them to the frontal motor cortex. In addition, the anterior nucleus of the thalamus sends radiations to the limbic cortex, and the dorsomedial nucleus receives fibers from the hypothalamus and other nuclei, and projects them to the prefrontal cortical field.

3. Specific elaborative systems (Fig. 5C). Fibers in this system arise from parts of the

dorsomedial, lateral dorsal, lateral posterior, and pulvinar nuclei. The dorsomedial nucleus projects to the prefrontal area. The lateral dorsal and lateral posterior nuclei project to the parietal lobe exclusive of the postcentral gyrus and limbic cortex, while the pulvinar projects to the superior parietal lobule, part of the adjoining occipital cortex, and the angular and supramarginal gyri in the parieto-temporal region.

The diffuse thalamic system is a polysynaptic system through which excitation spreads to all cortical areas. Its fibers originate in various thalamic nuclei, including the intralaminar, rhomboid, central medial, limitans, suprageniculatis, ventralis anterior and medialis, and reuniens. This system is capable of controlling the spontaneous rhythm of the brain within the 8–12 second frequencies. It cannot block the arrival of primary or secondary impulses to the cortex, but can inhibit cortical activity set in action by primary sensory stimuli. This may be a mechanism by which the thalamus influences differential cortical activity. Interaction between diffuse and specific systems occurs through collaterals from the principal sensory pathways that end in the intralaminar nuclei, collaterals from intralaminar to specific thalamic nuclei, overlapping cortical projections, and projections from the cortex to the thalamus.

The diffuse system, therefore, can receive afferent impulses through transcortical connections, spinothalamic tracts (Dusser de Barenne, 1935), and fibers within the reticular formation of the brain stem. Impulses affecting one nucleus eventually spread to affect all nonspecific nuclei. This allows for a diffuse cortical spread of ascending or descending impulses. Some authors do not even favor designating thalamic nuclei as specific or nonspecific, in view of current anatomical and physiological data which emphasize their close interrelation (Scheibel and Scheibel, 1967; Brodal, 1969).

It is convenient to divide the cortex into extrinsic and intrinsic sectors, based on the type of thalamic projections to specific cortical areas. The extrinsic areas of the cortex include the sensorimotor strip and the primary visual and auditory projection areas. These areas receive impulses from the peripheral sense organs, conducted through the primary sensory tracts, and relayed through specific thalamic nuclei. The intrinsic sectors of the cortex include the prefrontal, the anterior temporal, and the parieto-temporo-occipital cortex. These areas have been known collectively as association areas because they were formerly thought to receive no ascending afferent projections from subcortical areas. They were considered centers for elaboration and integration for adjacent sensory areas of the cortex. This, however, cannot be true, since we now know that they receive thalamocortical fibers from nonspecific thalamic nuclei, and from secondary afferent cortical fibers. The intrinsic sectors of man are considerably larger than those of the monkey. The cells and fibers of the intrinsic sectors mature at a slower rate than those of the extrinsic sectors. This is probably another reason why higher intellectual functions are not present at birth and are limited in early childhood.

Various modifications of speech have been observed following stimulation or lesions of subcortical connection. Electrical stimulation of the ventrolateral nucleus of the thalamus in patients with Parkinson's disease has resulted in simple arrest of speech, stuttering, or acceleration of the delivery of speech (Guiot et al., 1961; Sem-Jacobsen,

1966). Patients with Parkinsonism also have developed diminished voice volume and dysarthria following cryogenic lesions to the nucleus ventralis lateralis of either thalamus. Aphasia has followed thalamotomy done in the dominant hemisphere (Bell, 1968) and localized hemorrhages in the left thalamus of right-handed individuals (Coemins, 1970). In right-handed individuals, anomia has followed stimulation of the pulvinar and the deep parietal white substance in the paracallosal region of both hemispheres (Ojemann, et al., 1968).

THE RETICULAR FORMATION

The reticular formation of the brainstem is difficult to define. The term is used to describe an aggregate of cells, varying in size and shape, embedded in a network of fibers extending in all directions. The reticular cells in the brain stem cluster in nuclear formations that project to the spinal cord, the cerebellum, and the cerebral hemispheres, and in return receive fibers from these structures. Collaterals from the primary afferent pathways, such as those from the spinothalamic, trigeminial, optic, acoustic, and vestibular tracts, feed into the part of the reticular formation known as the reticular activating system. The medial lemniscus does not appear to send fibers into the reticular formation. Presumably, spinal influence on the reticular formation is mainly through direct spinoreticular fibers (Brodal, 1969).

According to Moruzzi and Magoun (1949), the fibers making up the reticular activating system are derived from the medial two-thirds of the reticular formation of the brain stem and the sensory nerve nuclei. Most of them ascend the brain stem within the central tegmental tract. Rostral projecting reticular fibers from the brain stem reticular formation bifurcate caudal to the thalamus into a dorsal and ventral bundle. A dorsal bundle can be traced to the thalamic intralaminar and dorsomedial areas. Intralaminar nuclei send a caudal group of fibers to the mesencephalic tegmental area and another to the orbitofrontal cortex. The ventral bundle bypasses the thalamus on its way to the frontal cortex and contributes to the desynchronization of spontaneous ongoing cortical activity. It also blocks recruiting responses subserved by intralaminar fibers which are under the influence of the reticular nucleus (Weinberger et al., 1965; Scheibel and Scheibel, 1967).

French and Magoun (1952) demonstrated that stimulation of the cephalic brain stem in monkeys can arouse them from sleep and desychnronize brain wave patterns recorded on the electoencephalogram. Lesions which destroy a major part of the reticular activating system produced a somnolent state in monkeys comparable to coma in man. Lesions that involve the ventral aspect of the pons can destroy the corticospinal, corticobulbar, and corticopontine tracts. The result is a severe quadriplegia and mutism. The patient remains conscious and alert, using eye blinks to communicate with others. Extension of the lesion into the reticular formation of the pons or midbrain will decrease awareness (Kemper and Romanul, 1960; Cravioto, et al., 1960; Neumann and Cohn, 1964; Feldman, 1971). In the syndrome of akinetic mutism, the patient is unresponsive even though he may show a superficial appearance of alertness. He is mute, immobile, and propositionally unresponsive. This condition has followed bilateral hemorrhagic lesions in the dorsomedial nucleus of the thalamus (Cairns, 1952) and infarction in bilateral midline and reticular thalamic nuclei (Segarra, 1970).

CEREBRAL CIRCULATION

A pair of internal carotids and two vertebral arteries supply the brain with blood. As both sets of vessels enter the intracranial cavity, they give off a series of branches that spread throughout the brain. These are shown in Fig. 6. The frontal, parietal, insular, and parts of the temporal lobe receive their main blood supply through branches of the internal carotid, while the occipital lobe, part of the temporal lobe, the brain stem, and the cerebellum are supplied by branches of the vertebral and basilar arteries. The most important branches of the internal carotid and vertebrobasilar systems—with the areas they supply, and the neurological deficit following occlusion (Davidson, *et al.*, 1934; Gray, 1959)—are shown in Table I.

The bifurcation of the common carotid gives rise to both the internal and external carotid arteries. In the dog and cat, the external carotid contributes more to cerebral circulation than does the internal carotid, and both animals have complex networks of vessels that connect the orbital portions of the external carotid with the intracranial portions of the internal carotid (Batson, 1944). In man, the internal and external carotids are also interconnected. Orbital groups of vessels belonging to the ophthalmic artery—which is a branch of the internal carotid—anastomose with twigs of the internal and external maxillary arteries—which are branches of the external carotid. This anastomosis may become an important source of collateral circulation when the internal carotid is occluded.

Another source of collateral circulation is the circle of Willis, which is a polygonal arrangement of blood vessels at the base of the brain. It includes the anterior and posterior communicating arteries, and the proximal portion of the anterior and posterior cerebral arteries, as shown in Fig. 7. Usually there is a mingling of blood from the two carotids by way of the circle of Willis. This is frequently demonstrated by cerebral angiography. In disease, however, the circle of Willis may become a source of collateral circulation for either hemisphere. Collateral circulation is far from perfect. The circle of Willis is frequently the site of developmental defects. One or both posterior communicating arteries may be absent, or the lumen of either may be extremely narrow. In addition, the cortical network of vessels may not provide enough blood to prevent necrosis within an area of infarction. There are many other sources of collateral circulation, some of them a result of developmental abnormalities. All intracranial cerebral arterial collaterals of any significant size occur on the surface of the brain (Kaplan, 1961).

Drainage of cerebral blood is accomplished by a system of cortical and intracerebral veins. Many of these veins drain into dural sinuses that join with the internal jugular veins. Blood may also leave by the forward anastomosis within the orbit and the pterygoid plexus of veins, by way of emissary vessels through the cranium, and by numerous channels which join the vertebral venous plexus (Batson, 1944).

Blood flow must be regular and continuous to meet cerebral metabolic requirements.

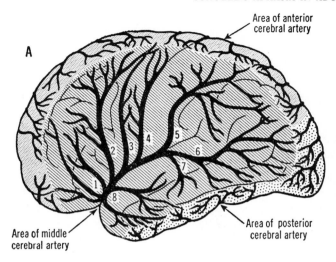

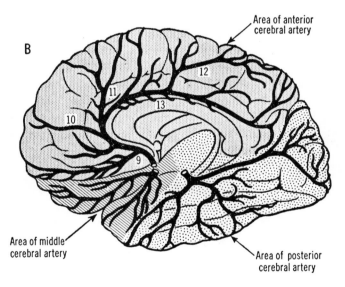

Fig. A–6. The cerebral circulation.

A. Dorsolateral aspect of the left cerebral hemisphere with its main arterial supply. The following numbers identify the branches of the middle cerebral artery:

1 = orbital artery	5 = posterior parietal artery
2 = ascending frontal artery	6 = angular gyrus
3 = prerolandic artery	7 = posterior temporal artery
4 = Rolandic artery	8 = anterior temporal artery

B. The mediobasilar aspect of the right cerebral hemisphere with its main arterial supply. The following numbers identify the branches of the anterior cerebral artery:

9 = orbital artery	12 = posterior internal frontal artery
10 = frontopolar artery	13 = pericallosal artery
11 = callosomarginal artery	

TABLE 1. Blood Supply to The Brain and Neurologic Deficits Following Occlusion of Main Vessels.

Main vessels	Region supplied	Neurologic deficit following occlusion
I. Internal carotid A. Branches of internal carotid	Most of the cerebral hemispheres, hypophysis	Contralateral hemiplegia Contralateral hemianesthesia Aphasia Hemianopsia or ipsilateral blindness
1. Anterior choroidal (ligation often fails to elicit obvious neurologic deficit)	Optic tract Cerebral peduncle Lateral geniculate body Posterior 2/3 posterior limb of internal capsule Infralenticular and retrolenticular portions internal capsule	Hemianopsia or upper quadrant defect Contralateral hemiplegia Partial thalamic sensory changes
2. Ophthalmic	Orbit and surrounding tissue Muscles and bulb of the eye	Unilateral blindness Optic atrophy
3. Anterior cerebral	Rostrum of corpus callosum Septum pellucidum Lower part of head caudate nucleus Lower part frontal pole of putamen Frontal pole globus pallidus Anterior limb internal capsule Orbital surface frontal lobe Superior frontal gyrus Cingulate gyrus Upper part of precentral gyrus Precuneus, adjacent lateral Surface of the hemispheres	Spastic monoparesis of the contralateral lower extremity Contralateral forced grasping and groping Cortical type sensory defects Transient aphasia Sluggish mentality, dementia Incontinence of bowel and bladder

4. Middle cerebral	Putamen except for lower anterior pole	Contralateral hemiplegia
	Upper part head and whole body caudate nucleus	Contralateral cortical sensory deficit
	Lateral part globus pallidus	Hemianopsia
	Internal capsule above level globus pallidus	Severe aphasia (if dominant hemisphere involved)
	Inferior and middle frontal gyrus	Stupor
	Lateral part orbital surface of frontal lobe	
	Precentral and postcentral gyri	
	Lower part superior parietal lobule	
	Supramarginal and angular gyri	
	Lateral surface of the temporal lobe	

B. Branches of middle cerebral

1. Pre-Rolandic branch	Contralateral lower facial and hypoglossal weakness
	Aphasia with dysarthria (if dominant hemisphere affected)
	Contralateral monoplegia
2. Anterior parietal branch	Decrease in deep sensibilities
	Ataxia
	Contralateral slight spastic hemiparesis
3. Posterior temporal and angular	Contralateral hemianopsia
	Severe aphasia
4. Posterior parietal and angular	Hemianopsia
	Contralateral cortical sensory defects
	Severe aphasia
5. Rolandic artery	Contralateral hemiplegia
6. Basilar branches	Total contralateral hemiplegia

II. Vertebrobasilar system

1. Posterior cerebral	Third temporal gyrus	Quadrant anopsia or
	Fusiform gyrus	hemianopsia
	Hippocampus	Bilateral central scotoma
	Uncus	Cortical blindness (both
	Lingula	branches involved)
	Cuneus	Aphasia
	All occipital gyri	Contralateral mild hemiparesis
	Part thalamus	Contralateral cerebellar ataxia
	Cerebral peduncle	Thalamic syndrome
	Superior cerebellar peduncle	
2. Basilar	Pons and territory supplied by posterior cerebral	Quadriplegia
		Dysphagia
		Diplopia
		Stupor or coma
		Dysarthria
		Rarely unilateral or bilateral deafness visual field defects, or blindness, etc.
3. Vertebral	Medulla	Dysphagia
	Posterior inferior region of cerebellum	Dysarthria
	Cervical portion of spinal cord	Hoarseness
		Ipsilateral cerebellar ataxia
		Contralateral or bilateral hemiparesis
		Contralateral hypaesthesia,
		Ipsilateral facial hypaesthesia, etc.

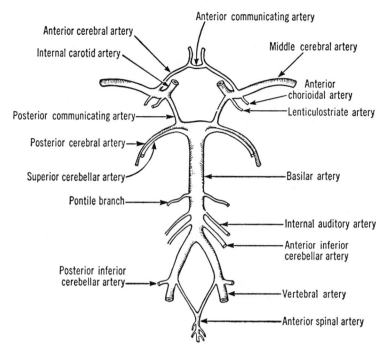

Fig. A–7. The circle of Willis.

This is accomplished through numerous physiological mechanisms, among the most important of which is systemic arterial pressure. However, as long as systemic blood pressure maintains an average value, cerebral blood flow is under the direct control of the brain. This regulatory effect is achieved by conditions that modify resistance to blood flow, such as intracranial pressure, viscosity of the blood, and changes in the diameter of the cerebral blood vessels. The latter is subject to neurogenic, humoral, hormonal, and drug effects. Under normal conditions, in an average size brain, cerebral blood flow in man has been estimated to be 650 cubic centimeters per minute. Oxygen consumed by the normal adult brain averages 3.5 cubic centimeters per 100 grams of brain weight per minute. A disturbance in this rate of flow may produce severe brain damage.

SUBSYSTEMS RELATED TO SPEECH AND LANGUAGE

THE AUDITORY SYSTEM

The auditory system includes the ear, the auditory nerve, the brain stem, and the cerebral cortex. It interacts with other cerebral systems in elaborate ways, and the organization of the speech and language is largely dependent on this system.

There are between 25 and 30 thousand auditory nerve cells in the spinal ganglion of each ear. The peripheral process from each neuron is associated with more than one hair cell. The central processes of the auditory nerve cells enter the internal auditory canal to form the auditory nerve. Intensity discrimination is determined by the number of active auditory nerve fibers.

The cochlear nerve follows a twisted course into the brain stem, where it divides into ascending and descending branches. Central auditory pathways are shown in Fig. 8. The ascending branches of the cochlear nerve enter the ventral cochlear nucleus, while

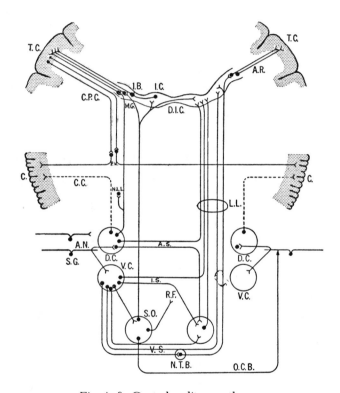

Fig. A–8. Central auditory pathways.

A.N.	= auditory nerve.		*L.L.*	= lateral lemniscus.
A.R.	= auditory radiations.		*M.G.*	= medial geniculate.
A.S.	= auditory striae.		*N.L.L.*	= nucleus lateral lemniscus.
C.	= cerebellum.		*N.T.B.*	= nucleus trapezoid body.
C.C.	= cerebello-cochlearis (proposed pathway).		*O.C.B.*	= olive cochlear bundle.
C.P.C.	= corticopontocerebellar fibers.		*P.N.*	= pontile nucleus.
D.C.	= dorsal cochlear nucleus.		*R.F.*	= reticular formation.
D.I.C.	= decussation inferior colliculi.		*S.G.*	= spiral ganglion.
I.B.	= inferior quadrigeminal brachium.		*S.O.*	= superior olive.
I.C.	= inferior colliculus.		*T.C.*	= temporal cortex.
I.S.	= intermediate striae.		*V.C.*	= ventral cochlear nucleus.
			V.S.	= ventral striae.

the descending branches of the cochlear nerve terminate in the dorsal cochlear nucleus. Fibers leaving the dorsal cochlear nucleus cross the midline (acoustic striae) of the brain stem and end in the contralateral superior olivary nucleus. Some fibers from the ventral cochlear nucleus cross the midline (intermediate striae) to end in the contralateral superior olivary nuclei. The existence of both crossed and uncrossed fibers insures that impulses from each ear reach the auditory cortex of each cerebral hemisphere, and explains why deafness does not result from unilateral destruction of auditory pathways rostral to this crossing.

Other fibers that arise from the ventral cochlear nucleus cross the midline and synapse with neurons of the trapezoid body, or the ventral striae. This group of striae is the most essential crossing for maximal representation of each ear in the opposite hemisphere. Many of its fibers, instead of entering the superior olivary nucleus, join the lateral lemniscus, which is a tract composed of fibers from all three groups of striae and the ipsilateral olivary nucleus. Some of its fibers end in the nucleus of the lateral lemniscus, and others in the nucleus of the inferior colliculus.

The efferent olivocochlear bundle is part of an auditory centrifugal system present at all levels of the auditory system. Its fibers, mostly from the superior olive, decussate as a midline bundle, join the auditory nerve, and end in the organ of Corti (Gacek, 1961). Presumably, its function is purely inhibitory, preventing unwanted auditory impulses from reaching the cochlear nucleus (Whitfield, 1967).

Neurophysiological studies have shown direct connections between the peripheral auditory system and the cerebellum (Snider and Stowell, 1944). The auditory system also sends collateral fibers into the reticular formation of the brain stem. Through this mechanism, auditory stimuli can produce cortical arousal and prolonged wakefulness. This response is still possible after destruction of all the lateral lemniscal fibers immediately caudal to the thalamus.

Fibers of the lateral lemniscus go to the inferior colliculi, and through the inferior quadrigeminal brachium to the medial geniculate nucleus of the thalamus. Fibers originating in the inferior colliculus also project by way of the inferior quadrigeminal brachium to the medial geniculate. In addition, the inferior colliculus sends fibers to the opposite inferior colliculus, superior colliculus, and the central gray matter of the mesencephalon. Some descending fibers originating in the inferior colliculus end in the dorsal cochlear nucleus and superior olive (Moore and Goldberg, 1966). The medial geniculate also receives fibers from the medial lemniscus, spinothalamic tract, cerebellum, and superior colliculus. This diverse input into the medial geniculate suggests a modulating function for this nucleus aside from being a relay station in the auditory system (Bowsher, 1961). Fibers from the medial geniculate proceed, by way of the auditory radiations, to the first transverse gyrus of Heschl of the supratemporal bank of the Sylvian fissure. Polyak's studies (1932) of primates have shown that lesions of the medial geniculate body produce degeneration of most of the posterior superior surface of the superior temporal gyrus, which represents the auditory projection cortex. Its boundaries are not sharply delineated.

Celesia *et al.* (1968), by studying evoked potentials to acoustic stimulation recorded from exposed human cortex, have demonstrated that in man the region responding to auditory stimulation is rather large. It includes not only the transverse gyrus of

Heschl, but also the posterior part of the superior temporal gyrus and the upper bank of the Sylvian fissure. We do not know how much of this represents primary auditory cortex. In addition, auditory responses evoked in the upper bank of the Sylvian fissure overlap the second somatosensory area, which in man is located at the base of the postcentral convolution. Cortical activity in this second somatosensory area may well be influenced by this direct auditory input.

The temporal lobe has transcortical projections to the third frontal convolution, the occipital lobe, and the cingulate gyrus of the limbic lobe. Its subcortical projections include the pulvinar nucleus, the lateral posterior complex of the thalamus, the medial geniculate body, the suprageniculate and intralaminar nuclei of the thalamus, the substantia nigra, and the mesencephalic reticular formation.

Animal experiments have shown that the auditory cortex is not essential for perceiving a pure tone (Bard and Rioch, 1937) or discriminating frequency of tones (Lorente De No, 1933; Magoun, 1952; Goldberg and Neff, 1962), The consensus, however, is that it is essential for pattern perception (Goldberg *et al.*, 1957; Neff and Diamond, 1958). Temporal cues for sound localization are analyzed at the medial superior olive (Masterton *et al.*, 1968).

Penfield and Rasmussen (1950) have outlined the primary auditory cortex in man, by electrical stimulation of the brain in patients undergoing surgery for temporal lobe lesions. Patients reported hearing ringing, buzzing, and clicking sounds when the electrode was applied. Bilateral ablation of the primary cortex resulted in cortical deafness. Electrical stimulation of the temporal cortex adjacent to the primary auditory area produced interpretive responses that seemed to indicate these areas were involved in a more complex response to sound. Wernicke (1908), Mills (1891), and others have stressed the importance of the first and second temporal gyri in relation to language.

THE VISUAL SYSTEM

The human retina contains about 125 million rods, and 4–7 million cones. The optic nerve, however, contains only 1,250,000 fibers. This means that each optic nerve fiber must be linked with many rods—since the ratio of rods to nerve fibers is 125:1—and to multiple cones—since the ratio of cones to nerve fibers is 4–7:1. These ratios suggest a discriminative function for the cones, versus an integrative one for the rods.

The optic nerves from each eye unite to form the optic chiasm. The fibers from the nasal half of each optic nerve cross the midline and join the temporal fibers of the opposite nerve to form the optic tract. Each optic tract sends fibers to the pretectal area, the superior colliculus, and the lateral geniculate body. The visual pathways are shown in Fig. 9.

The pretectal region and the superior colliculus are reflex centers. The pretectal region sends fibers to the oculomotor nuclei in the midbrain, and is involved in pupillary reflexes. The superior colliculus receives fibers from various sources which include the inferior colliculi, the spinotectal, and trigeminotectal tracts, as well as the frontal and occipital lobes and extrapyramidal structures. The superior colliculus sends efferent fibers to the brain stem and the spinal cord, which permit initiation of reflex head and eye movements.

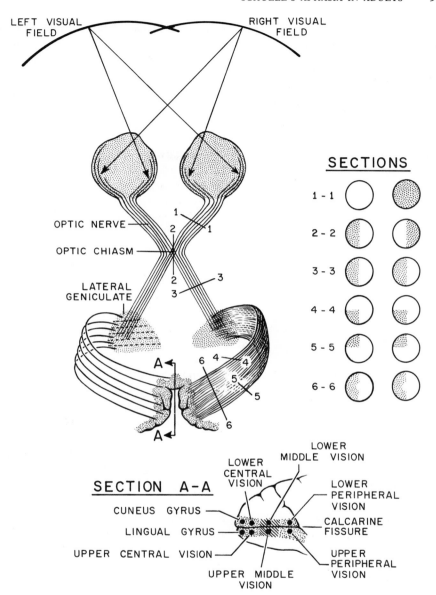

Fig. A–9. The visual pathways. The numerals represent typical deficits produced by lesions at different sites of the visual pathways.

      1–1 = total blindness, right eye.

      2–2 = bitemporal hemianopsia.

      3–3 = left homonymous hemianopsia.

      4–4 = left lower quadrant-anopsia.

      5–5 = left upper quadrant-anopsia.

      6–6 = left homonymous hemianopsia (no loss of central vision).

The figure in the lower left-hand corner shows the representation of the retina along the medial aspect of the occipital lobe.

Most fibers from the optic tract end in the lateral geniculate body. This nucleus also receives fibers from the occipital cortex. Some fibers originating in the lateral geniculate project rostrally and end in the retina. This group of centrifugal fibers function as modulators of visual impulses within th retina. Fibers leaving the lateral geniculate body form the geniculocalcarine tract, or the optic radiations. They follow an orderly course into the occipital lobe of each hemisphere, and end in the occipital cortex bordering the calcarine fissure. This cortex is known as the primary visual cortex. Polyak (1934) has demonstrated that lesions in the visual cortex result in retrograde degeneration of neurons in the lateral geniculate body. The primary visual cortex, or striate area, corresponds to area 17 of Brodmann. Areas 18 (parastriate) and 19 (peristriate) of Brodmann also receive geniculocortical projections (Garey and Powell, 1967). In addition, there are crossed geniculocortical pathways to the visual areas of the opposite hemisphere. The function of the geniculocortical pathways is unknown (Glickstein *et al.*, 1967).

The lower half of the optic radiations subserves vision in the upper temporal and nasal quadrants of the visual field, while the upper half subserves the lower quadrants. Destruction of the upper or lower radiations in either hemisphere is followed by corresponding upper or lower homonymous quadrantanopsia. The term *homonymous quadrantanopsia* simply means that the patient suffers a loss of vision in corresponding quarters of the visual field in both eyes. Complete destruction of the optic radiations in either hemisphere results in loss of left or right visual fields in both eyes. If the injury is in the left hemisphere, the patient has difficulty seeing to the right with each eye, and vice versa. Since the fibers representing the macula of the retina are usually spared, vision is retained in the center of the hemianoptic field. In some instances, patients with no visual-field defects demonstrate visual disorientation on homonymous half fields. They are unable to localize objects in space since stereoscopic vision has been impaired (Riddoch, 1935).

The topical representation of the retina in the striate area of the occipital lobe is very interesting. The macula is represented in the caudal end of the calcarine cortex, and the most peripheral part of the retina in the rostral end. The intermediate calcarine cortex represents the retinal layer between the macula and the peripheral retina. The representation of the upper half of the retina is found in the upper lip of the calcarine fissure, and that of the lower half upon the lower lip. Brain (1941) pointed out that: "when we perceive a two-dimensional circle we do so ·by means of an activity in the brain which is halved, reduplicated, transposed, inverted, distorted, and three-dimensional." Brouwer's studies (1939) in monkeys and men suggest a representation of the macula along the entire length of the calcarine fissure. This could explain the sparing of central vision in man after a substantial amount of the occipital lobe has been removed surgically.

Bonin, *et al.* (1942) have strychninized various parts of the visual cortex of the macaque and the chimpanzee. Strychninization of area 17, the primary visual cortex, produced spike activity within areas 17 and 18, but none in area 19. Strychninization of area 18 produced widespread firing in area 18, and spikes in area 19 as well as the anterior part of the middle temporal convolution, and area 18 of the opposite hemisphere. Strychninization of area 19, the preoccipital area, was followed by spikes confined to the area stimulated, followed by a wave of suppression of electrical activity which spread through the whole brain.

These results point to a close relationship between areas 17 and 18, the widespread connections of area 18, and a possible suppressor function of area 19 over incoming visual impulses. Traditional theory has regarded area 17 as the primary receptor of visual impulses, while area 18 was thought to subserve visual recognition, and area 19, association and elaboration of visual impulses. Present knowledge, however, does not support these assumptions for areas 18 and 19. Penfield and Rasmussen (1950) demonstrated that although excision of area 17 resulted in complete homonymous hemianoptic blindness, and excisions of areas 18 and 19 did not, either electrical or epileptic stimulation of all three areas produced identical visual phenomena. Patients reported sensations of light, color, movement, and forms variously described as balls, wheels, spots, or stars. The authors suggested that, "there is represented in the visual cortex no more than elements that go to make up the final image that reaches consciousness during normal vision."

The subcortical projections of visual cortex to the brain stem have been found with neurophysiological techniques. Jasper et al. (1952) found that the striate areas project to the lateral geniculate body, the pulvinar nucleus of the thalamus, the superior colliculus, and surrounding areas of the midbrain. The adjacent parastriate area sends fibers to the pulvinar and intralaminar nuclei of the thalamus, the mesencephalic reticular formation, the substantia nigra, and the subthalamic region. The peristriate area connects with the parastriate area, superior parietal lobule, opposite peristriate area, superior colliculus, and pretectal region.

In man, only the pupillary light reflex is mediated by the mesencephalon. All other optic functions appear to have been corticalized.

THE SENSORIMOTOR SYSTEM

Peripheral nerves convey afferent or sensory fibers from end organs in the muscle joints, tendons, fascia, and skin to the spinal cord, and cranial nerves carry impulses from the special sense organs to the brain stem. Present evidence seems to indicate that the stretch receptors in the muscles contribute little or nothing to the flow of proprioceptive information the brain recieves (Rose and Mountcastle, 1960). However, muscle contraction activates receptors in the joints and tendons, which in turn give rise to impulses that convey information about the movements and about the position of the body in space. Rose and Mountcastle maintain that proprioceptive impulses can also enter the central nervous system through the roots of the ninth and tenth cranial nerves, and that some of the chorda tympani fibers may be activated by mechanoreceptors.

The spinothalamic tracts conduct sensations of pain, temperature, and touch to the posterolateral ventral nucleus of the thalamus. Since most of the fibers within these tracts are crossed fibers, damage to the right spinothalamic tract impairs sensations of pain, temperature, and touch on the left side of the body, and vice versa. However, not all spinothalamic fibers end in the posterolateral ventral nucleus. Many end in the reticular formation of the brain stem, and others terminate in the diffuse thalamic nuclei (Rasmussen and Peyton, 1941; Gardner and Cuneo, 1945; Bowsher, 1961). It has been suggested that fibers entering the reticular formation aid in maintaining general sensory awareness.

Deep and superficial sensations from the face area are conveyed to the posteromedial nucleus of the thalamus through the secondary trigeminal tracts. These tracts are made up of crossed fibers; therefore, a lesion affecting the right secondary trigeminal tracts will lead to decrease or loss of temperature, touch, pain, and proprioceptive sensations to the left side of the face.

The dorsal fasciculi of the spinal cord conduct impulses associated with deep sensibility, localization, and spatial discrimination to the nucleus gracilis and cuneatus of the medulla. Fibers leaving these nuclei cross the midline, turn rostrally, and as the medial lemniscal pathway, ascend to the posterolateral nucleus of the thalamus. The nucleus gracilis and cuneatus receive corticofugal fibers from primary and secondary somatosensory cortices. Through these fibers the somatosensory cortices can excite or inhibit the activity within the dorsal column nuclei (Levitt, et al., 1964; Jabbur and Towe, 1961). Unilateral destruction of the medial lemniscal tract in monkeys and chimpanzees has produced loss of position sense, or discrimination of form, contour, and weight of objects held in the contralateral hand.

In summary, most sensory impulses ascend the brain stem by way of the spinothalamic tracts, the trigeminal pathways, and the medial lemniscal tracts, and relay impulses to the posterior ventral nucleus of the thalamus. This nucleus gives rise to the thalamocortical fibers, which project to the postcentral gyrus. This area of the parietal lobe is usually referred to as the primary somatosensory area of the cortex.

The sensory organization of the postcentral gyrus is similar to the organization of movements in the precentral motor strip, as shown in Fig. 10. The posteromedial ventral nucleus of the thalamus projects to the face area in the lower dorsolateral third of the postcentral gyrus. The medial portion of the posterolateral ventral nucleus projects to the arm and trunk area in the middle portion of the postcentral gyrus. The lateral portion projects to the leg area in the dorsomedial aspect of the postcentral gyrus and the posterior half of the paracentral area.

A secondary somatosensory area has been identified in man and in animals in the parietal opercular region. Fibers projecting to this area seem to arise from an area in the thalamus between the ventrobasal complex and the medial geniculate body. However, all somatosensory fibers do not reach either the primary or secondary sensory regions. Tactual and proprioceptive sensation, for example, can be evoked from a much larger cortical zone that includes areas 4, 5, 6, and 7 of Brodmann. It is possible that the somatosensory cortex may include the entire parietal and frontal lobe except for its most anterior part (Zollinger, 1935; Bard, 1956).

The primary and secondary somatosensory cortices project to the ipsilateral nucleus ventralis posterolateralis, nucleus ventralis posteromedialis, nucleus gracilis and cuneatus, and posterior horn of the spinal cord gray matter. Projections of the primary somatosensory cortex to the posterior horn of the spinal cord is mainly contralateral, while that of the secondary somatosensory cortex is bilateral. Physiological studies have demonstrated how these corticofugal fibers can alter afferent input (Rinvik, 1968;

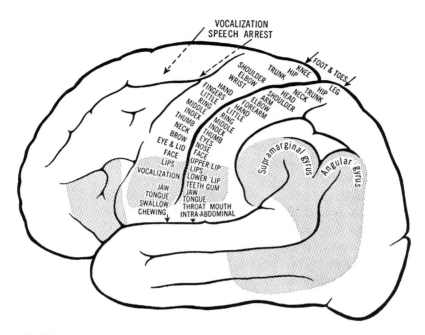

Fig. A–10. The sensorimotor system. Dorsolateral view of the left hemisphere (dominant) showing the motor-sensory representation of the human body on the cortex as mapped out by electrical stimulation. The darkened areas indicate regions which yield vocalization or alteration in language during cortical electrical stimulation. Broken arrows point to the medial surface of the cerebral hemisphere. The motor representation of the foot, ankle, and toes turns over the medial margin of the hemisphere into the paracentral lobule. (*Adapted from* Penfield and Rasmussen in Ranson, S. W., and Clark, S.L.: *The Anatomy of the Nervous System*, Ed. 10., Philadelphia, W. B. Saunders Company, 1959.)

Andersen, *et al.*, 1964; Lindbloom and Ottosen, 1957). Both somatosensory areas maintain reciprocal connections with each other and with the motor cortex (Jones and Powell, 1968).

Ranson and Clark (1959) believe the cerebral cortex plays a significant role in discriminating aspects of sensation such as "recognition of differences in weight, spatial discrimination of two closely juxtaposed points, tactile localization, appreciation of size and shape, of similarities or differences in temperature," An aphasic with parietal lobe damage may show impairment of ability to copy, draw, and write, due to impaired proprioceptive discrimination. Abalation of the postcentral gyrus results in disturbance of superficial sensation and poor return, if any, of deep sensation. The deficit is greatest in the distal ends of the involved extremities. The face is the only area which has strong ipsilateral as well as bilateral representation in the postcentral gyrus.

The sensory pathways, with their many synapses between the periphery and the cortex, are channels not only for conveying impulses that are stimulated by events in the environment, but also for conveying impulses stimulated by events that occur in the organism, including postural changes and movements of all kinds. Sensory events initiate, regulate, and control complex patterns of motor activity that supply further sensory stimulation in their turn. Motor responses have been evoked in man and animals from the cortex of the precentral gyri, the supplementary motor area in the frontal lobe, the postcentral gyri, and the secondary somatosensory area. In neither an anatomical, a physiological, or a psychological sense can sensory and motor mechanisms be considered apart from each other.

Penfield obtained both sensory and motor responses from electrical stimulation of the postcentral gyrus, although evoked sensations predominated. Similar results were obtained from stimulation of the precentral gyrus, although here evoked movements predominated (see Fig. 10). Thus, the precentral and postcentral gyri are actually a mixed sensorimotor region.

The somatotopic representations of the human body in the precentral motor strip have been reinvestigated by Penfield and his associates. The movements produced by stimulation of the motor strip are always contralateral, with the exception of midline structures such as the tongue (Riddoch, 1917; Penfield and Roberts, 1959).

Descending fibers from Brodmann area 4, the precentral motor strip, make up about 20% of the fibers found in the corticospinal or pyramidal tracts. The pyramidal tracts participate in the initiation of movements and in providing speed and agility to voluntary movements, especially those of the hands and fingers. An individual with pyramidal tract lesions may show impairment in such manual tasks as drawing, typing, or writing.

Other descending pathways such as the rubrospinal tract—long descending fibers from the pontine and medullary reticular formation—and the vestibular complex are directly involved in the maintenance of erect posture and integrated movements of the body and limbs, and in controlling the independent use of the extremities, particularly of the hands (Lawrence and Kuypers, 1968 a,b). Corticofugal fibers not passing through the pyramids in the medulla form part of what traditionally has been called the extrapyramidal system, which included the basal ganglia. Actually, neither the pyramidal nor the extrapyramidal system is a well-defined anatomical or physiological entity. Bucy (1957) has argued that both systems consist of fibers running through the cerebrum to the spinal cord with diverse origins, terminations, and functions, and has urged that the terms be discarded since they are both inaccurate and misleading. He added that at the present time, a complete understanding of the neural mechanisms responsible for muscular activity is impossible.

Cerebellar mechanisms also play a part in the integration and control of movement. The cerebellum receives afferents from the vestibular nerve, the spinocerebellar tracts, and the cerebral cortex. It functions to regulate balance, posture, and muscle tonus, and to facilitate smooth movements.

Destruction of area 4 or sectioning of the corticospinal tract at the level of the pyramids in monkeys and chimpanzees, produces flaccidity in all extremities, without increase in deep tendon reflexes or clonus (Fulton and Kennard, 1934). Total decortication, or bilateral removal of the motor and premotor cortex, Brodmann areas 4 and 6, incapacitates monkeys and baboons severely: All four extremities are permanently spastic; forced grasping is marked and permanent; and voluntary isolated movements of the hands are abolished.

Removal of the motor cortex in the dog or cat does not paralyze these animals; they can sit, run, or walk. Decorticated monkeys are still capable of righting reflexes, sitting, standing, and walking. Thus, these movements are not completely corticalized in lower-order mammals (Travis and Woolsey, 1956). In man, however, removal of area 4 produces more impairment of movement of the contralateral extremities: There is almost total paralysis of the distal muscles of the hands and feet. Almost no movement is present in the wrists, hands, and fingers. Only speech is not abolished, although a transitory dysarthria is produced. Recovery of speech movements may be due to the bilateral representation of the lower face area in the primary sensorimotor area.

Electrical stimulation of the lower two-thirds of the sensorimotor cortex of either hemisphere has produced arrest or slowing of speech. In the dominant hemisphere, these responses were also obtained from the posterior end of the third frontal gyrus, and from the parietal and posterior temporal areas. No arrest of speech followed stimulation of Broca's area in the nondominant hemisphere. The predominant response to stimulation of the sensorimotor strip was arrest or slowing of speech, while difficulty finding words was the predominant response to stimulation of the temporal and parietal areas.

Vocalization—in the form of an undifferentiated cry—has been obtained in man from electrical stimulation of the sensorimotor cortex, and of the medial aspect of the frontal cortex four centimeters anterior to the central fissure. However, vocalization does not require the complexity of a cerebral cortex. Woolsey (1943) reported vocalization in a decorticated monkey which survived surgery for 161 days. A human anencephalus without cortex, striatum or pallidum is still able to cry. The cry of a newborn human could well be equivalent to that of a decorticated animal, since man's brain is not fully matured at birth. Most of the newborn's activities indicate a lack of inhibitory control of subcortical structures by the immature cerebral cortex: There are no volitional movements. All movements are incoordinated and generalized. Isolated limb movements do not occur. Crying increases muscle rigidity. Grasping, sucking, and tonic neck reflexes are present.

DISCUSSION AND CONCLUSIONS

It is fascinating to observe how, in the process of evolution, many subcortical functions have gradually become encephalized. The partial and total decortication experiments in primates and subprimates have shown that subcortical structures are still capable of functioning without the discriminating and inhibitory influences of the cerebral cortex. Ambulation, although grossly impaired, is still possible in the decorticated monkey. After removal of the auditory cortex, cats can still localize sound, perceive a pure tone stimulus, and perform auditory frequency discrimination tasks. Bilateral removal of the occipital cortex in monkeys has not abolished the pupillary reflex, conjugate movements of the eyes, or brightness discrimination. Lower mammals such as cats and dogs exhibit better functional capabilities after decortication than do primates. Thus encephalization of functions has been greater in primates than in cats and dogs.

Together with the encephalization of function, newer groups of cells and tracts have appeared within the central nervous system of many species. Although fish have dorsal columns within their spinal cords, these columns are very small and are confined to the cord. The appearance of the nuclei gracilis and cuneatus mark the encephalization of the fasciculi gracilis and cuneatus within the dorsal columns of the spinal cord. The nuclei are present in reptiles and amphibians, but together with their fibers (medial lemnisci) attain their greatest development in man. They conduct proprioceptive impulses which are essential in man for proper maintenance of body posture and muscle tone. Also, the pyramidal tract is not a phylogenetically old structure. It is present only in mammals, and attains its greatest development in primates (Lassek, 1948). It is thought to be essential for all skilled digital movements.

In man, both the thalamus and the cortex have greatly increased in size, relative to other primates. Associational, commissural, and projective fibers have become more numerous. Thus, a multiplicity of pathways has become available through which ascending afferent fibers can reach the cerebellar and cerebral cortices. In return, the cerebellar and cerebral cortices send efferent fibers to subcortical structures, the brain stem, and the spinal cord. Most of the efferent and afferent pathways send collaterals to groups of neurons (nuclei) at different levels of the central nervous system. This creates the intricate network of connections that has made the central nervous system of man so difficult to study. In the newborn, early development of primary sensory cortical areas establishes receiving centers for afferent impulses. Thus light is seen, sound is heard, touch is felt. However, the primary sensory cortical areas of the newborn are not capable of higher visual, auditory, or tactile discriminations. They perceive stimuli, but cannot organize them into complex patterns in the absence of secondary sensory areas and much larger intrinsic sectors.

Cortifugal projections from many cortical regions overlap within the thalamus, the subthalamic area, and midbrain region. This arrangement emphasizes the importance of the mesodiencephalic area as coordinator, integrator, and relay center for ascending and descending afferent or efferent impulses. The cortex is essential for higher psychic functions; however, subcortical connections between intrinsic and extrinsic systems may be responsible for the lack of gross deficits observed after restricted cortical ablations in the left hemisphere (Penfield and Roberts, 1959).

In conclusion, the importance of cortical speech areas has been clearly demonstrated, by such experiments as Penfield's electrical stimulation of the human brain. However, in addition to functions assigned to different areas of the cortex, the contribution of subcortical structures as integrating mechanisms should never be forgotten.

TABLE 1. Principal Axes Factor Loadings*

Tests	1	2	3	4	5
AUDITORY					
1. Recognition words	82	−13	32	−34	10
2. Recognition letters	91	10	9	7	− 6
3. Items serially	88	14	30	− 6	− 6
4. Repetition sentences	82	53	−11	2	− 7
5. Repetition digits	90	33	−14	− 4	3
6. Directions	91	19	24	2	−14
7. Recognition errors	79	− 1	− 9	−12	−25
8. Short paragraph	79	− 9	9	11	−16
9. Long paragraph	74	13	− 5	− 4	−14
10. Ammons	69	−11	13	−12	−19
VISUAL-READING					
11. Subjective findings	−27	−45	7	2	50
12. Matching forms	60	−60	14	−48	−16
13. Matching letters	46	−48	3	−55	−31
14. Object categories	75	−37	1	0	0
15. Word to pictures	81	−25	17	−26	− 4
16. Printed to spoken word	90	2	21	− 7	− 5
17. Sentence comprehension	85	−12	19	− 8	6
18. Silent reading rate	82	− 9	21	8	−15
19. Short paragraph	85	−25	25	9	−11
20. Long paragraph	86	− 8	29	13	−18
21. Oral reading	92	16	14	− 1	−10
SPEECH AND LANGUAGE					
22. Phonation	34	−36	−57	8	−12
23. Tongue movements	73	−27	−42	8	− 6
24. Jaw movements	49	−51	−43	− 9	3
25. Palatal movements	37	−14	−61	−24	− 5
26. Pharyngeal movements	29	−27	−53	9	3
27. Alternating movements	64	8	−57	−13	− 7
28. Repetition words	87	20	−30	− 8	2
29. Sentence completion	88	38	− 8	−14	− 3
30. Counting to 20	85	22	−37	9	− 4
31. Days of week	91	27	−26	2	7
32. Months	90	34	−13	2	9

TABLE 1. (Continued)

Tests	1	2	3	4	5
33. Questions	83	49	− 8	−19	0
34. Naming	90	34	7	−17	14
35. Rhymes	82	24	−31	5	7
36. Definitions	90	34	− 9	− 4	16
37. Information	89	39	0	−12	2
38. Expressing ideas	87	33	−16	− 7	9
39. Picture description	87	38	− 9	−16	15
40. Similarities	88	39	− 3	− 7	11
41. Proverbs	76	39	21	−22	19
VISUO-MOTOR-WRITING					
42. Copying forms	58	−40	− 7	−10	0
43. Copying Greek letters	57	−61	− 1	−23	24
44. Drawing house	60	−56	10	− 1	11
45. Reproducing wheel	54	−49	7	− 1	17
46. Numerals to 20	73	−29	3	16	12
47. Reproducing letters	72	−44	3	− 9	25
48. Words, visual	91	0	19	13	− 2
49. Words, auditory	91	2	18	18	− 3
50. Letters, dictation	88	−10	13	20	−15
51. Written spelling	90	− 2	19	22	5
52. Oral spelling	89	31	−21	14	0
53. Sentences, dictation	92	5	12	26	− 2
54. Sentences, spontaneous	95	0	− 1	35	7
55. Spontaneous paragraph	90	8	− 6	35	6
NUMERICAL, ARITHMETIC					
56. Change	87	−13	1	−12	− 1
57. Setting clock	83	− 8	12	17	12
58. Simple combinations	80	−28	5	20	−17
59. Simple stated problems	91	− 2	− 1	13	−10
60. Addition	75	−36	0	28	−15
61. Subtraction	76	−23	7	31	−11
62. Multiplication	71	−21	5	13	65
63. Division	83	−31	−13	6	− 5
BODY IMAGE					
64. Naming body parts	89	34	− 6	−17	10
65. Recognition body parts	90	− 3	28	−19	7
66. Directions	92	15	20	− 9	3
67. Drawing man	56	−50	− 7	− 1	21
68. Assembling manikin	46	−78	−12	10	−13
69. Assembling head	44	−57	−18	4	0
Proportion of estimated common factor variance (cumulative)	.70	.81	.87	.90	.93

* Decimal points are omitted for all entries in the body of the table.

TABLE 2. Oblimin Factor Matrix*

Tests	1	2	3	4	5
AUDITORY					
1. Recognition words	22	13	1	− 2	46
2. Recognition letters	38	33	− 3	2	4
3. Items serially	42	29	− 4	−14	18
4. Repetition sentences	81	6	− 4	− 9	−10
5. Repetition digits	72	3	2	2	− 3
6. Directions	43	36	− 9	− 9	12
7. Recognition errors	39	16	9	3	20
8. Short paragraph	15	42	− 1	6	7
9. Long paragraph	43	16	3	0	7
10. Ammons (reflected)	8	32	−13	14	32
VISUAL-READING					
11. Subjective findings	−37	−16	23	7	− 8
12. Matching forms	− 4	2	38	− 5	61
13. Matching letters	− 6	− 1	16	11	71
14. Object categories	3	30	5	24	16
15. Word to picture	19	16	16	− 1	38
16. Printed to spoken word	35	28	6	−10	18
17. Sentence comprehension	25	25	4	3	20
18. Silent reading rate	23	39	11	−12	8
19. Short paragraph	5	49	6	0	14
20. Long paragraph	16	52	− 4	− 5	10
21. Oral reading	49	26	3	−12	8
SPEECH AND LANGUAGE					
22. Phonation	− 6	7	9	51	− 4
23. Tongue movements	14	21	−10	59	3
24. Jaw movements	− 4	4	− 1	64	17
25. Palatal movements	27	−25	6	48	15
26. Pharyngeal movements	− 1	3	− 8	61	− 7
27. Alternating movements	51	−15	10	31	2
28. Repetition words	66	− 3	4	17	− 1
29. Sentence completion	75	− 2	6	−10	6
30. Counting to 20	62	7	7	16	−16
31. Days of week	69	2	5	11	−11
32. Months	75	2	9	− 4	−12
33. Questions	82	− 8	− 4	− 7	8
34. Naming	73	− 1	1	− 9	10
35. Rhymes	67	− 1	12	8	−17
36. Definitions	69	4	−10	11	− 2
37. Information	72	5	− 7	− 4	7
38. Expressing ideas	75	− 4	5	1	− 5
39. Picture description	76	− 8	− 1	1	5
40. Similarities	72	3	− 8	1	1
41. Proverbs	58	3	−23	− 1	20
VISUO-MOTOR-WRITING					
42. Copying forms	11	3	51	−10	10
43. Copying Greek letters	4	−10	61	− 6	19
44. Drawing house	−12	20	46	− 7	10
45. Reproducing wheel	0	9	45	− 7	4

TABLE 2. (Continued)

Tests	1	2	3	4	5
46. Numerals to 20	12	28	22	6	− 8
47. Reproducing letters	12	4	45	− 3	9
48. Words, visual	33	39	1	− 3	1
49. Words, auditory	34	39	11	−12	− 6
50. Letters, dictation	20	48	7	− 2	− 2
51. Written spelling	26	44	3	− 2	− 9
52. Oral spelling	66	16	− 7	14	−17
53. Sentences, dictation	39	41	10	− 9	−17
54. Sentences, spontaneous	38	39	18	− 3	−30
55. Spontaneous paragraph	44	35	10	3	−32
NUMERICAL, ARITHMETIC					
56. Change	33	15	11	8	19
57. Setting clock	28	30	18	− 7	−11
58. Simple combinations	7	48	5	13	1
59. Simple stated problems	29	40	− 8	18	2
60. Addition	− 2	49	20	7	− 9
61. Subtraction	3	54	1	14	−10
62. Multiplication	16	8	20	13	−19
63. Division	17	29	− 2	36	9
BODY IMAGE					
64. Naming body parts	72	− 4	4	− 4	8
65. Recognition body parts	33	18	13	−15	28
66. Directions	52	18	9	−17	12
67. Drawing man	1	3	53	− 3	− 1
68. Assembling manikin	−35	33	31	26	11
69. Assembling head	−12	10	53	2	0

* Decimal points are omitted for all entries in the body of the table.

TABLE 3. Correlations Between Test Sections for 154 Aphasic and 50 Nonaphasic Subjects

	1 Auditory tests	2 Visual, reading tests	3 Speech, language tests	4 Visuo-motor, writing tests	5 Numerical, arithmetic tests	6 Tests for body image
1. Auditory tests						
aphasics		.81	.86	.81	.84	.80
nonaphasics		.32	.26	.28	.13	.28
2. Visual, read-ing tests						
aphasics	.81		.68	.84	.84	.83
nonaphasics	.32		.34	.49	.08	−.13
3. Speech, language tests						
aphasics	.86	.68		.70	.72	.71
nonaphasics	.26	.34		.52	.31	−.007
4. Visuomotor, writing tests						
aphasics	.81	.84	.70		.85	.84
nonaphasics	.28	.49	.52		.42	.11
5. Numerical, arith-metic tests						
aphasics	.84	.84	.72	.85		.86
nonaphasics	.13	.08	.31	.42		.39
6. Test for body image						
aphasics	.80	.83	.71	.84	.86	
nonaphasics	.28	−.13	−.007	.11	.39	

TABLE 4. Means and Standard Deviations of Errors for 178 Aphasic Subjects in Seven
Diagnostic Groups Over Five Sections of the Minnesota Test for Differential Diagnosis of Aphasia*

Type of Test	Simple (N 21)		Visual (N 27)		Dysfluent (N 7)		Scattered (N 65)		Sensorimotor (N 18)		Auditory (N 17)		Irreversible (N 33)	
Auditory tests	M 12.14	SD 11.57	M 12.44	SD 10.72	M 6.29	SD 2.25	M 26.81	SD 23.20	M 31.19	SD 16.95	M 52.65	SD 19.52	M 74.78	SD 14.69
Visual and reading tests	M 8.90	SD 6.93	M 16.00	SD 12.63	M 18.00	SD 3.22	M 25.58	SD 18.59	M 18.75	SD 9.71	M 68.06	SD 17.78	M 58.74	SD 19.64
Speech and language tests	M 28.19	SD 25.34	M 18.89	SD 24.02	M 34.57	SD 5.36	M 66.51	SD 53.52	M 95.38	SD 47.13	M 120.35	SD 39.59	M 159.17	SD 22.39
Visuomotor and writing tests	M 18.24	SD 20.84	M 37.96	SD 27.31	M 18.71	SD 3.47	M 60.88	SD 34.93	M 50.25	SD 22.45	M 65.53	SD 21.19	M 120.48	SD 22.82
Numerical relations and	M 3.10	SD 3.02	M 4.74	SD 4.56	M 3.14	SD 1.00	M 9.06	SD 5.58	M 6.63	SD 3.46	M 14.18	SD 6.13	M 18.57	SD 3.91
Body parts	M 3.67	SD 8.76	M 8.89	SD 9.78			M 20.43	SD 15.96	M 12.19	SD 8.15			M 52.17	SD 12.33
All Tests	M 74.24	SD 70.28	M 98.93	SD 77.54	M 80.71	SD 11.60	M 209.25	SD 124.84	M 214.38	SD 89.93	M 320.76	SD 41.37	M 483.91	SD 71.11

* Data in boldface were collected on the 1965 published test, which contains no tests on body parts.

TABLE 5.
Mean Percentage of Error for 69 Subjects in Seven
Diagnostic Categories over Five Sections of the Minnesota Test*

Group	Auditory tests (N 9)	Reading tests (N 6)	Language tests (N 14)	Writing tests (N 8)	Arithmetic tests (N 8)
Simple (N 17)					
Initial	21	24	27	32	14
Final	9	12	12	16	5
Visual (N 16)					
Initial	24	43	25	57	26
Final	12	26	14	37	15
Dysfluent (N 4)					
Initial	**6**	**17**	**28**	**21**	**9**
Final	**2**	**2**	**3**	**4**	**2**
Scattered (N 22)					
Initial	43	54	51	72	43
Final	29	43	36	60	36
Sensorimotor (N 14)					
Initial	35	39	87	65	36
Final	24	26	45	48	23
Auditory (N 12)					
Initial	**45**	**42**	**68**	**55**	**41**
Final	**23**	**25**	**26**	**38**	**29**
Irreversible (N 4)					
Initial	89	86	93	98	77
Final	67	81	84	98	55
Nonaphasic subjects (N 50)	2	4	1	6	2

* NOTE: Data in boldface were collected on the 1965 published test. See p.   for description of differences between test batteries.

TABLE 6.
Summary of Neurological and Medical Data by Diagnostic Groups

History and Etiology

Diagnostic Category	Total N (N 175)	Mean Age (N 175)	Mean Years Schooling (N 175)	Occupational level rank order (N 167)	% CVA's (N 171)	% Complete thrombosis among CVA's (N 146)
Simple	21	38.0	12+	2	76	19
Visual	27	45.0	10+	5	68	6
Dysfluent	7	41.0	13	2	43	29
Scattered	65	59.4	6−9	4	84	4
Sensorimotor	16	43.6	12	3	94	40
Auditory	16	52.6	12+	1	50	38
Irreversible	23	59.6	10+	1	96	27
TOTAL SAMPLE	175	48	11+	2.5	78	23

Indices of Severity

Diagnostic Category	% Involvement extremities (N 175)	% Paralysis only (N 175)	% Facial paralysis (N 175)	% Sensory loss (N 143)	% Focal EEG findings (N 113)
Simple	67	14	62	50	47
Visual	67	15	63	74	52
Dysfluent	86	14	72	57	100*
Scattered	89	45	68	69	41
Sensormotor	94	56	75	67	55
Auditory	62	50	66	42	80
Irreversible	100	96	91	93	76
TOTAL SAMPLE	79	42	67	63	58

* This value is likely to be misleading. There were EEGs for only three Dysfluent patients. All showed focal findings in the frontal lobe.

TABLE 6 (Continued)

Course and Outcome

Diagnostic category	% Self-care, admission (N 129)	% Self-care, discharge (N 128)	% Ambulation, discharge (N 128)	% Ambulation, admission (N 129)	% Adverse sequelae (N 148)	% Training, employment (N 148)
Simple	87	100	73	100	24	33
Visual	87	96	83	91	15	35
Dysfluent	86	86	57	86	0	25
Scattered	57	85	43	70	34	0
Sensorimotor	94	100	94	100	13	60
Auditory	81	81	50	62	18	6
Irreversible	41	65	32	65	44	0
TOTAL SAMPLE	83	86	55	79	28	9

TABLE 6 (Continued)

Complicating Conditions

Diagnostic Category	% Hypertension (N 167)	% Cardiac involvement (N 165)	% Previous episodes (N 168)	% Bilateral weakness (N 175)	% Bilateral Neurological Findings (N 175)	% Palatal, laryngeal pharyngeal involvement (N 170)	% Tongue involvement (N 166)	% Visual field defects (N 102)	% Abnormal mental status (N 169)
Simple	5	48	14	0	14	0	0	31	5
Visual	28	35	19	0	14	0	0	75	0
Dysfluent	29	42	14	0	14	33	75	0	0
Scattered	45	63	30	14	35	53	69	38	68
Senseori Motor	7	33	7	0	6	4	0	36	0
Auditory	0	19	12	0	45	27	5	53	37
Irreversible	32	74	35	0	17	61	64	40	50
TOTAL SAMPLE	28	46	25	4	27	32	39	45	33

REFERENCES

Akelaitis AJ, (1943): Studies on the corpus callosum VII. Study of language functions (tactile and visual lexia and graphia) unilaterally following section of the corpus callosum. J Neuropath Exp Neurol 2:226–262

Akelaitis AJ (1944): A study of gnosis, praxis, and language following section of the corpus callosum and anterior commissure. J Neurosurg 1:94–102

Alajouanine T (1948): Aphasia and artistic realization. Brain 71:229–241

Alajouanine T, Ombredane A, Durand M (1939): Le Syndrome de Désintégration Phonétique dans l'Aphasie. Paris, Masson

Ammons RB, Ammons HS (1948): Full-Range Picture Vocabulary Test. Missoula, Montana, Psychological Test Specialists

Andersen P, Eccles JC, Sears TA (1964): Cortically evoked depolarization of primary afferent fibers in the spinal cord. J Neurophysiol 27:63–77

Arbib MA (1964): Brains, Machines and Mathematics. New York, McGraw-Hill

Arbib MA (1972): The Metaphorical Brain. New York, Wiley

Ashby RW (1960): Design for a Brain. New York, Wiley

Bailey P, Bonin G von (1957): Evolution of the cerebral cortex organ of the mind. What's New 198:13–19

Baldwin M, Frost LL, Wood CD (1954): Investigation of the primate amygdala. Neurology 4:586–598

Bard P (1956): Medical Physiology. 10th ed., St. Louis, Mosby, pp. 1147–1206

Bard P, Rioch DMCK (1937): A study of four cats deprived of neocortex and additional portions of the forebrain. Bull Hopkins Hosp. 60:73–125

Basser LS (1962): Hemiplegia of early onset and the faculty of speech with special reference to the effects of hemispherectomy. Brain 85:427–460

Bastian HC (1887): On different kinds of aphasia, with special reference to their classification and ultimate pathology. Br Med J 2:931–936, 985–990

Bastian HC (1898): A Treatise on Aphasia and Other Speech Defects. London, Lewis

Batson OV (1944): Anatomical problems concerned in the study of cerebral blood flow. Fed Proc 3:139–144

Bay E (1953): Disturbances of visual perception and their examination. Brain 76:515–550

Bay E (1962): Aphasia and non-verbal disorders of language. Brain 85:411–426

Bell DS (1968): Speech functions of the thalamus inferred from the effects of thalamotomy. Brain 91 (IV):619–638

Bender L (1952): Child psychiatric techniques. Springfield, Illinois: Charles C. Thomas

Benton AL, Joynt RJ (1960): Early descriptions of aphasia Arch Neurol 3:205–222

Berkeley EC (1961): Giant Brains: Or Machines That Think. New York, Science House

Bernstein N (1967): The Co-ordination and Regulation of Movements. New York, Pergamon Press

Beyn ES (1958): Peculiarities of thought in patients with sensory aphasia. Lang Speech 1:233–249

Birch HG, Lee J (1955): Cortical inhibition in expressive aphasia. Arch Neurol 74:514–517

Bogen JE (1969): The other side of the brain: I, Dysgraphia and dyscopia following cerebral commissurotomy. Bull Los Angeles Neurol Soc 34:73–105 (a)

Bogen JE (1969): The other side of the brain: II, An appositional mind. Bull Los Angeles Neurol Soc 34:135–161 (b)

Bogen JE, Bogen GM (1969): The other side of the brain: III, The corpus callosum and creativity. Bull Los Angeles Neurol Soc 34:191–220

Bonin G von (1960): Some Papers on the Cerebral Cortex. Springfield, Illinois, Thomas

Bowsher D (1961): The termination of second somatosensory neurons within the thalamus of Macaca Mulatta: An experimental degeneration study. J Comp Neurol 117:213–222

Brain R (1941): Visual disorientation with special reference to lesions of the right cerebral hemisphere. Brain 64:244–272

Brain R (1961): Speech Disorders. Washington, DC, Butterworths

Breasted JH (ed) (1930): The Edwin Smith Surgical Papyrus, Vol. I. Chicago, Univ of Chicago Press

Bremer F (1950): Physiology of the corpus callosum. Res Publ Ass Res Nerv Ment Dis 36:424–448

Bricker A, Schuell HM, Jenkins JJ (1964): Effect of word length and word frequency on spelling errors of aphasic patients. J Speech Hear Res 7:183–192

Broca P (1861): Remarques sur le siège de la faculté du langage articulé, suives d'une observation d'aphémie. Bull Soc Anat (Paris) 330–357 (a)

Broca P (1861): Nouvelle observation d'aphémie produite par une lésion de la mortié posterieure des deuxième et troisième circonvolutions frontales. Bull Soc Anat (Paris) 398–407 (b)

Brodal A (1969): Neurological Anatomy in Relation to Clinical Medicine, 2nd ed. New York, Oxford Univ Press

Brooke R (1915): The soldier *in* Collected Poems. New York, Dodd, Mead

Brouwer B (1934): Projection of the retina on the cortex in man. Res Publ Ass Res Nerv Ment Dis 13:529–534

Brown JR, Schuell HM (1950): Preliminary report of a diagnostic test for aphasia. J Speech Hear Disord 15:21–28

Browning R (1845): Home thoughts, from abroad *in* Collected Poems. New York, Dodd, Mead (1915)

Bryngelson B, Glaspey E (1941): Speech Improvement Cards. Chicago, Scott, Foresman

Bucy PC (1957): Is there a pyramidal tract? Brain 80:1376–1392

Cairns H (1952): Disturbances of consciousness with lesions of the brain stem and diencephalon. Brain, 75:109–146

Castiglioni A (1941): A History of Medicine. Krumbhaar, E.B. (Trans.), New York, Knopf

Celesia GG, Broughton RJ, Rasmussen T, Branch C (1968): Auditory evoked responses from the exposed human cortex. Electroencephalogr Clin Neurophysiol 24:458–466

Chafe WL (1970): Meaning and the Structure of Language. Chicago, Univ of Chicago Press

Chomsky N (1957): Syntactic Structures. The Hague, Mouton

Chomsky N (1959): Review of Skinner's verbal behavior. Language 35:26–58

Chomsky N (1965): Aspects of the Theory of Syntax. Cambridge, Massachusetts, MIT Press

Chomsky N (1967): The formal nature of language *in* Biological Foundations of Language. By EH Lenneberg. New York, Wiley, pp. 397–442

Ciardi JL (1963): Manner of speaking. Sat. Rev, 46:16

Clapesattle H (1941): The Doctors Mayo. Minneapolis: University of Minnesota Press

Cobb IS (1915): Speaking of Operations. New York, Doran

Coemins VA (1970): Localized thalamic hemorrhage. Neurology (Minneap), 20:776–782

Cravioto H, Silberman J, Feigin I (1960): A clinical and pathological study of akinetic mutism. Neurology (Minneap) 10:10–21

Critchley M (1953): The Parietal Lobes. London, Arnold

Critchley M (1964): The origins of aphasiology. Scott Med J 1:274–290

Crosbie SB (1952): Retrospectroscope. Seriograph

Crosby EC, Humphrey T, Lauer EW (1962): Correlative Anatomy of the Nervous System. New York, Macmillan, pp. 343–350

Darley FL, Aronson AE, Brown JE (1969): Differential diagnostic patterns of dysarthria. Speech Hear Res 12:246–269

Davison C, Goodhart P, Needles W (1934): Cerebral localization in cerebrovascular diseases. Res Publ Ass Res Nerv Ment Dis 13:435–465,

Dempsey EW, Morison RS (1942): The production of rhythmically recurrent cortical potentials after localized thalamic stimulation. Amer J Physiol 135:293–300 (a)

Dempsey EW, Morison RS (1942): The interaction of certain spontaneous and induced cortical potentials. Amer J Physiol 135:301–308 (b)

De Renzi E, Pieczuro A, Vignolo LA (1966): Oral apraxia and aphasia. Cortex 2:50–73

de Reuck AVS, O'Connor M (eds) (1964): Disorders of Language. Boston, Little, Brown

Dolch EW (1949): Basic Sight Vocabulary Cards. Champaign, Illinois, Garrard (a)

Dolch EW (1949): Picture-Word Cards. Champaign, Illinois, Garrard (b)

Downer JL de C (1962): Interhemispheric integration in the visual system in Interhemispheric Relations and Cerebral Dominance. Edited by VB Mountcastle. Baltimore, Johns Hopkins Press

Draper MH, Ladefoged P, Whitteridge D (1957): Expiratory muscles involved in speech. J Physiol (Lond) 138:17 P

Draper MH, Ladefoged P, Whitteridge D (1959): Respiratory muscles in speech. J Speech Hear Res 2:16–27

Draper MH, Ladefoged P, Whitteridge D (1960): Expiratory pressures and air flow during speech. Br Med J I:1837–1843

Dusser de Barenne JG (1934): The labyrinthine and postural mechanisms. In C. A. Murchison (Ed.), Handbook of General Experimental Psychology. Worcester, Massachusetts: Clark University Press

Dusser de Barenne JG, McCulloch WS (1938): Functional organization in the sensory cortex of monkey (Macca mullata). J Neurophysiol 1:69–85

Ebstein E (1923): Gall in defense of his theory. Med Life 30:369–372

Eimas PD, Siqueland ER, Jusczyk P, Vigorito J (1971): Speech perception in infants. Science 171:303–306

Eisenson J (1954):Examining for Aphasia, rev ed. New York, New York Psychological Corp

Eisenson J (1957): Aphasia in adults in Handbook of Speech Pathology. Edited by LE Travis. New York, Appleton, pp. 436–502

Eisenson J (1960): When and what is aphasia. Monogr Soc Res Child Dev 25:90–95

Ettlinger G (1956): Sensory deficits in visual agnosia. J Neurol Neurosurg Psychiatry 19:297–307

Fairbanks G (1954): A theory of the speech mechanism as a servosystem. J Speech Hear Disord 19:133–139

Feldman MH (1971): Physiological observations in a chronic case of locked-in syndrome. Neurology (Minneap) 21:459–478

Feyerabend PK (1970): Consolations for the specialist in Criticism and the Growth of Knowledge. Edited by I Lakatos, A Musgrave. Cambridge: Cambridge Univ Press, pp. 197–230

Fisher RA (1935): The Design of Experiments. London, Oliver and Boyd

French JD, Magoun HW (1952): Effects of chronic lesions in central cephalic brain stem of monkeys. Arch Neurol 68:591–604

Freud S (1891): On Aphasia. Translated by E Stengel. New York, International Univ Press (1953)

Froeschels E (1954): Some voice problems in aphasia. Overdruk Logopaedie Phoniatrie 4:1–8

Froeschels E (1955): Grammar, a basic function of language-speech. Am J Psychother 9:43–53

Froeschels E, Dittrich O, Wilheim I (1932): Psychological Elements in Speech. Translated by N Ferre. Boston, Expression

Frontera JG (1956): Some results obtained by electrical stimulation of the cortex of the island of Reil in the brain of the monkey (Macaca mulatta). J Comp Neurol 105:365–394

Fry DB (1958): Phonemic substitutions in an aphasic patient. Lang Speech 1:52–61

Fulton JF (1949): Physiology of the Nervous System, 3rd ed. New York, Oxford Univ Press

Fulton JF, Kennard MA (1934): A study of flaccid and spastic paralysis produced by lesions of the cerebral cortex in primates. Res Publ Ass Res Nerv Ment Dis 13: 158–210

Gabor D (1946): Theory of communication. J Inst Elec Eng 93:429

Gacek RR (1961): The efferent cochlear bundle in man. Arch. Otolaryng 74:102–106

Gammon SA, Smith P, Daniloff R, Kim C (1971): Articulation and stress/juncture production under oral anesthetization and masking. J Speech Hear Res 14:271–282

Gardner E, Cuneo HM (1945): Lateral spinothalamic tract and associated tracts in man. Arch Neurol 53:423–430

Garey LJ, Powell TPS (1967): The projection of the lateral geniculate nucleus upon the cortex in the cat. Proc R Soc Lond [Biol]169:107–126

Gazzaniga MS, Bogen JE, Sperry RW (1965): Observations on visual perception after disconnection of the cerebral hemispheres in man. Brain 88:221–236

Gazzaniga MS, Sperry RW (1967): Language after section of the cerebral commissures. Brain 90:131–148

Geschwind N (1965): Disconnection syndromes in animals and man. Brain 88:585–644

Geschwind N, Kaplan E (1962): A human cerebral deconnection syndrome. Neurology 12:675–685

Glees P (1961): Experimental Neurology. London, Oxford Univ Press

Glickstein M, King RA, Miller J, Berkley M (1967): Cortical projections from the dorsal lateral geniculate nucleus of cats. J Comp Neurol 130:55–76

Goldberg JM, Diamond IT, Neff WD (1957): Auditory discrimination after ablation of temporal and insular cortex in cat. Fed Proc 16:47–48

Goldberg JM, Neff WD (1962): Frequency discrimination after bilateral ablation of cortical auditory areas. J Neurophysiol 24:119–128

Goldman-Eisler F (1954): On the variability of the speed of talking and on its relation to the length of utterances in conversations. Br J Psychol 45:94–107

Goldstein K (1939): The Organism, New York, American Book Co

Goldstein K (1942): Aftereffects of Brain Injuries in War. New York, Grune & Stratton

Goldstein K (1948): Language and Language Disturbances. New York, Grune & Stratton

Goldstein K, Scheerer M (1941): Abstract and concrete behavior. Psychol Monogr 53: No. 1, 110–130

Goldstein MR, Joynt AJ (1969): Long-term follow-up of a callosal-sectioned patient. Arch Neurol 20:96–102

Gooddy W (1956): Cerebral representation. Brain 79:167–187

Goodglass H, Kaplan EF (1963): Disturbance of gesture and pantomime in aphasia. Brain 86:703–720

Gray H (1959): The Arteries, in Gray's Anatomy. 27th edition, Goss, C.M., (Ed.), Philadelphia, Lea & Febiger pp 631–646

Greenblatt M, Solomon HC (1958): Studies of lobotomy. Res Publ Ass Res Nerv Ment Dis 36:19–34

Guiot G, Hertzog E, Rondot P, Molina P (1961): Arrest or acceleration of speech evoked by thalamic stimulation in the course of stereotaxic procedures for parkinsonism. Brain 84:363–379

Guttman L (1950): The basis for scalogram analysis in Studies in Social Psychology in World War II. Edited by SA Stouffer, L Guttman, EA Suchman, PR Lazersfield, SA Star, JA Clausen. Princeton, New Jersey, Princeton Univ Press pp. 60–90

Halwes T, Jenkins JJ (1971): Problem of serial order in behavior is not resolved by context-sensitive associative memory models. Psychol Rev 78:122–129

Harris CM (1953): A study of the building blocks in speech. J Acoust Soc Am 25:962–969

Haymaker W, Baer KA (eds) (1953): The Founders of Neurology. Springfield, Illinois, Thomas

Head H (1915): Hughlings Jackson on aphasia and kindred affections of speech. Brain 38:1–27

Head H (1926): Aphasia, and Kindred Disorders of Speech. New York, Macmillan

Heimer L, Ebner FF, Nauta WJH (1967): A note on the termination of commissural fibers in the neocortex. Brain Res 5:171–177

Henschen SE (1920–1922): Klinische und anatomische Beiträge zur Pathologie des Gehirns. Uppsala, Sweden, Almquist

Howes D (1964): Application of the word-frequency concept to aphasia in Disorders of language. Edited by AVS de Reuck, M O'Connor.Boston, Little, Brown, pp. 47–78

Howes D, Geschwind N (1960): Statistical properties of aphasic language. Progr Rep, NIH grant M-1802

Howes D, Geschwind N (1964): Quantitative studies of aphasic language In Disorders of Communication. Edited by DM Rioch, EA Weinstein. Baltimore, Williams & Wilkins, pp. 229–244

Humphrey ME, Zangwill OL (1951): Cessation of dreaming after brain injury. J Neurol Neurosurg Psychiatry 14:322–325

Jabbur SJ, Towe AL (1961): Cortical excitation of neurons dorsal column nuclei of cat, including an analysis of pathways. J Neurophysiol 24:499–509

Jackson JH (1864): Loss of speech: its association with valvular disease of the heart and with hemiplegia on the right side. Brain 38:28–42 (1915)

Jackson JH (1868): On the physiology of language. Brain 38:59–64 (1915)

Jackson JH (1874): On the nature and duality of the brain in Selected Writings, Vol. 2. New York, Basic Books, pp. 129–145 (1958)

Jackson JH (1879): On affection of speech from disease of the brain *in* Selected Writings, Vol 2. New York, Basic Books, pp. 184–204 (1958)

Jackson JH (1882): On some implications of dissolution of the nervous system *in* Selected Writings, Vol. 2. New York, Basic Books, pp. 29–44 (1958)

Jackson JH (1887): Remarks on evolution and dissolution *in* Selected Writings, Vol. 2. New York, Basic Books, pp. 76–118 (1958)

Jackson JH (1888): Remarks on the diagnosis and treatment of diseases of the brain *in* Selected Writings, Vol. 2. New York, Basic Books, pp. 365–392 (1958)

Jackson JH (1893): Words and other symbols in mentation *in* Selected Writings, Vol. 2. New York, Basic Books, pp. 205–212 (1958)

Jackson JH (1958): Selected Writings, Vol. 2. New York, Basic Books

Jakobson R (1962): Kindersprache, aphasie und allgemeine lautgesetze *in* Selected Writings, Vol. I. S'Gravenhage, Mouton

Jasper HH (1949): The integrative action of the thalamic reticular system. Electroenceph Clin Neurophysiol 1:405–419

Jasper HH, Ajmone-Marsan C, Stoll J (1952): Symposium on brain and mind; corticofugal projections to the brain stem. Arch Neurol 67:155–166

Jenkins JJ, Schuell HM (1964): Further work on language deficit in aphasia. Psychol Rev 71:87–93

Jones EG, Powell TPS (1968): Cortical connections of the somatic sensory area. Brain Res 9:71–94

Jones EG, Powell TPS (1969): Connections of the somatic sensory cortex of the Rhesus monkey II—contralateral cortical connections. Brain 92:717–730

Kaplan HA (1961): Collateral circulation of the brain. Neurology (Minneap) 11 (II): 9–15

Kappers CUA, Huber GC, Crosby EC (1960): The Comparative Anatomy of the Nervous System of Vertebrates Including Man, Vol. 3. New York, Hafner, pp. 1517–1713

Karlin IW, Eisenson J, Hirschenfang S, Miller MH (1959): A multievaluational study of aphasic and non-aphasic right-hemiplegic patients. J Speech Hear Disord 24: 369–379

Katz JJ, Fodor JA (1963): The structure of a semantic theory. Language 39:170–210

Katz JJ, Postal PM (1964): An Integrated Theory of Linguistic Descriptions. Research Monograph, No. 26. Cambridge, Massachusetts, MIT Press

Kemper TL, Romanul FCA (1960): State resembling akinetic mutism in basilar artery occlusion. Neurology (Minneap) 17:74–80

Kluever H, Bucy PC (1939): Preliminary analysis of functions of the temporal lobes in monkeys. AMA Arch Neurol Psychiatry, 42:979–1000

Kuhn TS (1962): The Structure of Scientific Revolutions. Chicago, Univ of Chicago Press

Kussmaul A (1887): Disturbances of speech: An attempt in the pathology of speech *in* Cyclopedia of the Practice of Medicine, Vol. 14. Edited by H von Ziemssen. New York, Wood, pp. 581–875

Lakatos I (1970): Falsification and the methodology of scientific research programs *in* Criticism and the Growth of Knowledge. Edited by I Lakatos, A Musgrave. Cambridge, Cambridge Univ Press, pp. 91–196

Langworthy OR (1933): Development of behavior patterns and myelinization of the nervous system in the human fetus and infant, *in* Contributions to Embryology. Washington, D.C., Carnegie Inst. of Washington, pp. 3–57

Lashley KS (1951): The problem of serial order in behavior *in* Cerebral Mechanisms in Behavior. Edited by LA Jeffress. New York, Wiley, pp. 112–131

Lashley KS (1958): Cerebral organization and behavior.Res Publ Assoc Res Nerv Ment Dis 36:1–18

Lassek AM (1948): The pyramidal tract: basic considerations of corticospinal neurons. Res Publ Ass Res Nerv Ment Dis 27:106–128

Lawrence DG, Kuypers HGJM (1968): The functional organization of the motor system in the monkey (I). The effects of bilateral, pyramidal lesions. Brain 91:1–14 (a)

Lawrence DG, Kuypers HGJM (1968): The functional organization of the motor system in monkey (II). The effects of lesions of the descending brain stem pathways. Brain 91:15–36 (b)

Le Gros Clark WE (1940–41): Observations of the association fibre system of the visual cortex and the central representation of the retinae. J Anat 75:225–235

Lehman RAW (1968): Motor co-ordination and hand preference after lesions of the visual pathway and corpus callosum. Brain 91:525–538

Lenneberg EH (1967): Biological Foundations of Language. New York, Wiley

Levitt M, Carreras M, Liu CN, Chambers WW (1964): Arch Ital Bio 102:197–229

Levy-Agresti J, Sperry RW (1968): Differential perceptual capacities in major and minor hemispheres. Proc Nat Acad Sci USA 61:1151

Liberman AM (1957): Some results of research on speech perception. J Acoust Soc Am 29:117–123

Liberman AM, Cooper FS, Shankweiler DP, Studdert-Kennedy M (1967): Perception of the speech code. Psychol Rev 74:431–461

Liberman AM, Ingemann F, Lisker L, Delattre P, Cooper FS (1959). Minimal rules for synthesizing speech. J Acoust Soc Am 31:1490–1499

Lindbloom UF, Ottosen JO (1957): Influence of pyramidal stimulation upon the relay of coarse cutaneous afferents in the dorsal horn. Acta Physiol Scand 38:309–318

Lindsley DB (1938): Electrical potentials of the brain in children and adults. J Genet Psychol 19:285–306

Locke S, Yakovlev PI (1965): Transcallosal connections of the cingulum of man. Arch Neur 13:471–476

Loevinger J (1957): Objective tests as instruments of psychological theory. Psychiatr Res Rep Am Psychiatr Ass 3:635–694

Longerich MC (1959): Aphasia Therapy Sets. Los Angeles, California, Longerich

Lorente De Nó R (1933): The anatomy of the eighth nerve. Laryngoscope 43:1–38

Luria AR (1958): Brain disorders and language analysis. Lang Speech 1:14–34

Luria AR (1966): Higher Cortical Functions in Man. New York, Basic Books

MacKay DM (1950): The nomenclature of information theory; quantal aspects of scientific information; and entropy,time and information *in* the Procedures of Information-Theory Symposium, London, September, 1950 (Lithoprinted American Institute of Radio Engineers, 1953)

MacNeilage PF, Rootes TP, Chase RA (1967): Speech production and perception. Speech Hear Res 10:449–467

Magoun HW (1952): The ascending reticular activating system. Res Publ Ass Res Nerv Ment Dis 30:480–492

Marie P (1906): Revision de la question de l'aphasie: la troisième circonvolution frontale gauche ne joue aucun rôle spéciale dans la fonction du language. La Simaine Médicale 26:241–247 (a)

Marie P (1906): Revision de la question de l'aphasie: l'aphasie de 1861 à 1866: Essai de critique historique sur la genèse de la doctrine de Broca. La Simaine Médicale 26:565–571 (b)

Maspes PE (1948): Le syndrome expérimental chez l'homme de la section du splénium du corps calleux; alexie visuelle pure hémianopsique. Rev Neurol 80:100–113

Masterton RB, Jane JA, Diamond IT (1968): Role of the brain stem auditory structures in sound localization II: Inferior colliculus and its branches. J Neurophysiol 31:96–107

Meynert T (1881): On the collaboration of parts of the brain *in* Some Papers on the Cerebral Cortex. Translated by G von Bonin. Springfield, Illinois, Thomas, pp. 159–180 (1960)

Milisen R (1963): Personal communication

Miller GA, Galanter E, Pribram KH (1960): Plans and the Structure of Behavior. New York, Holt, Rhinehart & Winston

Millikan CH, Darley FL (eds) (1967): Brain Mechanisms Underlying Speech and Language. New York, Grune & Stratton

Mills CK (1891): On the localisation of the auditory centre. Brain *14*:465–472

Moffitt AR (1968): Speech Perception by Infants. Ph D Thesis, Univ of Minnesota

Moore P, Schuell HM (1954): The Language Master-Handbook for Aphasia. Language Stimulation Series. New York, McGraw-Hill

Moore RY, Goldberg JM (1966): Projections of the inferior colliculus in the monkey. Exp Neurol 14:429–438

Morison RS, Dempsey EW (1942): A study of thalamo-cortical relations. Amer J Physiol *135*:281–292

Moruzzi G, Magoun H (1949): Brain stem reticular formation and activation of the EEG. EEG Clinical Neurophysiology I:455–473

Munk H (1881): On the functions of the cortex *in* Some Papers on the Cerebral Cortex. Translated by G von Bonin. Springfield, Illinois, Thomas, pp. 97–117 (1960)

Myers RE (1956): Function of corpus callosum in interocular transfer. Brain 79:358–363

Nathan PW (1947): Facial apraxia and apraxic dysarthria. Brain 70:449–478

Neff WD, Diamond IT (1958): The neural basis of auditory discrimination, *in* Biological and Biochemical Bases of Behavior. Edited by HF Harlow, CN Woolsey, (Eds.), Madison, Wis., Univ Wisc Press, pp. 101–126

Neumann J von (1958): The Computer and the Brain. New Haven, Connecticut, Yale Univ Press

Neumann MA, Cohn R (1964): The reticular formation and coma in man. Trans Am Neurol Assoc 235–237

Newcomb FB, Oldfield RC, Wingfield A (1965): Object-naming by dysphasic patients. Nature 207:1217–1218

Nielsen JM (1946): Agnosia, Apraxia, Aphasia: Their Value in Cerebral Localization, 2nd ed. New York, Hoeber

Nielsen JM, Fitzgibbon JP (1936): Agnosia, apraxia, Aphasia: Their Value in Cerebral Location. Los Angeles, California, Los Angles Neurological Society

Nielsen JM, Sult CW (1939): Agnosias and the body scheme; five clinical cases. Bull Los Angeles Neurol Soc 4:69–76

Ojemann GA, Fedio P, Van Buren JM (1968): Anomia from pulvinar and subcortical parietal stimulation. Brain 91:99–116

Osgood CE (1963): On understanding and creating sentences. Am Psychol 18:735–751

Osgood CE, Miron MS (1963): Approaches to the Study of Aphasia. Urbana, Illinois, Univ of Illinois Press

Papez JW (1953): Theodore Meynert in Founders of Neurology. Edited by W Haymaker, KA Baer. Springfield, Illinois, Thomas, pp. 64–67

Pearson GHJ, Alpers BJ, Weisenburg TH (1928): Aphasia: A study of normal control cases. Arch Neurol Psychiatry 19:281–295

Peele TL (1944): Acute and chronic parietal lobe ablations in monkeys. J Neurophysiol 7:267–286

Penfield W, Faulk ME, Jr (1955): The insula. Brain 78:445–470

Penfield, W, Rasmussen T (1950): The Cerebral Cortex of Man: A Clinical Study of Localization of Function. New York, Macmillan

Penfield W, Roberts L (1959): Speech and Brain Mechanism. Princeton, New Jersey, Princeton Univ Press

Pick A (1913): Die agrammatischen Sprachstörungen. Berlin, Springer

Pick A, Thiele R (1931): Aphasie in Handbuch der normalen und pathologischen Physiologie, Vol. 15. Edited by A Bethe, G von Bergmann, G Embden, A Ellinger. Berlin, Springer, pp. 1416–1524

Pitres A (1895): Etude sur l'aphasie chez les pologlottes. Rev Med 15:873–899

Polyak S (1932): The Main Afferent Fiber System of the Cerebral Cortex in Primates. Berkeley, Univ Cal Press

Popper KR (1961): The Logic of Scientific Discovery. New York, Science House

Pribram KH (1971): Languages of the Brain. Englewood Cliffs, New Jersey, Prentice-Hall

Ranson SW, Clark SL (1959): The Anatomy of the Nervous System, 10th ed. Philadelphia, Saunders

Rasmussen AT, Peyton WT (1941): The location of the lateral spinothalamic tract in the brain stem of man. Surgery 10:699–710

Reader's Digest Reading Skill Builder Series (1951): Edited by LA Thomas. New York, Reader's Digest Educational Service

Ribot TA (1883): Les Maladies de la Memoire, 2nd ed. Paris, Libraire Germer Bailliere

Riddoch G (1917): Dissociation of visual perception due to occipital injuries, with especial reference to appreciation of movement. Brain 40:15–57

Riddoch G (1935): Visual disorientation in homonymous half fields. Brain 58:376–382

Rinvik E (1968): The corticothalamic projection from the second somatosensory cortical area in the cat: An experimental study with silver impregnation methods. Exp Brain Res 5:153–172

Rochford G, Williams M (1962): Studies in the development and breakdown of the use of names; I. The relationship between nominal dysphasia and the acquisition of vocabulary in childhood. J Neurol Neurosurg Psychiatry 25:222–233

Rochford G, Williams M (1963): Studies in the development and breakdown of the use of names; III. Recovery from nominal dysphasia. J Neurol Neurosurg Psychiatry 26:377–381

Rolnick M, Hoops HR (1969): Aphasia as seen by the aphasic. J Speech Hear Disord 34:48–53

Rose JE, Mountcastle VB (1960): Touch and Kinesthesis, in Handbook of Physiology. Edited by J Field, HW Magoun, VE Hall, Baltimore, Williams & Wilkins pp. 387–429

Rosenbek JC (1971): Oral sensation and perception in apraxia of speech and aphasia. Dissertation Abstracts International 32:1271 (2–B)

Russell B (1948): Human Knowledge: Its Scope and Limits. New York, Simon & Schuster

Russell B (1903): The Principles of Mathematics, 2nd ed. London, Allen & Unwin (1950)

Russell WA, Jenkins JJ (1954): The complete Minnesota norms for responses to 100 words from the Kent-Rosanoff word association test. Technical Report No. 11, ONR Contract N8 onr-66216. University of Minnesota

Russell WR, Espir MLE (1961): Traumatic Aphasia. London, Oxford Univ Press

Rylander G (1948): Personality analysis before and after frontal lobotomy. Res Publ Ass Res Nerv Ment Dis 27:691–705

Sarno MT (ed) (1972): Aphasia: Selected readings. New York: Appleton-Century-Crofts

Scheibel ME, Scheibel AB (1967): Structural organization of nonspecific thalamic nuclei and their projection toward cortex. Brain Res 6:60–94

Schneider RC, Crosby EC (1954): Stimulation of "second" motor areas in the macaque temporal lobe. Neurology 4:612–622

Schuell HM (1965): Differential diagnosis of aphasia with the Minnesota test. Minneapolis: University of Minnesota Press

Schuell HM (1957): A short examination for aphasia. Neurology 7:625–635

Schuell HM (1955): Minnesota Test for Differential Diagnosis of Aphasia, Research ed. Minneapolis, University of Minnesota Printing Department

Schuell HM (1966): Some dimensions of aphasic impairments in adults considered in relation to investigation of language disturbances in children. British Journal of Disorders of Communication 1:33–45

Schuell HM (1950): Paraphasia and paralexia. J Speech Hear Disord 15:291–306

Schuell HM (1953): Aphasic difficulties understanding spoken language. Neurology (Minneap) 3:176–184

Schuell HM (1960): Review of the month: Speech and brain mechanisms. RehabilLit 21:181–184

Schuell HM, Jenkins JJ (1959): The nature of language deficit in aphasia Psychol Rev 66:45–67

Schuell HM, Jenkins JJ (1961): Reduction of vocabulary in aphasia. Brain 84:243–261

Schuell HM, Jenkins JJ, Carroll JB (1962): A factor analysis of the Minnesota test for differential diagnosis of aphasia. J Speech Hear Res. 5:349–369

Schuell HM, Jenkins JJ, Jimenez-Pabon E (1964): Aphasia in Adults: Diagnosis, Prognosis and Treatment. New York, Harper & Row

Schuell HM, Jenkins JJ, Landis L (1961): Relationship between auditory comprehension and word frequency in aphasia. J Speech Hear Res 4:30–36

Schuell HM, Nagae K (1969): Aphasia studies. Geriatrics, October 141–152

Schuell HM, Shaw R, Brewer W (1969): A psycholinguistic approach to aphasia. A methodological study. J Speech Hear Res 12:794–806

Scott CM, Ringel RL (1971): Articulation without oral sensory control. J Speech Hear Res 14:804–818

Sefer JW, Henrikson EH (1966): The relationship between word association and grammatical classes in aphasia. J Speech Hear Res 9:529–541

Segarra JM (1970): Cerebral vascular disease and behavior. I. The syndrome of the mesencephalic artery (basilar artery bifurcation). Arch Neurol 22: 408–418

Sem-Jacobsen CW (1966): Depth-electrographic observations related to Parkinson's disease. J Neurosurg 24:388–402

Shankweiler D (1971): An analysis of laterality effects in speech perception *in* The Perception of Language. Edited by DL Horton, JJ Jenkins. Columbus, Ohio, Merrill, pp. 185–215

Shankweiler D, Harris KS (1966): An experimental approach to the problem of articulation in aphasia. Cortex 2:277–292

Shannon CE (1948): A mathematical theory of communication. Bell Sys Tech J 27: 379–423, 623–656

Siegel GM (1959): Dysphasic speech responses to visual word stimuli. J Speech Hear Res 2:152–167

Simon HA (1969): The Sciences of the Artificial. Cambridge, Massachusetts, MIT Press

Smith JR (1938): The electroencephalogram during normal infancy and childhood. I: Rhythmic activities present in the neonate and their subsequent development. J Genet Psychol 53:431–543

Smith KU (1951): Learning and the associative pathways of the human cerebral cortex. Science 114:117–120

Smith RA, Smith WA (1966): Loss of recent memory as a sign of focal temporal lobe disorder. J Neurosurg 24:91–95

Smythies JR (1967): Brain mechanisms and behavior. Brain 90:697–706

Snider R, Stowell J (1944): Receiving areas of the tactile, auditory, and visual systems in the cerebellum. J Neurophysiol 7:331–357

Sperry RW (1947): Cerebral regulation of motor coordination in monkeys following multiple transection of sensorimotor cortex. J Neurophysiol 10:275–294

Sperry RW (1958): Physiological plasticity and brain circuit theory *in* Biological and Biochemical Bases of Behavior. Edited by HF Harlow, CN Woolsey. Madison, Wisconsin, Univ of Wisconsin Press

Sperry RW (1961): Some developments in brain lesion studies of learning. Fed Pro 20:609–616

Sperry RW (1964): Problems Outstanding in the Evolution of Brain Function. James Arthur Lecture, American Museum of Natural History, New York

Spreen O (1968): Psycholinguistic aspects of aphasia. J Speech Hear Res 11:467–480

Spreen O, Benton AL, Fincham RW (1965): Auditory agnosia without aphasia. Arch Neurol 13:84–92

Stevens KN (1971): Perception of phonetic segments: Evidence from phonology, acoustics and psychoacoustics in The Perception of Language. Edited by DL Horton, JJ Jenkins. Columbus, Ohio, Merrill, pp. 216–235

Taylor, H, Marks, M. (1959): Aphasia Rehabilitation Manual and Therapy Kit. New York, McGraw-Hill

Templin MC (1957): Certain Language Skills of Children. Minneapolis, Minnesota, Univ of Minnesota Press

Teuber HL (1965): Postcript: Some needed revisions of the classical views of agnosia. Neuropsychologia 3:371–378

Travis AM, Woolsey CN (1956): Motor performance of monkeys after bilateral partial and total cerebral decortications. Amer J Phys Med 35:273–310

Trevarthen CB (1962): Double visual learning in split-brain monkeys. Science 136: 258–259

Van Buren JM (1963): Confusion and disturbance of speech from stimulation in the vicinity of the head of the caudate nucleus. J Neurosurg 20:148–157

Vogt MO (1898): Sur la myelinization de l'hémispherê cérebral du chat. C R Soc Biol (Paris) 50:54–56

Von Bonin G, Garol HW, McCullock WS (1942): Functional organization of occipital lobe. Biol. Symposia 7:165–192

Weinberger NM, Velasco M, Lindsley DB (1965): Effects of lesions upon thalamically induced electrocortical desynchronization and recruiting. Electroencephalogr Clin Neurophysiol 18:369–377

Weisenburg TH, McBride KE (1935): Aphasia. New York, Commonwealth Fund of New York

Wepman JM (1972): Aphasia therapy: Some "relative" comments and some purely personal prejudices in Aphasia: Selected readings. Edited by MT Sarno New York: Appleton-Century-Crofts pp. 436–444

Wepman JM (1951): Recovery from Aphasia. New York, Ronald Press

Wepman JM, Bock RD, Jones LV, Van Pelt D (1956): Psycholinguistic study of aphasia: A revision of the concept of anomia. J Speech Hear Disord 21:468–477

Wepman JM, Jones LV (1961): Studies in Aphasia: An Approach to Testing. Chicago, Education-Industry Service

Werner H (1965): Microgenesis and aphasia. J Abnorm Social Psychol 52:347–353

Wernicke C (1874): The symptom-complex of aphasia in Diseases of the Nervous System. Edited by A Church. New York, Appleton, pp. 265–324 (1908)

White HH (1961): Cerebral hemispherectomy in the treatment of infantile hemiplegia. Confin Neurol 21:1–50

Whitfield IC (1967): The Auditory Pathway. Baltimore, Williams & Wilkins

Wickelgren WA (1969): Context sensitive coding, associative memory, and serial order in (speech)behavior. Psychol Rev 76:1–15

Wiener N (1961): Cybernetics, 2nd ed. New York, Wiley

Wigan AL (1847): A Few More Words on the Duality of the Mind and Some of Its Corollaries. London, Savil

Woolsey CN (1943): A monkey which survived bilateral decortication for 161 days. Fed Proc 2:56 (b).

Zipf GK (1935): The Psychobiology of Language. Boston, Houghton Mifflin

Zollinger R (1935): Removal of left cerebral hemisphere. Arch Neurol 34:1055–1064

AUTHOR INDEX

SUBJECT INDEX

76 77 78 79 80 9 8 7 6 5 4 3 2